T0324892

CURRENT CLINICAL UROLOGY

Eric A. Klein, MD, Series Editor
Professor of Surgery
Cleveland Clinic Lerner College of Medicine Head
Section of Urologic Oncology
Glickman Urological and Kidney Institute
Cleveland, OH, USA

More information about this series at http://www.springer.com/series/7635

Dr Klein Series Editor

Led by Eric Klein of the Cleveland Clinic, Current Clinical Urology presents timely topics from world famous urologists at that institution and many others. Topics include the management of prostate cancer, urinary stone disease, male sexual function, chronic prostatitis, urologic robotic surgery, and bladder cancer. Urologists are enabled to stay current with rapid advances in urology. Current Clinical Urology is the leading reference source for clinical research and practice.

From the Editor of this issue
Jihad H. Kaouk, MD FACS

I am excited to present to you this unique book on an evolving and promising approach in laparoscopy. LESS or single port laparo-endoscopic surgery is an attempt to further minimize minimally invasive surgery. Awaiting significant modifications to current laparoscopic and robotic tools, LESS and robotic LESS remains in evolution. Future purpose built robotic systems my hold the key to adopting this new approach in minimally invasive surgery.

Jihad H. Kaouk

Editor

Robert J. Stein • Georges-Pascal Haber

Associate Editors

Atlas of Laparoscopic and Robotic Single Site Surgery

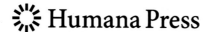 Humana Press

Editor
Jihad H. Kaouk, MD, FACS
Professor of Surgery
Department of Urology
Cleveland Clinic Lerner
College of Medicine
Zagarek Pollock Chair in Robotic
Surgery, Center for Robotic and Image
guided Surgery
Glickman Urologic Institute
Cleveland, OH
USA

Associate Editors
Robert J. Stein, MD
Associate Professor of Surgery
Department of Urology
Center for Robotic and Image
Guided Surgery
Glickman Urological and Kidney Institute
Cleveland Clinic
Cleveland, OH
USA

Georges-Pascal Haber, MD, PhD
Associate Staff
Department of Urology
Center for Robotic and Image
Guided Surgery
Glickman Urological Institute
Cleveland Clinic
Cleveland, OH
USA

ISSN 2197-7194   ISSN 2197-7208   (electronic)
Current Clinical Urology
ISBN 978-1-4939-3573-4   ISBN 978-1-4939-3575-8   (eBook)
DOI 10.1007/978-1-4939-3575-8

Library of Congress Control Number: 2017933966

Printed on acid-free paper

This Humana Press imprint is published by Springer Nature
The registered company is Springer Science+Business Media LLC
The registered company address is: 233 Spring Street, New York, NY 10013, U.S.A.

Contents

Contributors

Editors

Jihad H. Kaouk, MD, FACS Professor of Surgery, Department of Urology, Cleveland Clinic Lerner College of Medicine, Zagarek Pollock Chair in Robotic Surgery, Center for Robotic and Image guided Surgery, Glickman Urologic Institute, Cleveland, OH, USA

Associate Editors

Robert J. Stein, MD Associate Professor of Surgery, Department of Urology, Center for Robotic and Image Guided Surgery, Glickman Urological and Kidney Institute, Cleveland Clinic, Cleveland, OH, USA

Georges-Pascal Haber, MD, PhD Associate Staff, Department of Urology, Center for Robotic and Image Guided Surgery, Glickman Urological Institute, Cleveland Clinic, Cleveland, OH, USA

Authors

Oktay Akca, MD Department of Urology, Glickman Urological and Kidney Institute, Cleveland Clinic, Cleveland, OH, USA

Antonio Alcaraz, MD, PhD Department of Urology, Hospital Clinic, Barcelona, Spain

Mohamad E. Allaf, MD James Buchanan Brady Urological Institute and Department of Urology, The Johns Hopkins University School of Medicine, Baltimore, MD, USA

Javier C. Angulo, MD, PhD Jefe de Servicio de Urología, Department of Urology, Hospital Universitario de Getafe, Profesor Titular de Urología, Universidad Europea de Madrid, Laureate Universities, Madrid, Spain

Riccardo Autorino, MD, PhD, FEBU Department of Urology, University Hospitals Urology Institute, Richmond Heights, Cleveland, OH, USA

Mark W. Ball, MD James Buchanan Brady Urological Institute and Department of Urology, The Johns Hopkins University School of Medicine, Baltimore, MD, USA

Eric Barret, MD Department of Urology, Institut Montsouris Université Paris-Descartes, Paris, France

Liu Bing, MD The Department of Urology, Changhai Hospital, Second Military Medical University, Shanghai, China

Luis Felipe Brandao, MD Department of Urology, Paulista Medicine School from the Federal University of São Paulo, São Paulo, Brazil

Robert D. Brown, MD Department of Urology, Cleveland Clinic, Cleveland, OH, USA

Pedro M. Cabrera, MD Department of Urology, Hospital Universitario de Getafe, Madrid, Spain

Marino Cabrera Fierro, MD Robotics and Minimal Invasive Surgery, Urology Department, Instituto Medico La Floresta, Caracas, Venezuela

Felipe Cáceres, MD Department of Urology, Hospital Universitario de Getafe, Madrid, Spain

Jeffrey A. Cadeddu, MD Department of Urology, J8.106, UT Southwestern Medical Center, Dallas, TX, USA

Urology and Radiology, University of Texas Southwestern Medical Center, Dallas, TX, USA

Andrea Cestari, MD Urology Department, Scientific Institute "Istituto Auxologico Italiano", Milan, Italy

Antonio Cicione, MD Clinical and Experimental Medicine, Magna Graecia University of Catanzaro, Catanzaro, Italy

Ernesto R. Cordeiro Feijoo, MD, FEBU Department of Urology, Institut Montsouris Université Paris-Descartes, Paris, France

Rocco Damiano, MD, PhD Clinical and Experimental Medicine, Magna Graecia University of Catanzaro, Catanzaro, Italy

Rodrigo Donalisio da Silva, MD Department of Urology, Denver Health Hospital and Authority, Denver, CO, USA

Ithaar H. Derweesh, MD Urology, UCSD Medical Center, San Diego, CA, USA

Robert F. Elder, MD Women's and Children's Health, Obstetrics and Gynecology Surgery, University of Tennessee Medical Center, Knoxville, TN, USA

Sammy E. Elsamra, MD Department of Surgery, Division of Urology, Rutgers - Robert Wood Johnson Medical School, New Brunswick, NJ, USA

Fabio Fabbri, MD Urology Department, Scientific Institute "Istituto Auxologico Italiano", Milan, Italy

Matteo Ferrari, MD Urology Department, Scientific Institute "Istituto Auxologico Italiano", Milan, Italy

Cristian Fiori, MD Division of Urology, Department of Oncology, School of Medicine-University of Turin, "San Luigi Gonzaga" Hospital, Orbassano, Turin, Italy

Jeffrey C. Gahan, MD Department of Urology, UT Southwestern Medical Center, VA North Texas Health System, Dallas, TX, USA

Vishnuvardhan Ganesan Department of Urology, Center for Laparoscopic and Robotic Surgery, Glickman Urological and Kidney Institute, Cleveland Clinic Foundation, Cleveland, OH, USA

Massimo Ghezzi, MD Urology Department, Scientific Institute "Istituto Auxologico Italiano", Milan, Italy

Diedra Gustafson, BS Department of Urology, Denver Health Hospital and Authority, Denver, CO, USA

Marios Hadjipavlou, BSc, MBBS, MRCS Department of Urology, Darent Valley Hospital, Dartford, Kent, UK

Önder Kara, MD Department of Urology, Laparoscopic and Robotic Surgery, Glickman Urological and Kidney Institute, Cleveland Clinic, Cleveland, OH, USA

Shahid Aziz Anwer Khan, FRCS (Urol), FEBU Department of Urology, East Surrey Hospital, Redhill, UK

Fernando J. Kim, MD, MBA/MHA, FACS Surgery/Urology, Denver Health Medical Center, Denver, CO, USA

Minimally Invasive Urological Oncology, University of Colorado Denver, Denver, CO, USA

Christos Komninos, MD, MSc, PhD Urology Department, Severance Hospital, Yonsei University College of Medicine, Seoul, South Korea, Korea

Humberto Laydner, MD Department of Urology, University Hospitals Urology Institute, Richmond Heights, Cleveland, OH, USA

Hak J. Lee, MD Robotics/Minimally Invasive Surgery and Urologic Oncology, Gordon Urology, Gordon Hospital, Calhoun, GA, USA

Wang Linhui, MD, PhD The Department of Urology, Changhai Hospital, Second Military Medical University, Shanghai, China

Matthew J. Maurice, MD Department of Urology, Laparoscopic and Robotic Surgery, Glickman Urological and Kidney Institute, Cleveland Clinic, Cleveland, OH, USA

Mireia Musquera, MD, PhD Department of Urology, Hospital Clinic, Barcelona, Spain

Luciano A. Nuñez Bragayrac, MD Robotics and Minimal Invasive Surgery, Urology Department, Instituto Medico La Floresta, Caracas, Venezuela

Idir Ouzaid, MD Department of Urology, Center for Laparoscopic and Robotic Surgery, Glickman Urological and Kidney Institute, Cleveland Clinic Foundation, Cleveland, OH, USA

Sung Yul Park, MD Department of Urology, Hanyang University College of Medicine, Seongdong-gu, Seoul, South Korea

Luís Peri, MD Department of Urology, Hospital Clinic, Barcelona, Spain

Ryan B. Pickens, MD Division of Urology, Department of Surgery, University of Tennessee Medical Center, Knoxville, TN, USA

Francesco Porpiglia, MD Department of Oncology, Division of Urology, School of Medicine-University of Turin, "San Luigi" Hospital, Turin, Italy

Soroush Rais-Bahrami, MD Urology and Radiology, University of Alabama at Birmingham, Birmingham, AL, USA

Abhay Rane, MS, OBE, FRCS (Urol) Department of Urology, East Surrey Hospital, Redhill, UK

Koon Ho Rha, MD, PhD Urology Department, Severance Hospital, Yonsei University College of Medicine, Seoul, South Korea

Department of Urology and Urological Science Institute, Yonsei University College of Medicine, Seoul, South Korea

Lee Richstone, MD Urology Department, The Hofstra – North Shore LIJ School of Medicine, Lake Success, NY, USA

Patrizio Rigatti, MD Urology Department, Scientific Institute "Istituto Auxologico Italiano", Milan, Italy

Estevao Augusto Rodrigues Lima, MD, PhD Urology Department, Hospital de Braga, Braga, Portugal

Selcuk Sahin, MD Urology Department, Bakırkoy Research and Training Hospital, Bakırkoy Dr. Sadi Konuk Training and Research Hospital, Istanbul, Turkey

Dinesh Samarasekera, BSc, MD, FRCSC Urology, Surrey Memorial Hospital, Surrey, BC, Canada

Rafael Sanchez-Salas, MD Department of Urology, Institut Montsouris Université Paris-Descartes, Paris, France

Mattia Sangalli, MD Urology Department, Scientific Institute "Istituto Auxologico Italiano", Milan, Italy

Tae Young Shin, MD Department of Urology, ChunCheon Sacred Heart Hospital, Hallym University, Chuncheon, Kangwon, South Korea

Rene J. Sotelo Noguera, MD Robotics and Minimal Invasive Surgery, Urology Department, Instituto Medico La Floresta, Caracas, Venezuela

Francesco Sozzi, MD Urology Department, Scientific Institute "Istituto Auxologico Italiano", Milan, Italy

Yinghao Sun, MD, PhD The Department of Urology, Changhai Hospital, Second Military Medical University, Shanghai, China

Volkan Tugcu, MD Urology Department, Bakırkoy Research and Training Hospital, Bakırkoy Dr. Sadi Konuk Training and Research Hospital, Istanbul, Turkey

Michael A. White, DO, FACOS Department of Urology, Urology San Antonio, San Antonio, TX, USA

Wesley M. White, MD Department of Urology, Laparoscopic and Robotic Urologic Surgery, The University of Tennessee Medical Center, Knoxville, TN, USA

Matteo Zanoni, MD Urology Department, Scientific Institute "Istituto Auxologico Italiano", Milan, Italy

Homayoun Zargar, MBChB, FRACS Department of Urology, Glickman Urology and Kidney Institute, Cleveland Clinic, Cleveland, OH, USA

Wang Zhixiang The Department of Urology, Changhai Hospital, Second Military Medical University, Shanghai, China

Part I

Introduction to LESS

History and Evolution of LESS

Marios Hadjipavlou, Shahid Aziz Anwer Khan, and Abhay Rane

Introduction

From very humble beginnings, roughly a century ago, laparoscopic surgery has now become the standard of care for many surgical procedures. Its application in various surgical specialities has helped patients tremendously by replacing traditional open surgical procedures with laparoscopic techniques that have the added benefit of better cosmesis, significantly improved operative and post-operative outcomes without compromising on oncological outcomes. Within the field of urology, laparoscopy has evolved significantly from initially being a diagnostic tool to now providing the means for performing complex extirpative and reconstructive procedures intra-corporally. Rapid advancements made in technology, the incorporation of robotics and the development of laparoendoscopic single-site surgery (LESS) and natural orifice translumenal endoscopic surgery (NOTES) have now made truly 'scarless' surgery achievable.

M. Hadjipavlou, BSc, MBBS, MRCS
Department of Urology, Darent Valley Hospital, Dartford, Kent, UK
e-mail: marioshad@doctors.org.uk

S.A.A. Khan, FRCS (Urol), FEBU (✉)
A. Rane, MS, OBE, FRCS (Urol)
Department of Urology,
East Surrey Hospital, Redhill, UK
e-mail: saak_2000@yahoo.co.uk;
a.rane@btinternet.com

Non-urological LESS

While LESS is thought to be a novel technique in laparoscopy, the use of a single port for diagnostic and simple interventions has been in place in the fields of gynaecology and general surgery for many decades. Basic laparoscopic procedures performed via a single transabdominal port for diagnostic laparoscopy and punch biopsies of solid organs date back to over 50 years ago [1]. Gynaecologists to this day have been using a similar approach for tubal ligation; Wheeless reported a large series of 'single trocar operative laparoscopy using a 12 mm laparoscope with one operative working channel' in 1969 [2]. Advancements in surgery and the need to perform more complex and technically demanding procedures led to the introduction of additional ports that not only would prove both safe and effective but also provided viable alternative laparoscopic approaches to traditional open surgical procedures. The addition of ports that allowed triangulation, improved visualisation and reduced instrument clashing enabled surgeons to perform complex extirpative and reconstructive procedures safely. Using multi-port laparoscopic techniques developed in the 1980s and 1990s, procedures like cholecystectomy, appendectomy, gastric bypass and hysterectomy have stood the test of time and still remain gold standard interventions.

© Springer Science+Business Media New York 2017
J.H. Kaouk et al. (eds.), *Atlas of Laparoscopic and Robotic Single Site Surgery*,
Current Clinical Urology, DOI 10.1007/978-1-4939-3575-8_1

Following over 20 years of dormancy in the evolution of single-site laparoscopy, in 1991 the American gynaecologist Dr. Marco Pelosi performed a hysterectomy with bilateral salpingo-oophorectomy via a single transumbilical port which was the first complex extirpative procedure using this approach [4]. It was followed by a supracervical hysterectomy the next year [5]. In 1992 the same group reported the first series of appendectomies performed through a single puncture ('minilaparoscopy') [6]. Five years later Navarra et al. reported the first 'one-wound' laparoscopic cholecystectomy [7]. In 2001 the first paediatric case using LESS was reported with an ovarian cystectomy performed in a 2-month-old infant through a 10 mm transumbilical trocar using a 3 mm laparoscope with no complications [8]. Four years later Ghezzi et al. reported a ten-patient series of salpingectomy for management of tubal pregnancy through a single transumbilical trocar [9]. They reported the procedure to be 'not technically demanding' and recommended it as 'feasible and safe'. In 2007 LESS Meckel's diverticulectomy was reported in nine patients; a short bowel segment was brought to the skin through the transumbilical incision to excise the diverticulum [10]. The fascial incision had to be extended to assist exteriorisation and to avoid ileal vascular congestion.

LESS, however, initially failed to gain popularity, largely due to the technical challenges associated with the procedure. Compared to multi-port laparoscopy, the main difficulties encountered were loss of triangulation and depth perception, reduced range of instrument movements, limited extra-abdominal working space for the surgeon and compromised views due to the parallel arrangement of instruments [3]. However, with exciting innovations in instrument design, rapid advancements in optics incorporating high-definition (HD) cameras with the possibility of incorporating 3D vision to improve depth perception, a renewed interest in LESS has been generated.

LESS in Urology

In 2005, Hirano et al. reported a 54-patient series of retroperitoneoscopic adrenalectomy via a single port using a 4 cm large cylinder without carbon dioxide insufflation [11]. Significant complications were reported including pulmonary embolism, fulminant hepatitis and one death. The authors did not describe the technique as 'laparoscopic' owing to the lack of carbon dioxide insufflation and the size of the skin incision.

The past decade has seen a revival of single-site laparoscopic surgery forming the next stepping stone towards scarless surgery. Research performed in parallel in urological centres across the globe has led to the creation of a wide variation in terminology and overlapping nomenclature such as single-incision laparoscopic surgery (SILS), single port access (SPA), single-site laparoscopy (SSL), one-port umbilical surgery (OPUS), single laparoscopic port procedure (SLAPP), single-port laparoscopic surgery (SPLS), single laparoscopic incision transabdominal (SLIT) surgery and single-instrument port laparoscopic (SIMPL) surgery. To avoid confusion, the collective term laparoendoscopic single-site surgery (LESS) has now been adopted [12].

In 2007, Rane et al. presented at the 25th World Congress of Endourology in Cancun the first successful LESS case in urology [13]. The group used a purpose-built multichannel port (R-PORT®, Advanced Surgical Concepts, Wicklow, Ireland) to introduce a 5 mm telescope and two 5 mm working instruments while also allowing a 10 mm clip applier. By introducing the port in a flank incision, the first LESS simple nephrectomy was performed on a 36-year-old man with a non-functioning right kidney. Using the same multichannel port through an umbilical incision, the group also performed a ureterolithotomy for a 25 mm proximal ureteric calculus, an orchidopexy and an orchidectomy without the use of accessory ports [14]. A revolution therefore began, and LESS was increasingly been seen as a viable step towards achieving 'scarless surgery'.

Raman et al. performed the first multi-trocar single-incision transumbilical nephrectomy in three patients [15]. For the two benign cases (non-functioning kidneys due to chronic infection), three trocars were inserted via a single umbilical incision through which articulating laparoscopic graspers were used for dissection.

The third nephrectomy was performed for a 4.5 cm renal tumour where a 3 mm accessory instrument was introduced for liver retraction. In 2008 Desai et al. reported a single-port nephrectomy and pyeloplasty for the first time using specially designed curved instruments introduced via a transumbilical incision through the R-PORT® [16]. A 2 mm needle port was inserted to facilitate suturing thereby avoiding an additional skin incision. The operative time was 3.4 and 2.7 h, respectively, and no complications were reported.

The same year, a group from the Cleveland cClinic led by Dr Jihad Kaouk used a single-port transumbilical platform (Uni-X®, Pnavel Systems, Morganville, NJ, USA) to perform renal cryoablation, wedge kidney biopsy and sacrocolpopexy [17]. To achieve this, a 5 mm flexible scope and bent laparoscopic instruments, along with conventional ones, were used. The same group reported the first experience of LESS advanced reconstructive procedures such as psoas hitch, bilateral single-session Anderson-Hynes pyeloplasty, ileal ureter and ureteroneocystostomy with excellent results [18]. LESS approach was used for a live donor nephrectomy in four patients with no complications and excellent allograft function following transplantation, results promising for this typically younger altruistic population [19]. The group used the same platform to subsequently perform single-site transumbilical radical prostatectomy [20] and transvesical simple prostatectomy [21] uneventfully.

By 2008, robotic-assisted surgery had been well established in many US centres, and there was no delay in an attempt to complement the platform with LESS. Using the da Vinci-S® robotic system (Intuitive Surgical, Sunnyvale, CA, USA), Desai et al. illustrated the technical feasibility of performing a transvesical robotic radical prostatectomy on two human cadavers [22]. Technical difficulties, most notably clashing of the robotic arms, were recognised especially with the single-port compared to the multi-port approach. Using a transumbilical approach, the platform was subsequently used to successfully complete radical prostatectomy, radical nephrectomy and pyeloplasty [23]. The benefit of articulating robotic instruments to overcome the laparoscopic principles of triangulation for suturing was stressed. More complex LESS procedures were subsequently attempted such as subtotal cystectomy and augmentation enterocystoplasty [24], radical cystectomy and pelvic lymph node dissection [25] and repair of retrocaval ureter [26] (Table 1.1).

Table 1.1 Highlights of laparoendoscopic single-site surgery (LESS) procedures

Year	Procedure	Comments	Reference
1969	Tubal ligation	Single transumbilical trocar	Wheeless [2]
1991	Hysterectomy with bilateral salpingo-oophorectomy	Single transumbilical trocar	Pelosi et al. [4]
1992	Supracervical hysterectomy with bilateral salpingo-oophorectomy	Single transumbilical trocar	Pelosi et al. [5]
1992	Appendectomy	Single transumbilical trocar	Pelosi et al. [6]
1997	Cholecystectomy	–	Navarra et al. [7]
2001	Ovarian cystectomy	Single transumbilical trocar	Kosumi et al. [8]
2005	Salpingectomy for ectopic pregnancy	Single transumbilical trocar	Ghezzi et al. [9]
2005	Retroperitoneal adrenalectomy	Single retroperitoneal port. No insufflation used	Hirano et al. [11]
2006	Meckel's diverticulectomy	Single transumbilical trocar	Cobellis et al. [10]
2007	Simple nephrectomy, radical nephrectomy	Single transumbilical incision, multiple ports	Raman et al. [15]
2008	Simple nephrectomy	Single port through a flank incision	Rane et al. [14]
2008	Orchidectomy, orchidopexy, ureterolithotomy	Transumbilical R-port	Rane et al. [14]
2008	Simple nephrectomy	Single transumbilical port	Desai et al. [16]

(continued)

Table 1.1 (continued)

Year	Procedure	Comments	Reference
2008	Pyeloplasty	Transumbilical port and 2 mm needle port	Desai et al. [16]
2008	Renal cryotherapy, radical nephrectomy, wedge kidney biopsy, sacrocolpopexy	Single transumbilical port	Kaouk et al. [17]
2008	Live donor nephrectomy	Transumbilical port and 2 mm needle port	Gill et al. [19]
2008	Paediatric varicocelectomy	First experience in paediatric urology	Kaouk et al. [27]
2008	Radical prostatectomy	Single transumbilical port exclusively	Kaouk et al. [20]
2008	Transvesical simple prostatectomy		Desai et al. [21]
2008	Transvesical robotic radical prostatectomy (cadaveric)		Desai et al. [22]
2008	Robotic single-port (RSP) surgery (radical prostatectomy, pyeloplasty, radical nephrectomy)	Single transumbilical port	Kaouk et al. [23]
2009	Ileal ureter, psoas hitch ureteroneocystostomy	Transumbilical port and 2 mm needle port	Desai et al. [18]
2009	Transumbilical simple prostatectomy	Single transumbilical trocar	Sotelo et al. [28]
2009	Subtotal cystectomy and augmentation enterocystoplasty	Single transumbilical port	Sotelo et al. [24]
2010	Radical cystectomy and pelvic lymph node dissection	Single transumbilical port	Kaouk et al. [25]
2010	Repair of retrocaval ureter	Single transumbilical port	Autorino et al. [26]

Adapted and edited from Canes et al. [29]

Conclusion

In recent years minimally invasive surgery research has been centred on the development of techniques that will ultimately be 'scarless'. Since its revival in the twenty-first century, the history of LESS is relatively short, but, nevertheless, the field is rapidly evolving. The laparoscopic instrument industry has played a crucial role in the development of LESS by introducing purpose-built multichannel ports, roticulating instruments, high-definition cameras and multi-length working instruments. Solutions to the technical challenges associated with LESS are becoming available allowing more complex surgery through virtually non-visible wounds.

References

1. Platteborse R. Laparoscopy, laparophotography, punch biopsy of the liver, gallbladder punch biopsy and collection of specimens of the peritoneal organs through a single trocar. Acta Gastroenterol Belg. 1961;24:696–700.
2. Wheeless C. A rapid inexpensive and effective method of surgical sterilization by laparoscopy. J Reprod Med. 1969;3:65.
3. Gill IS, Advincula AP, Aron M, et al. Consensus statement of the consortium for laparoendoscopic single-site surgery. Surg Endosc. 2010;24:762–8.
4. Pelosi MA. Laparoscopic hysterectomy with bilateral salpingo-oophorectomy using a single umbilical puncture. N J Med. 1991;88:721–6.
5. Pelosi MA. Laparoscopic supracervical hysterectomy using a single-umbilical puncture (mini-laparoscopy). J Reprod Med. 1992;37:777–84.

6. Pelosi MA. Laparoscopic appendectomy using a single umbilical puncture (minilaparoscopy). J Reprod Med. 1992;37:588–94.

7. Navarra G, Pozza E, Occhionorelli S, Carcoforo P, Donini I. One-wound laparoscopic cholecystectomy. Br J Surg. 1997;84:695.

8. Kosumi T, Kubota A, Usui N, Yamauchi K, Yamasaki M, Oyanagi H. Laparoscopic ovarian cystectomy using a single umbilical puncture method. Surg Laparosc Endosc Percutan Tech. 2001;11:63–5.

9. Ghezzi F, Cromi A, Fasola M, Bolis P. One-trocar salpingectomy for the treatment of tubal pregnancy: a "marionette-like" technique. BJOG. 2005;112: 1417–9.

10. Cobellis G, Cruccetti A, Mastroianni L, Amici G, Martino A. One-trocar transumbilical laparoscopic-assisted management of Meckel's diverticulum in children. J Laparoendosc Adv Surg Tech A. 2007;17:238–41.

11. Hirano D, Minei S, Yamaguchi K, et al. Retroperitoneoscopic adrenalectomy for adrenal tumors via a single large port. J Endourol. 2005;19:788–92.

12. Box G, Averch T, Cadeddu J, et al. Nomenclature of natural orifice translumenal endoscopic surgery (NOTES) and laparoendoscopic single-site surgery (LESS) procedures in urology. J Endourol. 2008;22:2575–81.

13. Rane A, Kommu S, Eddy B, Bonadio F, Rao P, Rao P. Clinical Evaluation of a novel laparoscopic port (R-Port) and evolution of the single laparoscopic port procedure (SLiPP). J Endourol. 2007;21:A22–3.

14. Rané A, Rao P, Rao P. Single-port-access nephrectomy and other laparoscopic urologic procedures using a novel laparoscopic port (R-port). Urology. 2008;72:260–3; discussion 263–4.

15. Raman JD, Bensalah K, Bagrodia A, Stern JM, Cadeddu JA. Laboratory and clinical development of single keyhole umbilical nephrectomy. Urology. 2007;70:1039–42.

16. Desai MM, Rao PP, Aron M, Pascal-Haber G, Desai MR, Mishra S, Kaouk JH, Gill IS. Scarless single port transumbilical nephrectomy and pyeloplasty: first clinical report. BJU Int. 2008;101:83–8.

17. Kaouk JH, Haber G-P, Goel RK, Desai MM, Aron M, Rackley RR, Moore C, Gill IS. Single-port laparoscopic surgery in urology: initial experience. Urology. 2008;71:3–6.

18. Desai MM, Stein R, Rao P, Canes D, Aron M, Rao PP, Haber G-P, Fergany A, Kaouk J, Gill IS. Embryonic natural orifice transumbilical endoscopic surgery (E-NOTES) for advanced reconstruction: initial experience. Urology. 2009;73:182–7.

19. Gill IS, Canes D, Aron M, Haber G-P, Goldfarb DA, Flechner S, Desai MR, Kaouk JH, Desai MM. Single port transumbilical (E-NOTES) donor nephrectomy. J Urol. 2008;180:637–41; discussion 641.

20. Kaouk JH, Goel RK, Haber G-P, Crouzet S, Desai MM, Gill IS. Single-port laparoscopic radical prostatectomy. Urology. 2008;72:1190–3.

21. Desai MM, Aron M, Canes D, et al. Single-port transvesical simple prostatectomy: initial clinical report. Urology. 2008;72:960–5.

22. Desai MM, Aron M, Berger A, Canes D, Stein R, Haber G-P, Kamoi K, Crouzet S, Sotelo R, Gill IS. Transvesical robotic radical prostatectomy. BJU Int. 2008;102:1666–9.

23. Kaouk JH, Goel RK, Haber G-P, Crouzet S, Stein RJ. Robotic single-port transumbilical surgery in humans: initial report. BJU Int. 2009;103:366–9.

24. Noguera RJS, Astigueta JC, Carmona O, De Andrade RJ, Luis S, Cuomo B, Manrique J, Gill IS, Desai MM. Laparoscopic augmentation enterocystoplasty through a single trocar. Urology. 2009;73:1371–4.

25. Kaouk JH, Goel RK, White MA, White WM, Autorino R, Haber G-P, Campbell SC. Laparoendoscopic single-site radical cystectomy and pelvic lymph node dissection: initial experience and 2-year follow-up. Urology. 2010;76:857–61.

26. Autorino R, Khanna R, White MA, Haber G-P, Shah G, Kaouk JH, Stein RJ. Laparoendoscopic single-site repair of retrocaval ureter: first case report. Urology. 2010;76:1501–5.

27. Kaouk JH, Palmer JS. Single-port laparoscopic surgery: initial experience in children for varicocelectomy. BJU Int. 2008;102:97–9.

28. Sotelo RJ, Astigueta JC, Desai MM, Canes D, Carmona O, De Andrade RJ, Moreira O, Lopez R, Velásquez A, Gill IS. Laparoendoscopic single-site surgery simple prostatectomy: initial report. Urology. 2009;74:626–30.

29. Canes D, Desai MM, Aron M, Haber G-P, Goel RK, Stein RJ, Kaouk JH, Gill IS. Transumbilical single-port surgery: evolution and current status. Eur Urol. 2008;54:1020–9.

Consent and IRB Requirements

Humberto Laydner, Luis Felipe Brandao, and Jihad H. Kaouk

Introduction

Over the last 20–30 years, the urology operating suite has undergone significant changes with the incorporation of new technologies, instruments, and innovative techniques aiming to decrease the invasiveness of surgical procedures. After the pioneering work of Clayman et al. in early 1990s, laparoscopic surgery spread quickly in the urological field [1]. Since the early 2000s, robot-assisted surgery has also been increasingly adopted and even replaced standard laparoscopy in some instances [2, 3]. Laparoendoscopic single-site surgery (LESS) was developed with the goal to reproduce the same operative steps of laparoscopic surgery through a single incision, maximizing the cosmetic results and potentially causing less pain [4]. More than 1,000 LESS urological procedures have been reported worldwide, encompassing almost the whole spectrum of urological surgery [5]. With appropriate case selection, the safety of this approach appears to be similar to standard laparoscopy [6].

The regulations for the introduction of new drugs and medical devices are very strict and well defined [7, 8]. Several phases of experimental studies and thorough scrutiny by regulatory agencies are required before they can obtain approval for clinical use. However, the same is not necessarily true for innovative surgical techniques [9]. Obtaining patient's consent to a procedure is required even outside the context of clinical trials, but there is no legal obligation to inform the innovative nature of the procedure [9]. The Belmont Report summarized the basic ethical principles identified by the National Commission for the Protection of Human Subjects of Biomedical and Behavioral Research, which was created after the signature of the National Research Act (Pub. L. 93-348) into law in 1974 [10, 11]. The Belmont Report recommends that only "radically new procedures" should prompt formal evaluations of safety and efficacy [10]. Unlike natural orifice translumenal endoscopic surgery (NOTES), for example, LESS is not a radically new procedure in comparison to standard laparoscopic surgery. Although technically more demanding for the surgeon, it is

H. Laydner, MD
Department of Urology, University Hospitals Urology Institute, Richmond Heights, Cleveland, OH, USA
e-mail: laydner@icloud.com

L.F. Brandao, MD
Department of Urology, Paulista Medicine School from the Federal University of São Paulo, São Paulo, Brazil
e-mail: drluisbrandao@gmail.com

J.H. Kaouk, MD, FACS (✉)
Professor of Surgery, Cleveland Clinic Lerner College of Medicine, Zagarek Pollock Chair in Robotic Surgery, Center for Robotic and Image guided Surgery, Glickman Urologic Institute, Cleveland, OH, USA
e-mail: kaoukj@ccf.org

© Springer Science+Business Media New York 2017
J.H. Kaouk et al. (eds.), *Atlas of Laparoscopic and Robotic Single Site Surgery*,
Current Clinical Urology, DOI 10.1007/978-1-4939-3575-8_2

essentially the same laparoscopic procedure with all the instruments introduced through the same skin incision.

Whenever there is doubt whether a surgical innovation should undergo a formal research protocol or not, the approach we use and recommend is to obtain an opinion from the local institutional review board (IRB). In this chapter, we discuss the requirements for the informed consent process and IRB protocols.

Consent

The informed consent process has been largely incorporated into the clinical routine. The consent is extremely important for the protection of patients, healthcare personnel, and health institutions. Ideally, the informed consent should be a communication process in which the patient obtains an explanation about his disease, therapeutic options and alternatives, as well as information about possible risks and complications.

It is important to give time to the patient to think about the information just received, ask additional questions that may arise, and get further information from other sources. The surgeon should document in the patient's chart all the discussions and information provided. The documentation of the whole information process has much more value than a signed sheath of paper collected just before the procedure. A simple signature may have its validity questioned because it does not prove that the consent process was appropriately conducted, and, despite being apparently tedious, the informed consent process is much less complicated than experiencing a lawsuit [12].

The consent process should take into account the patient's level of understanding, impairment or disability, as well as his language and cultural characteristics. Some of the points to discuss include: (a) nature and severity of the pathology; (b) what the planned treatment entails; (c) who will be the responsible for the treatment; (d) possible risks and benefits, including the likelihood that the benefit may not be achieved;

(e) most common side effects, potential long-term physical, emotional, sexual, or other disability that could result from the treatment; (f) what is the level of doubt about the diagnosis and possible treatment outcomes; (g) whether the procedure is experimental or not; (h) the estimated costs associated with the treatment; (i) the right to refuse treatment and withdraw at any time; and (j) alternatives of treatment available and the presumed outcome of not having any treatment.

For a valid consent, the patient must be able to: (1) understand the information, including risks, benefits, and alternatives, (2) retain the information, (3) make a judgment based on the information, and (4) communicate his decision. When the patient is not capable of making a decision, it may be necessary to obtain a psychiatric evaluation or even a legal opinion.

It is not practical to mention all the possible complications that may occur in the informed consent. But, at least the most common complications should be clearly explained, as well as serious and life-threatening complications. Although rare, such complications are more susceptible to litigious issues [12].

If there is no change in the patient's circumstances, the consent remains valid until the patient withdraws it. Such changes include: improvement or worsening of the condition; new treatment alternatives that may become available after the consent was first signed; or review of the treatment's objectives, secondary to modifications on the stage of the disease.

Research Consent

The consent form used for research has similar principles to those mentioned above. However, there are additional requirements that must be included.

The patient should be explained in plain language about the reasons why the study is being conducted, why the patient was invited to join the study, possible risks and benefits that could result from the research treatments, and the planned follow-up visits. Likewise, the research consent must be explained well in advance before the proposed treatment effectively starts. The patient should have the right to receive standard treatment even if he decides to withdraw the research at any time.

Brehaut et al. evaluated the informed consent documents of 139 trials registered in ClinicalTrials.gov. They concluded that existing informed consent documents do not meet validated standards for encouraging good decision-making. They identified that consent documents could improve some specific aspects: presenting outcome probabilities, clarifying and expressing values and structured guidance, and using evidence [13]. Enama et al. randomized 111 patients to one of the two IRB-approved consents, either a standard or a concise form, which had in average 63 % fewer words. All other characteristics of the consent were similar. They did not observed significant differences in study comprehension or satisfaction using either a standard or a concise consent form [14]. The use of simplified informed consent versions, maintaining its most important aspects and acceptable standards, could potentially help to minimize the risk of unintentional protocol violations.

IRB Requirements

The fact that a surgical intervention is innovative does not immediately require its classification as research from a bioethics perspective [15]. The Belmont Report recommends that only "radically new procedures" should elicit a formal research protocol process [10]. The decision whether a surgical innovation is considered research or practice is set within a culture that usually values innovation. Patients commonly look out surgeons who are on the "cutting edge" of knowledge and skill within their field. Scientific journals dedicate sections to report new techniques; professional society meetings highlight innovations and award its creators. Advertisements from hospitals commonly

reference "innovation," and the news media stimulates consumer demand for high-profile innovation. Such demand puts pressure on surgeons to rapidly adopt the latest technology [9]. Moreover, surgical techniques undergo quick evolution and refinement. Depending on its duration, a randomized trial designed to evaluate a new surgical technique could become obsolete by advances in surgical technology. In the absence of explicit guidance, the decision whether a surgical technique innovation is radically different and should be evaluated by a research protocol falls to the individual surgeon within the context of his respective institution's culture [9].

When the surgeon decides to submit his innovation to a formal research study, the next step is to prepare a protocol and research informed consent according to his local IRB standards. An IRB is a group under FDA regulations formally designated to review and monitor biomedical research involving human subjects. An IRB has the authority to approve, require modifications, or disapprove research protocols. The IRB review process helps to protect the rights and welfare of humans participating as subjects in the research [16].

All IRBs in the United States are regulated by the FDA and Department of Health and Human Services, but each institution may have specific requirements in its application process. General IRB requirements include: the identification of personnel involved in the research; the study sponsor, if any; a summary of the proposed research, describing the scientific rationale and research aims; information detailing research procedures, data collection, and statistical analysis; details of study recruitment; description of the study population, with inclusion and exclusion criteria; study locations; details about how the confidentiality of data will be preserved; description of how adverse events, unanticipated problems, safety, and efficacy data will be monitored; research costs; and whether the study involves investigational or marketed drugs or devices. An example of the main IRB requirements is shown:

1. *Study staff*
2. *Study sponsor*
3. *Study abstract and protocol*
   (a) Provide a summary of the proposed research and upload a complete copy of the protocol on the document tab.
   (b) Describe the scientific or scholarly rationale for this research.
   (c) Does this research involve a grant application to a federal or non-federal agency?
4. *Study aims*
   Primary objective
   Secondary objectives
5. *Research procedures*
   (a) Describe the research interventions, procedures, tests, or materials associated with this research that subjects would not be receiving as routine care.
   (b) Describe where the research interventions will take place, and ensure they are performed in a private manner and setting.
   (c) Identify the level of risks to subjects and what steps will be taken to protect the safety and welfare of participants. For example, exclusion/inclusion criteria, additional study visits, and special monitoring.
   (d) Do other nursing and/or technical personnel need to be made aware of this research?
   If yes, describe how the research protocol information will be shared.
   (e) Does this research involve genetic testing?
   If yes, do you intend to share the results with participants?
   If the results will be shared with participants, the protocol and consent must detail the use of a CLIA (*Clinical Laboratory Improvement Amendments*)-approved lab and the availability of a genetic counselor to explain the results.
   If the results are not shared, the protocol and consent must specifically state that the results will not be documented in the medical record or shared with participants.
   (f) Describe your communication plan to inform and share information among the research team regarding study implementation including who is responsible for determining subject eligibility, data collection, safety reports, consenting, maintenance of study files, etc. How often will these meetings be held?
   (g) Describe how you will ensure protocol tests/procedures; eligibility criteria and obtaining consent will be completed according to the approved protocol and consent process (i.e., use of checklists, secondary review, and internal quality monitoring programs).
6. *Study statistics and analysis*
   (a) Number of subjects anticipated to be enrolled.
   (b) If this is a multicenter study, total number of subjects anticipated to be enrolled.
   (c) Describe how this sample size was determined.
   (d) Describe the data analysis plan including how the data will be measured and analyzed and by whom.
7. *Study recruitment*
   (a) Describe how participants will be identified, selected, and recruited. Specifically address how, when, where, and by whom subjects will be identified and approached about participation.
   (b) Do you plan to use any advertisements?
   If yes, upload on the documents tab.
   (c) Will research participants receive any payments?

If yes, identify the amount and the method of distribution to ensure payments are prorated and not contingent upon study completion.

Note: If payments total $600 or greater, the IRS (Internal Revenue Service) reporting is required, and participants will receive an IRS 1099 form. This information should be included in the consent.

8. *Study population*
   (a) Describe the study population including the control groups:
   Eligibility criteria
   Exclusion criteria
   (b) Does this research involve vulnerable persons (e.g., children under the age of 18, pregnant women, fetuses or neonates, seriously/terminally ill, cognitive/mentally impaired or unable to provide consent, employees as healthy volunteers, and non-English-speaking persons). If yes, what additional safeguards will be taken to protect vulnerable persons?
   (c) Does this research deny minorities and women or children opportunities to participate in research if they would likely benefit from the research?
   If yes, provide justification for exclusion.
   (d) Do you intend to recruit employees as healthy volunteers?
   If yes, describe how employees would be informed of the research and confirm that no direct face-to-face solicitation is planned.

9. *Informed consent*
   (a) Are you using a written consent document that includes all of the required elements?
   If yes, upload a copy of the consent on the document tab.
   (b) Describe the consent process including where the consent interview takes

place to ensure it is conducted in a private manner and setting, when the consenting interview take place to ensure sufficient time is given to prospective subjects to make an informed decision, who conducts the consent interview, and how will it be documented.
   (c) If the language of the prospective subject is different from English, describe how the information about the research, and the consent process will be communicated.

10. *Waiver of informed consent*
    (a) Is a waiver or alteration of the written consent form being requested?
    If yes, explain why written consent cannot be used, and describe how patients will be informed of this research and what information will be provided in place of the written consent.
    Note: The following criteria must be met for a waiver or alteration of written informed consent:
    1. The research involves no more than minimal risk and the research is not FDA regulated.
    2. The rights and welfare of the participants will not be adversely affected by the waiver or alteration.
    3. The research could not practicably be conducted without the waiver or alteration; or the only record linking the participant and the research would be the consent document, and the principle risk would involve a breach of confidentiality.
    (b) Will an information sheet, cover letter, or phone script be used?
    If yes, upload these forms/letters/scripts as consent documents.

11. *Study sites*
    (a) Will this study be conducted at the main campus?

(b) Will this study be performed at one or more of the Family Health Centers?

If yes, identify all applicable sites.

(c) Will this study be performed at one of the Regional Hospitals?

(d) Is this study being conducted at any other sites such as nursing homes, schools, and community-based organizations?

If yes, provide contact information and a letter of authorization allowing this research to be conducted at their site.

12. *Confidentiality of data*

(a) Will the study data collection forms contain direct identifiers (patient name, address, SS #, hospital #, etc.)?

If yes, explain why identifiers cannot be replaced with study codes.

(b) Describe how study data is kept and securely maintained, including who will have access and where it will be stored.

(c) Will any data be stored on laptop computers or removable devices?

If yes, describe what precautions will be taken to protect confidentiality including verification that encryption software is being used and patient identifiers have been removed.

(d) Will identifiable study data be disclosed or shared with outside third parties?

If yes, will written consent be obtained to allow the release of data that includes direct identifiers?

13. *Safety and data monitoring*

(a) Describe how adverse events, unanticipated problems, safety data, and efficacy data will be monitored, assessed, and reported to the IRB and sponsor.

(b) Will a Data Safety Monitoring Board/Committee (DSMB) be used to review safety data involving adverse events?

If yes, describe the composition and review process for the DSMB.

(c) Will a data monitoring committee (DMC) be used to review the research data?

If yes, describe the composition and review process for the DMC.

14. *Research costs*

(a) Does this research involve any costs or expenses to the subject that are over and above the costs incurred for routine care?

If yes, specifically identify the costs associated with the research and identify who is responsible for payment (i.e., subject or subject's insurance, sponsor, and department).

Note: The cost section of the consent document must clearly identify all costs associated with the research and who is responsible for payment.

15. *Investigational drug*

Does this study involve an investigational drug?

If yes:

(a) Name of investigational drug.

IND #.

(b) Do you have a copy of the FDA IND assignment letter *or* equivalent documentation from the sponsor's regulatory official to verify that no conditions, restrictions, limitations, or holds were identified by FDA?

If yes, upload this document.

(c) Is the PI the holder of the IND?

If yes, there may be additional review requirements, and you will need to describe your external monitoring plan.

(d) Do you have an Investigator's Brochure (IB)?

If yes, upload the Investigator Brochure, and ensure risks of the drug are adequately described in the consent in lay terms.

(e) Will Investigational Drug Services (IDS) be responsible for storage, monitoring, and dispensing of study drugs?

   If no, describe your inventory control procedures, and provide approval from the IDS for ordering and dispensing research medications.

16. *Investigational device*

Does this study involve an investigational device?

If yes:

(a) Name of investigational device.

   IDE #.

(b) Do you have a copy of the FDA IDE letter or equivalent documentation from the sponsor's regulatory officer to verify whether any conditions, restrictions, or limitations were identified by FDA?

   If yes, upload this document. Note: IRB review cannot be completed without this document.

(c) Is the PI the holder of the IDE?

   If yes, there may be additional review requirements, and you will need to describe your external monitoring plan.

(d) What type of risk does this device represent?

   If NSR, describe the rationale for this classification, and provide documentation from the sponsor to justify this device as nonsignificant risk.

(e) Does this investigational device qualify for exemption from IDE regulations?

   If yes, identify the exemption category under IDE regulations 21 CFR 812.2(c), and provide a description of the device, reports of prior investigations with the device, the nature of the harm that may result from use of the device (life-threatening, permanent impairment, or potential for serious risk), and the sponsor assessment of the device's risk and rationale used in

making its risk determination. You may also seek a determination whether this is SR or NSR from the FDA.

(f) Describe your inventory control procedures for storage, monitoring, and distribution of study devices.

(g) Describe the procedures for training investigators and other research personnel to ensure the safe handling of this device.

17. *Marketed drugs/devices*

(a) Does this study involve an approved drug/device for an indication different from the approved labeling or instruction for use?

   If yes, describe the new indication and upload a copy of the approved drug insert/labeling or instructions for use.

(b) Does the use of this drug/device qualify for an exception from the requirements to obtain an IND/IDE?

   Provide sufficient documentation to prove this investigational use: (1) does not involve a route of administration or dosage level, use in a subject population, or other factor that significantly increase the risks associated with the use of this drug; (2) that this use is not intended to be reported to FDA in support of a new indication or any other significant change in labeling, advertising or promotion for the drug; or (3) submit documentation that the FDA has determined this use qualifies for IND exemption.

18. *Additional requirements*

(a) *Radiation safety*

   Does this study involve any additional radiation exposure solely for the research?

   If yes, complete the Subject Radiation Exposure Estimate form. Note: The consent should identify the cumulative risks of radiation exposure from both standard of care and the additional research-related tests.

Does this research involve the use of radioactive drugs?

If yes, identify the risks and the amount to be administered.

(b) *Biosafety*

Does this research involve the use of infectious agents, recombinant DNA, and gene transfer?

If yes, approval from the Institutional Biosafety Committee is required.

(c) *Point of care testing*

Does this research involve laboratory testing at the patient bedside outside of the main lab (such as urine pregnancy)?

If yes, POC testing requires prior approval by the POCT Compliance Council.

(d) *Tissue procurement*

Does this research involve the use of redundant/residual biological specimens accessioned to the Department of Anatomic Pathology for diagnostic or therapeutic purposes?

If yes, approval of the Director of Tissue Procurement is required.

(e) *New investigator*

Is the PI a new or first-time investigator?

If yes, obtain assistance with regulation elements and study start-up instructions.

19. *Additional documents*

Are there any additional documents other than the protocol and consent to be uploaded, for example, a second consent, an advertisement, a questionnaire, investigator brochure, patient information sheet, etc.? If yes, how many additional documents (other than the protocol and consent) are you uploading?

References

1. Clayman RV, Kavoussi LR, Soper NJ, et al. Laparoscopic nephrectomy. N Engl J Med. 1991;324(19):1370–1.
2. Abbou CC, Hoznek A, Salomon L, et al. Remote laparoscopic radical prostatectomy carried out with a robot. Report of a case. Prog Urol. 2000;10(4):520–3. Article in French.
3. Su LM. Robot-assisted radical prostatectomy: advances since 2005. Curr Opin Urol. 2010;20:130–5.
4. Box G, Averch T, Cadeddu J, Urologic NOTES Working Group, et al. Nomenclature of natural orifice translumenal endoscopic surgery (NOTES) and laparoendoscopic single-site surgery (LESS) procedures in urology. J Endourol. 2008;22(11):2575–81.
5. Kaouk JH, Autorino R, Kim FJ, et al. Laparoendoscopic single-site surgery in urology: worldwide multi-institutional analysis of 1076 cases. Eur Urol. 2011;60(5):998–1005.
6. Autorino R, Cadeddu JA, Desai MM, et al. Laparoendoscopic single-site and natural orifice transluminal endoscopic surgery in urology: a critical analysis of the literature. Eur Urol. 2011;59(1):26–45.
7. http://www.fda.gov/Drugs/DevelopmentApproval Process/HowDrugsareDevelopedandApproved/ ApprovalApplications/InvestigationalNew DrugINDApplication/default.htm#. Accessed on 13 Dec 2013.
8. http://www.fda.gov/MedicalDevices/ DeviceRegulationandGuidance/Overview/default. htm. Accessed on 13 Dec 2013.
9. Mastroianni AC. Liability, regulation and policy in surgical innovation: the cutting edge of research and therapy. Health Matrix Clevel. 2006;16(2):351–442.
10. Nat'l comm'n for the protection of human subjects of biomedical & behavioral research, The Belmont Report: ethical principles and guidelines for the protection of human subjects of research. 1979.
11. National Research Act, Pub. L. No. 93–348, 88 Stat. 342. 1974.
12. Kirby R, Challacombe B, Dasgupta P, et al. The importance of obtaining truly consensual informed consent. BJU Int. 2012;109(12):1743–4.
13. Brehaut JC, Carroll K, Elwyn G, et al. Informed consent documents do not encourage good-quality decision making. J Clin Epidemiol. 2012;65(7):708–24.
14. Enama ME, Hu Z, Gordon I, VRC 306 and 307 Consent Study Teams, et al. Randomization to standard and concise informed consent forms: development of evidence-based consent practices. Contemp Clin Trials. 2012;33(5):895–902.
15. Frader J, Caniano DA. Research and innovation in surgery. In: McCullough LB et al., editors. Surgical ethics. New York: Oxford University Press; 1998. p. 216. 220–21.
16. http://www.fda.gov/regulatoryinformation/guidances/ ucm126420.htm. Accessed on 13 Dec 2013.

Laboratory and Experimental Foundation for LESS

Antonio Cicione, Rocco Damiano, and Estevao Augusto Rodrigues Lima

Introduction

Analyzing the history of urology, urologists have traditionally comprised the vanguard of medical professionals who want to implement the usage of new technologies in their disciplines. Take into consideration the exponential development of video endoscopy and its routine use for the diagnosis and treatment of lower and upper urinary tract disease or the transurethral approach or shockwave lithotripsy and its prominent impact on urinary stones. Also, consider laparoscopy and, subsequently, robotic surgery that have deeply modified surgical approaches to many urological diseases, overcoming the open laparotomy approach in some cases.

In the case of urologists, they focus on procedures inside the urinary cavities and on the minimally invasive animus which have proved challenging to them for a long time.

Overall, the entire urologist community has been looking forward to the development of minimally invasive surgery with quickly perceivable benefits and limited invasiveness (including minimal or no scarring, reduced pain, fewer complications, and faster recovery time).

As a result of recent technological advancement and "urologist pioneer animus," two new minimally invasive surgeries have been developed [1, 2]: natural orifice transluminal endoscopic surgery (NOTES) and laparoscopic single-site surgery (LESS). They both mark a major milestone in the evolution of laparoscopic surgery.

NOTES involves an incision of the hollow viscera (e.g., stomach, colon, urinary tract, and/or vagina) with an endoscope in order to access the abdominal cavity and to perform intra-abdominal surgical procedures [3]. Using this method of accessing the target surgical organ helps to mostly, or sometimes completely, avoid skin incisions, as well as reduce discomfort to the patient and the invasiveness of the procedure as a whole [4].

Likewise, laparoscopic single-site surgery (LESS) represents minimally invasive surgical procedures that are carried out with a single incision [1]. LESS also offers the potential advantages of a more rapid recovery, fewer adhesions, a smaller chance of developing hernias, and less postoperative ileum [5]. From an aesthetical point of view, using a single incision instead of three to five incisions of 5–12 mm in width should minimize the palpable evidence of a surgical procedure. This is even more effective when the natural scar of the umbilicus is used as the port site [2].

A. Cicione, MD (✉) • R. Damiano, MD, PhD
Clinical and Experimental Medicine,
Magna Graecia University of Catanzaro,
Catanzaro, Italy
e-mail: cicione@unicz.it; damiano@unicz.it

E.A.R. Lima, MD, PhD
Urology Department, Hospital de Braga,
Braga, Portugal
e-mail: estevaolima@ecsaude.uminho.pt

© Springer Science+Business Media New York 2017
J.H. Kaouk et al. (eds.), *Atlas of Laparoscopic and Robotic Single Site Surgery*,
Current Clinical Urology, DOI 10.1007/978-1-4939-3575-8_3

Both LESS and NOTES belong to the next generation of standard laparoscopic surgery in which a reduction in the number of trocars has been tested; although there have been differing opinions regarding LESS and NOTES within the scientific community, those both surgical approaches generate interest for the notion that they should promote surgery with limited invasiveness and scarring. The possibility that such a surgical procedure might be possible continues to animate an increasing number of dreamers and skeptics.

In the following section, the experimental foundations of LESS and NOTES have been summarized.

The Underlying Basic Principles

LESS and NOTES represent the next step in the field of traditional laparoscopic surgery in which the use of multiple incisions (usually between 3 and 5) for the insertion of trocars has been replaced with the use of one singular incision at umbilical scar or at the hollow viscera in order to reduce the surgical trauma and the residual scarring of the patient.

Furthermore, not only does the principle of reducing the number of incisions present an aesthetic advantage to the patient but it also reduces the risk of organ damage and the occurrence of the undesired triad of "hernia, pain, and infection." Although the data demonstrating the effects of using LESS or NOTES procedures to reduce this risk is inconclusive, one should bear in mind that the laparoscopic approach has reduced the risk of wound infection from approximately 25 % in open surgeries to 5.8 % in laparoscopic urological surgeries [6, 7]; infection still tends to primarily occur at the site of specimen extraction [8]. Similarly, the risk of developing a hernia after an urological laparoscopic procedure is reduced compared to the open surgery approach (3 % and 18 %, respectively [5]), and Schafer [9] reported the risk related to the use of ports for both visceral and vascular injuries to be between 0.003 % and 0.3 %. Finally, the incisional pain after laparoscopic surgery has been

found to exceed that of visceral and shoulder pain in both level of occurrence and intensity during the first postoperative week [10]. To date, there is insufficient evidence to prove a significant reduction in incisional pain [11–13]; however, in a single-incision transumbilical laparoscopic cholecystectomy, using the periumbilical port incision method alone reduced the level of pain caused by traditional 4-port laparoscopic surgery [14].

Regarding the aesthetic benefits, Harrell [15] concluded his review by stating that surgeons concur in saying that small incisions associated with laparoscopic surgery, in general, produce a better "cosmetic" outcome and cause less pain than open surgery. Nevertheless, aesthetic benefits remain problematic to assess. Plastic surgeons are still investigating this difficult clinical outcome for the many confounding variables, such as the right scar assessment measure [16], the time at which scar evaluation should be carried out, and the evaluation of patient's scarring process [17]. It should be noted, however, that there is a consensus regarding the notion that a single periumbilical incision, or lack thereof in the case of NOTES, should be more aesthetically pleasing than three or four 5–10-mm incisions.

Another question to be asked is whether the NOTES and LESS procedures are viewed in a positive light by patients. Navarra et al. [18] reported in their study that NOTES cholecystectomy has gained a significant interest, while Strickland [19] showed that 75 % of 300 women surveyed were neutral or unhappy about the prospect of NOTES. However, a recent survey gauging public opinion on LESS and NOTES demonstrated that the concept of scar-free surgery associated with these new surgical techniques did appeal to the public, with LESS being the treatment of choice in a scenario of acute appendicitis [20]. Previously, Bucher et al. [21] surveyed medical and paramedic staff, surgical patients, and the general population regarding their treatment method of choice (LESS and NOTES were juxtaposed with laparoscopy) provided the surgical risk in all procedures is similar. 90 % of the participants (irrespective of sex) preferred a scar-free approach over a laparoscopy – a preference which was even more predominant among the younger participants. The support for the LESS and NOTES procedures diminished when an increased procedural risk was assumed.

With the aim of estimate, the perception and performance of urological surgeons when first applying scarless surgical techniques, Autorino et al. [22] evaluated the perception of urological surgeons; 14 naïve mini invasive surgical approaches surgeons who performed LESS, NOTES, and a mini-laparoscopy porcine nephrectomy. Subjective perception of the degree of difficulty trended in favor of the mini-laparoscopy, which was perceived to be technically less difficult to perform than the LESS and NOTES nephrectomy. Furthermore, no difference was detected between the surgeons' perceptions and expectations on the above minimal invasive techniques.

Subjective perception of the degree of difficulty trended in favor of the mini-laparoscopy, which was perceived to be technically less difficult to perform than the LESS and NOTES nephrectomy. Furthermore, no difference was detected between the surgeons' perceptions and expectations on the above minimal invasive techniques.

Regardless of unresolved issues, minimal invasive surgical therapy in the form of NOTES and LESS also provides an interesting road of discovery for urologists.

The Consortiums for Assessment and Research

In the era of evidence-based medicine, language standardization is of primary importance in urology as well as in other branches of medicine. Using standardized and unanimously accepted nomenclature while performing the relevant trials provides an opportunity to collect and analyze homogenized scientific data from a wider array of sources. However, early interest in LESS and NOTES methods in the medical and corporate world has led to the escalation of clinical applications within a relatively short period of time. Consequently, various terminologies and acronyms have been used to describe surgical procedures performed through a single incision or surgical site (Table 3.1).

In order to standardize the terminology related to scientific communications and the performing of clinical trials, a consortium comprised of experts from various surgical specialties was organized in Cleveland, Ohio, on July 2008 [23]. This multidisciplinary consortium of experts (the *LaparoEndoscopic Single-Site Surgery Consortium for Assessment and Research*- LESSCAR), having summarized the most important limitations (Table 3.2), produced a set of guidelines which define the usage of common appropriate nomenclature.

More recently, in an attempt to further simplify and clarify the nomenclature, as well as to discuss the emerging role of NOTES within the urologic community, a group of experts from the Endourological Society formed the *Urology Working Group on NOTES* in 2007 [2]. The objectives of this group were to amplify awareness of NOTES among professionals working in the field of urology, to create a platform on which to share discoveries related to urological NOTES, to direct the scientific evaluation and implementation of urological NOTES, to assist in creating learning opportunities related to urological NOTES, and to define the nomenclature of urological NOTES.

In order to address the final point, the aforementioned group presented a definition of urological NOTES, dividing it into (Table 3.1) *pure NOTES* (access through one natural orifice), *combined NOTES* (access through two natural orifices), and *hybrid NOTES* (access through a natural orifice and a transabdominal point).

Furthermore, the Urologic NOTES Group mainly adopted the LESSCAR group terminology and endorsed LESS surgery as the name for a single-port surgery [23].

Lastly, the *European Society of Urotechnology* also formed a working group dedicated to LESS and NOTES, proposing new recommendations for the future of both procedures [5, 11] and achieving a consensus on the most appropriate name for the single-site approach in the field of urology.

Notably, all the above research groups established a common nomenclature; this proves as a universal terminology remains a basic requirement so that research can be explained more consistently in literature and so that ideas and results can be quickly disseminated.

Table 3.1 Acronyms used to describe single-incision surgery and natural orifice surgery

The past		The present
NOTES	Natural orifice transluminal endoscopic surgery	
E-NOTES	Embryonic natural orifice transumbilical endoscopic surgery	
NOTUS	Natural orifice transumbilical surgery	
OPUS	One-port umbilical surgery	
SPA	Single-port access	
SILS	Single-incision laparoscopic surgery	
SSA	Single-site access	NOTES
SAS	Single-access-site laparoscopic surgery	Pure no additional port
SPL	Single-port laparoscopy	Combined using two different orifices
SITUS	Single-incision triangulated umbilical surgery	*Hybrid* additional transabdominal port
TULA	Transumbilical laparoscopic assisted	
TUES	Transumbilical endoscopic surgery	
LESS	Laparoendoscopic single-site surgery	
Mini-laparoscopy		
MISPORT	Minimally invasive single-port surgery	LESS
SLiP	Single laparoscopic port procedure	Pure no additional port[a]
SPA	Single-port access	Hybrid additional transabdominal port[b]
SPELS	Single-port endoscopic and laparoscopic surgery	Robotic use of VeSpA system
SPEARS	Single-port endoscopic and robotic surgery	
SPE	Single-port endoscopic surgery	
SPIs	Single-port intracorporeal surgery	
SPLS	Single-port laparoscopic surgery	
SPS	Single-port surgery	
TULAs	Translumenal laparoscopic-assisted surgery	
TUPS	Transumbilical universal port surgery	

[a]In urology mainly used transumbilical access (uLESS = LESS = pure LESS)
[b]With port ≤3 mm size

Table 3.2 Main limits and solutions underlined by LESSCAR group [23] on initial LESS experiences

Limits	Solutions
Terminology	A broader term was introduced: *laparoscopic single-site surgery* (LESS)
	It encompasses the following concepts: (1) a single entry port; (2) applicability to multiple locations (abdomen, pelvis, thorax); (3) laparoscopic, endoscopic, or robotic surgery; (4) umbilical or extraumbilical access; and (5) intra- and transluminal (percutaneous single-port access) approaches
Manuscript title	It would require a "mandatory descriptive second line" that succinctly provides: location and length of incision, approach, number and type of port used, type of surgery, laparoscope, and instruments used
Technology	An improvement in instruments field in order to overcome current drawback of LESS tools: triangulation-retraction-instrument crowding
Small case series	Developing a collaborative, international, web-based, registry database

Experimental Studies for LESS

A clear advantage of LESS is that surgeon access is achieved though the abdominal wall, which is more familiar to surgeons with prior laparoscopic experience. For that reason, the clinical application of LESS is occurring quickly and frequently, and few preliminary evaluations using animal models have been considered necessary.

Nevertheless, preliminary experimental studies involving LESS have been performed because physicians are also researchers, and new techniques or technologies need to be assessed for safety, usability, and reproducibility.

Raman and colleagues [24] performed a LESS nephrectomy on four female pigs followed by three human procedures. All the eight porcine kidneys were removed using a single 25-mm trocar and 10-mm with two 5-mm adjacent trocars in three renal units and in the remaining five, respectively. Articulating laparoscopic graspers, conventional endoshears, clips, and a stapler were used for dissection. Similarly, the three human LESS nephrectomies were successfully carried out with a mean operative time of 133 min (range, 90–160) and estimated blood loss of 30 ml. The kidneys were extracted through a solitary 2–4.5-cm periumbilical incision. No perioperative complications were recorded and all three patients were discharged on hospital day 2.

Before performing a LESS robot-assisted radical prostatectomy, Barret [25, 26] reported his experience with a LESS extraperitoneal radical prostatectomy in a cadaver model using both standard and articulated laparoscopic instruments. The author concludes that a robot-assisted LESS radical prostatectomy can feasibly be performed but that a human cadaver is an inadequate model for a LESS extraperitoneal radical prostatectomy.

Boylu et al. [27] determined the feasibility, instrumentation, and learning curve for a LESS partial nephrectomy in a pig model by performing ten transumbilical procedures using the R-port multichannel port, a 5-mm flexible laparoscope,

and custom-engineered articulating needle drivers, graspers, and scissors. Either the upper or lower pole of the kidney was scored and excised after placing a bulldog clamp on the renal pedicle. Bolsters were prepared with an absorbable hemostat which was placed at the site of excision and secured with polyglactin sutures. Modified suturing techniques were developed to achieve reconstruction in a small working space. There was no need for an additional port for triangulation. The total ischemia time decreased from 50 min in the first case to 27 min in the last. The authors concluded that the procedure is feasible; however, they also recognized that further refinement of instrumentation and techniques is needed.

Following this, animal studies have been required for the development and evaluation of LESS surgery-specific technology and instruments made to overcome technical limitations related to this surgical approach, i.e., the absence of triangulation, internal and external clashing, and poor range of movement [28]. Stolzenburg et al. [29] compared, in a dry animal laboratory, the efficacy of prebent instruments with conventional laparoscopic and flexible instruments in terms of time required, maneuverability, and ease of handling. An experienced laparoscopic surgeon performed 24 nephrectomies on 12 pigs using all sets of instruments through a single port, with the exception of the conventional instruments which were inserted through three ports. They showed that prebent instruments were less time consuming and had better maneuverability in comparison to flexible instruments in experimental single-port access surgery.

Regarding the prebent instruments, Autorino et al. [30] assessed a reusable access device (X-CONETM, Karl Storz, Tuttlingen, Germany) and four sets of prebent reusable instruments originally designed for gallbladder removal. Three surgeons with previous LESS experience performed 12 LESS nephrectomies (four per surgeon) on six pigs. In all procedures, the same reusable multichannel access device (X-CONE), a 5-mm extra-long telescope, and one out of every four sets were consecutively employed. Measuring the access device and set performances by objective and subjective parameters, the authors deduced that the standard set, consisting of straight scissors and a curved grasper, was found to be the easiest to use, while the reusable access device was an efficient and economical alternative.

By using a porcine model, Zeltser et al. [31] tested the feasibility of a single trocar nephrectomy using a novel transabdominal magnetic anchoring and guidance system platform through a 15-mm umbilical portal of entry. The porcine abdominal wall allowed the fixation of both a camera and a robotic cautery arm using magnetic couplers. Both of these were hardwired to external guidance systems, and light was provided by fiber-optic cables surrounding the umbilical trocar itself. The standard laparoscopic graspers and vascular stapler were manipulated through the umbilical trocar for the retraction and transaction of the renal vein and artery, while tissue dissection was accomplished with the robotic arm. Two non-survival nephrectomies were successfully completed with specimen extraction through the solitary umbilical incision.

Recently Haber et al. [32] reported their initial laboratory experience using the new flexible SPIDER platform (TransEnterix, Morrisville, NC, USA) for laparoendoscopic single-site surgery urologic procedures and its first clinical application. This platform was tested in a laboratory setting and used for a clinical case of renal cyst decortication. Three tasks were performed during the dry lab session, and different urologic procedures were conducted on a porcine model. Although surgeons deemed retraction to be the most labored task, the device provided good triangulation without instrument clashing during the clinical case.

Experimental Studies for NOTES

A natural orifice approach was decrypted in 1901 by Dimitri Ott [33] who performed a "ventroscopy" by introducing a speculum through an incision in the posterior vaginal fornix. However, the first porcine transvaginal extirpative procedure was only performed in 2002 by Gettman et al. [34] who used a single 5-mm trocars to carry out a radical nephrectomy in five female pigs. Some years later, Kalloo et al. [35], using a porcine model, introduced the technique of inserting a flexible endoscope into the peritoneum cavity, therefore overcoming a transgastric approach. The cavity was fully examined, liver biopsies were performed, and all pigs recovered and gained weight. Having transorally removed the organ, the gastric wall was closed with an intraluminal suturing technique. Following this, the transgastric route was adopted for various intraperitoneal procedures [36], but some indicated that limitations put human subjects at risk. Some of those limitations were primarily linked to the flexible gastroscope instruments used, which resulted in surgeons having to abandon the principles of classic and laparoscopic surgery.

Some years later, Lima et al. [37] tested on a porcine model the use of the transvesical port to approach the peritoneal cavity, demonstrating its feasibility. This naturally sterile approach allowed the introduction of rigid instruments above the bowel loops for easier retracting structure, and, in some cases, the vesicostomy was left open with just a bladder catheter. However, the only disadvantage seems to be urethra diameter compliance which limits the number of instruments which can be used and the success of specimen retrieval. Given the encouraging results of their first study, Lima et al. [38] tested the possibility of reaching the thoracic cavity, after passing the diaphragm. This study showed that NOTES was able to be extended from peritoneal to thoracic cavity, although the researchers were only able to perform limited thoracoscopy and lung biopsies.

While continuing to use the transvesical approach, a group from Harvard University [39, 40] developed the transcolonic access to perform a transcolonic cholecystectomy. However, the transcolonic port did not resolve many of the transgastric port limitations because it is not sterile and requires a reliable and effective closure device that is not available to this day.

In order to resolve the difficulties in finding safe devices for endoscopic closure, several investigators tried to rediscover the transvaginal access (posterior colpotomy), which had been used by gynecologists for many years to perform pelvic interventions. This access is easily closed by surgical stitches from the outside and allows both the introduction of rigid tools and organ retrieval of large dimensions [34]. After that, human cholecystectomies were performed [41–43]. However, the approach is seriously limited in that it is only available to women.

Training for LESS

In addition to technological improvement, surgeon training remains an important consideration when guaranteeing the secure implementation of novel techniques. Similar to most laparoscopic surgery, training for LESS is fundamental when it comes to the acquisition of skills needed to perform it on humans. That said, this technique has been considered less difficult to perform than NOTES due to its close similarity to a conventional laparoscopy. From this point of view, previous laparoscopy experience is an advantage when beginning LESS surgery. However, some peculiarities are noted in this approach, such as the difficulty and sometimes the impossibility of displaying surgical instruments in the center of the screen and the need to move both the camera and instruments together, which requires more delicate and precise movements than in a laparoscopy [44]. Furthermore, a conventional laparoscopy, as well as open surgery, was taught using the Halstedian apprenticeship model of "see one, do one, teach one" [45] whereby, during open surgery, an experienced surgeon guides the assistants and controls the surgery almost completely. During a laparoscopy, the surgeon loses some of this control and has to rely, at least in part, on an assistant with in-depth knowledge of surgery. At advanced minimally invasive procedures such as LESS, not only the surgeon requires precise training but also the rest of the team, as

maximum accuracy and coordination are needed from both the surgeon and the assistants.

To date, the optimal method for acquiring skills in LESS is yet to be clearly determined. Unlike the proliferation of literature published on initial clinical LESS experience, little has been written about the training and implementation of this approach [46]. Kravetz et al. [47] estimated a learning curve of approximately five cases for LESS cholecystectomy for a surgeon who is an expert in laparoscopic surgery.

Muller et al. [44] illustrated five different surgical procedures to be performed in an animal model as part of a training program for the LESS technique ((1) single-port transumbilical laparoscopic cholecystectomy, (2) single-incision transumbilical laparoscopic cholecystectomy, (3) right-sided single-incision laparoscopic radical nephrectomy, (4) single-incision transumbilical laparoscopic radical nephrectomy, (5) single-port transumbilical laparoscopic nephrectomy). Each of them has different degrees of difficulty associated with the use or not of intracorporeal sutures; these sutures already present some challenges during laparoscopic surgeries which become intensified when performing it with the LESS technique. The authors concluded by emphasizing that LESS is an approach which requires high levels of coordination between surgeons and their assistant, as well as a high degree of familiarity with the procedure by whole working team.

Stroup [46] described the LESS training program adopted at the University of California, San Diego. They suggested beginning by using a common training box (easily adaptable to a single-port platform or "Manhattan" multiport approach) and to perform the four training tasks of the Society of American Gastrointestinal Endoscopic Surgeons [48]. Subsequently, animal training protocols should focus on establishing access, kidney mobilization and medial visceral rotation, hilar dissection and ligation, and specimen extraction.

Also having the necessary clinical experience, initially using two basic straight instruments was suggested to be beneficial in ensuring operator familiarity due to their marked difference from other instruments; they are flexible and reticulating, for example. Finally, the authors also agree with Muller [44] that these techniques require close coordination between the operating surgeon, their assistant, and the entire operating room team.

Interestingly, Ramalingam [49] suggested the modification of a conventional self-made multiport endotrainer into a single-port endotrainer for LESS in order to reduce costs. Following this suggestion, this box trainer was tested by three expert laparoscopic surgeons. Again, the clashing of instruments and difficulty in positioning them were the main disadvantages reported by the surgeons, despite the fact they were able to perform pig nephrectomies.

Training for NOTES

Simulators and virtual reality mechanisms have been reported as effective in the acquisition of laparoscopic skills, and there may be a new role for simulators which are specifically designed for teaching transluminal surgery. Using simulators, the trainer can practice tasks and learn to manage all possible complications in a risk-free environment.

However, animal models do improve the authenticity of the training environment. Although porcine anatomy is not absolutely identical to that of a human, animal models are important tools in the learning of NOTES skills. Using the porcine model, surgeons can perform a range of approaches into the peritoneal cavity (transgastric, transvesical, transvaginal, and transcolonic), and carrying out several surgical procedures, at the same time, the difficulties of NOTES procedures should be appreciated. Stroup et al. [46] recommended the chief basis for successful NOTES training. The authors emphasized that instrument familiarization is also an important step for urologists who are otherwise familiar with endoscopic procedures. Moreover, a knowledge of NOTES principles and institutional environment support is essential in the progression of NOTES.

References

1. Box G, Averch T, Cadeddu J, Cherullo E, Clayman R, Desai M, et al. Nomenclature of natural orifice translumenal endoscopic surgery (NOTES) and laparoendoscopic single-site surgery (LESS) procedures in urology. J Endourol. 2008;22(11):2575–81.
2. Gettman MT, Box G, Averch T, Cadeddu JA, Cherullo E, Clayman RV, et al. Consensus statement on natural orifice transluminal endoscopic surgery and single-incision laparoscopic surgery: heralding a new era in urology? Eur Urol. 2008;53(6):1117–20.
3. Autorino R, Stein RJ, Lima E, Damiano R, Khanna R, Haber GP, et al. Current status and future perspectives in laparoendoscopic single-site and natural orifice transluminal endoscopic urological surgery. Int J Urol. 2010;17(5):410–31.
4. Pearl JP, Ponsky JL. Natural orifice translumenal endoscopic surgery: a critical review. J Gastrointest Surg. 2008;12(7):1293–300.
5. Georgiou AN, Rassweiler J, Herrmann TR, Stolzenburg JU, Liatsikos EN, Do EM, et al. Evolution and simplified terminology of natural orifice transluminal endoscopic surgery (NOTES), laparoendoscopic single-site surgery (LESS), and mini-laparoscopy (ML). World J Urol. 2012;30(5):573–80.
6. Bratzler DW, Houck PM, Richards C, Steele L, Dellinger EP, Fry DE, et al. Use of antimicrobial prophylaxis for major surgery: baseline results from the National Surgical Infection Prevention Project. Arch Surg. 2005;140(2):174–82.
7. Bratzler DW, Houck PM. Antimicrobial prophylaxis for surgery: an advisory statement from the National Surgical Infection Prevention Project. Am J Surg. 2005;189(4):395–404.
8. George AK, Srinivasan AK, Cho J, Sadek MA, Kavoussi LR. Surgical site infection rates following laparoscopic urological procedures. J Urol. 2011;185(4):1289–93.
9. Schafer M, Lauper M, Krahenbuhl L. Trocar and Veress needle injuries during laparoscopy. Surg Endosc. 2001;15(3):275–80.
10. Joshi GP, White PF. Management of acute and postoperative pain. Curr Opin Anaesthesiol. 2001;14(4):417–21.
11. Gettman MT, White WM, Aron M, Autorino R, Averch T, Box G, et al. Where do we really stand with LESS and NOTES? Eur Urol. 2011;59(2):231–4.
12. Autorino R, Cadeddu JA, Desai MM, Gettman M, Gill IS, Kavoussi LR, et al. Laparoendoscopic single-site and natural orifice transluminal endoscopic surgery in urology: a critical analysis of the literature. Eur Urol. 2011;59(1):26–45.
13. Rao PP, Rao PP, Bhagwat S. Single-incision laparoscopic surgery – current status and controversies. J Minim Access Surg. 2011;7(1):6–16.

14. Bresadola F, Pasqualucci A, Donini A, Chiarandini P, Anania G, Terrosu G, et al. Elective transumbilical compared with standard laparoscopic cholecystectomy. Eur J Surg. 1999;165(1):29–34.

15. Harrell AG, Heniford BT. Minimally invasive abdominal surgery: lux et veritas past, present, and future. Am J Surg. 2005;190(2):239–43.

16. Draaijers LJ, Tempelman FR, Botman YA, Tuinebreijer WE, Middelkoop E, Kreis RW, et al. The patient and observer scar assessment scale: a reliable and feasible tool for scar evaluation. Plast Reconstr Surg. 2004;113(7):1960–5.

17. Rassweiler JJ. Is LESS/NOTES really more? Eur Urol. 2011;59(1):46–8.

18. Navarra G, Curro G. SILS and NOTES cholecystectomy: a tailored approach. ANZ J Surg. 2010; 80(11):769–70.

19. Strickland AD, Norwood MG, Behnia-Willison F, Olakkengil SA, Hewett PJ. Transvaginal natural orifice translumenal endoscopic surgery (NOTES): a survey of women's views on a new technique. Surg Endosc. 2010;24(10):2424–31.

20. Chow A, Purkayastha S, Dosanjh D, Sarvanandan R, Ahmed I, Paraskeva P. Patient reported outcomes and their importance in the development of novel surgical techniques. Surg Innov. 2012;19(3):327–34.

21. Bucher P, Pugin F, Ostermann S, Ris F, Chilcott M, Morel P. Population perception of surgical safety and body image trauma: a plea for scarless surgery? Surg Endosc. 2011;25(2):408–15.

22. Autorino R, Kim FJ, Rassweiler J, De SM, Ribal MJ, Liatsikos E, et al. Mini-laparoscopy, laparoendoscopic single-site surgery and natural orifice transluminal endoscopic surgery-assisted laparoscopy: novice surgeons' performance and perception in a porcine nephrectomy model. BJU Int. 2012;110(11 Pt C):E991–6.

23. Gill IS, Advincula AP, Aron M, Caddedu J, Canes D, Curcillo PG, et al. Consensus statement of the consortium for laparoendoscopic single-site surgery. Surg Endosc. 2010;24(4):762–8.

24. Raman JD, Bensalah K, Bagrodia A, Stern JM, Cadeddu JA. Laboratory and clinical development of single keyhole umbilical nephrectomy. Urology. 2007;70(6):1039–42.

25. Barret E, Sanchez-Salas R, Kasraeian A, Benoist N, Ganatra A, Cathelineau X, et al. A transition to laparoendoscopic single-site surgery (LESS) radical prostatectomy: human cadaver experimental and initial clinical experience. J Endourol. 2009;23(1):135–40.

26. Barret E, Sanchez-Salas R, Watson J, Vallancien G. NOTES-LESS. Radical prostatectomy. Arch Esp Urol. 2009;62(5):336–8.

27. Boylu U, Oommen M, Thomas R, Lee BR. Transumbilical single-port laparoscopic partial nephrectomy in a pig model. BJU Int. 2010; 105(5):686–90.

28. Canes D, Desai MM, Aron M, Haber GP, Goel RK, Stein RJ, et al. Transumbilical single-port surgery: evolution and current status. Eur Urol. 2008;54(5):1020–9.

29. Stolzenburg JU, Kallidonis P, Oh MA, Ghulam N, Do M, Haefner T, et al. Comparative assessment of laparoscopic single-site surgery instruments to conventional laparoscopic in laboratory setting. J Endourol. 2010;24(2):239–45.

30. Autorino R, Kim FJ, Rane A, De SM, Stein RJ, Damiano R, et al. Low-cost reusable instrumentation for laparoendoscopic single-site nephrectomy: assessment in a porcine model. J Endourol. 2011;25(3):419–24.

31. Zeltser IS, Bergs R, Fernandez R, Baker L, Eberhart R, Cadeddu JA. Single trocar laparoscopic nephrectomy using magnetic anchoring and guidance system in the porcine model. J Urol. 2007; 178(1):288–91.

32. Haber GP, Autorino R, Laydner H, Yang B, White MA, Hillyer S, et al. SPIDER surgical system for urologic procedures with laparoendoscopic single-site surgery: from initial laboratory experience to first clinical application. Eur Urol. 2012;61(2):415–22.

33. Ott DO. Ventroscopic illumination of the abdominal cavity in pregnancy. Akush Zhenskikl Boleznei. 1901;15:7–8.

34. Gettman MT, Lotan Y, Napper CA, Cadeddu JA. Transvaginal laparoscopic nephrectomy: development and feasibility in the porcine model. Urology. 2002;59(3):446–50.

35. Kalloo AN, Singh VK, Jagannath SB, Niiyama H, Hill SL, Vaughn CA, et al. Flexible transgastric peritoneoscopy: a novel approach to diagnostic and therapeutic interventions in the peritoneal cavity. Gastrointest Endosc. 2004;60(1):114–7.

36. Autorino R, Haber GP, White MA, Khanna R, Altunrende F, Yang B, et al. Pure and hybrid natural orifice transluminal endoscopic surgery (NOTES): current clinical experience in urology. BJU Int. 2010;106(6 Pt B):919–22.

37. Lima E, Rolanda C, Pego JM, Henriques-Coelho T, Silva D, Carvalho JL, et al. Transvesical endoscopic peritoneoscopy: a novel 5 mm port for intra-abdominal scarless surgery. J Urol. 2006;176(2):802–5.

38. Lima E, Henriques-Coelho T, Rolanda C, Pego JM, Silva D, Carvalho JL, et al. Transvesical thoracoscopy: a natural orifice translumenal endoscopic approach for thoracic surgery. Surg Endosc. 2007;21(6):854–8.

39. Pai RD, Fong DG, Bundga ME, Odze RD, Rattner DW, Thompson CC. Transcolonic endoscopic cholecystectomy: a NOTES survival study in a porcine model (with video). Gastrointest Endosc. 2006;64(3):428–34.

40. Fong DG, Pai RD, Thompson CC. Transcolonic endoscopic abdominal exploration: a NOTES survival study in a porcine model. Gastrointest Endosc. 2007;65(2):312–8.

41. Zorron R, Maggioni LC, Pombo L, Oliveira AL, Carvalho GL, Filgueiras M. NOTES transvaginal cholecystectomy: preliminary clinical application. Surg Endosc. 2008;22(2):542–7.
42. Bessler M, Stevens PD, Milone L, Parikh M, Fowler D. Transvaginal laparoscopically assisted endoscopic cholecystectomy: a hybrid approach to natural orifice surgery. Gastrointest Endosc. 2007;66(6):1243–5.
43. Marescaux J, Dallemagne B, Perretta S, Wattiez A, Mutter D, Coumaros D. Surgery without scars: report of transluminal cholecystectomy in a human being. Arch Surg. 2007;142(9):823–6.
44. Muller EM, Cavazzola LT, Machado Grossi JV, Mariano MB, Morales C, Brun M. Training for laparoendoscopic single-site surgery (LESS). Int J Surg. 2010;8(1):64–8.
45. Al-Akash M, Boyle E, Tanner WA. Training on N.O.T.E.S.: from history we learn. Surg Oncol. 2009;18(2):111–9.
46. Stroup SP, Bazzi W, Derweesh IH. Training for laparoendoscopic single-site surgery and natural orifice transluminal endoscopic surgery. BJU Int. 2010;106(6 Pt B):934–40.
47. Kravetz AJ, Iddings D, Basson MD, Kia MA. The learning curve with single-port cholecystectomy. JSLS. 2009;13(3):332–6.
48. Peters JH, Fried GM, Swanstrom LL, Soper NJ, Sillin LF, Schirmer B, et al. Development and validation of a comprehensive program of education and assessment of the basic fundamentals of laparoscopic surgery. Surgery. 2004;135(1):21–7.
49. Ramalingam M, Senthil K, Murugesan A, Pai MG. Cost reductive laparoendoscopic single site surgery endotrainer and animal lab training-our methodology. Diagn Ther Endosc. 2010;2010:598165.

Part II

Instruments for LESS

LESS: Ports, Optics, and Instruments

4

Sammy E. Elsamra, Soroush Rais-Bahrami, and Lee Richstone

Introduction

Laparoendoscopic single-site surgery (LESS) represents a progression in the evolution of minimally invasive surgery. The goal of LESS is to minimize the number of incisions necessary to conduct a given procedure, without compromising outcomes. Proponents of the technique postulate that the decreased number of surgical scars may translate to a decrease in pain, convalescence time, and port site complications such as risk of injury to viscera upon entry, bleeding, or hernia [1]. Ongoing studies continue to help define the extent of such potential benefits. Further, cosmetic benefit is likely if the port sites are hidden within the umbilicus or the extraction site. Further still, LESS is considered a step in the progression toward natural orifice transluminal endoscopic surgery, often referred to as NOTES. While LESS has been applied to simple general surgical and gynecologic cases, such as appendectomies and fallopian tube ligations, its application to urology has flourished in the last several years, with nearly every retroperitoneal and pelvic urologic case deemed feasible with LESS.

The first urologic application of LESS was described in 2007 [2]. Since its advent there has been an abundance of research and development involving LESS in urology [3]. Recently, in a worldwide multi-institutional analysis, Kaouk et al. detailed the outcomes of over 1,000 cases done with this approach [4]. The trend within this paper revealed significant increase in number of cases performed from 234 before 2009 to 842 after. Clearly, the expansion of this approach has occurred in tandem with development of accessories necessary to facilitate this approach. New approaches to access with various ports, novel camera technology, and augmentation to instruments and platforms have all played a role in overcoming some of the technical challenges inherent to performing complex surgery through a single access point. Such developments are ever advancing and will likely allow for the adaptation of LESS into the community. Herein we provide a detailed review of ports, cameras, and instrumentation utilized in LESS urologic surgery.

S.E. Elsamra, MD
Department of Surgery, Division of Urology,
Rutgers – Robert Wood Johnson Medical School,
New Brunswick, NJ, USA
e-mail: elsamrsa@rutgers.edu

S. Rais-Bahrami, MD
Departments of Urology and Radiology, University of
Alabama at Birmingham, Birmingham, AL, USA
e-mail: sraisbahrami@uabmc.edu

L. Richstone, MD (✉)
Urology Department, The Hofstra – North Shore LIJ
School of Medicine, Lake Success, NY, USA
e-mail: lrichsto@nshs.edu

© Springer Science+Business Media New York 2017
J.H. Kaouk et al. (eds.), *Atlas of Laparoscopic and Robotic Single Site Surgery*,
Current Clinical Urology, DOI 10.1007/978-1-4939-3575-8_4

Access: Location

The central benefit of LESS to the patient is likely to be cosmesis based, and therefore it is obvious that the point of access is of critical importance. While surgery performed through a single incision may be more difficult, patients, particularly those who are younger, of female gender, and with benign surgical indications, tend to prefer a scarless surgical approach in order to avoid external pain and scarring [5]. In fact, in a prospective randomized trial evaluation on cosmetic satisfaction of patients who were undergoing either multiport or LESS surgery, patients in the LESS cohort reported significantly higher cosmetic satisfaction both shortly after surgery (1 week) and after nearly 6 months [6]. Hence, many patients desire improved cosmetic results, and LESS can provide such improvement in aesthetic outcomes.

The most common location for access during LESS is within the umbilicus. The elastic nature of skin allows for increased spacing of ports and a larger fasciotomy than the incision on the skin. Hence, a 2.5-cm skin incision may allow for access to a 5-cm fasciotomy. This property is often manipulated to allow for greater working room and decreased clustering of instruments within the surgical field.

The umbilicus is a ubiquitous, naturally occurring, aesthetically pleasing, congenital scar that can allow for the facile concealment of periumbilical or transumbilical incisions. In fact, transumbilical surgery is considered by some to be on the spectrum toward NOTES as evidenced by some of its acronyms: TUES (transumbilical endoscopic surgery), SPA (single-port access), SILS (single-incision laparoscopic surgery), E-NOTES (embryonic-NOTES), or NOTUS (natural orifice transumbilical surgery) [7]. Incisions may be placed either within the umbilical fold or through its center to allow for incisions as large as 5 cm. Peri- or transumbilical skin incisions may be separate stab incisions for each port or in contiguity. A single larger contiguous incision may allow for a single port to be placed at the extremes of exposed fascia or for the placement of a multichannel port. Such larger contiguous incisions may also be preferred for extirpative cases.

When an extraction incision is necessary, such as a partial nephrectomy, adrenalectomy, prostatectomy, donor nephrectomy, etc., the extraction site may be utilized for port placement. As described above, a periumbilical incision is often well concealed and suitable for the extraction of small or morcellated specimens. However, due to the limits of the fasciotomy length, extraction of large specimens (e.g., un-morcellated kidneys, large renal masses, or adrenal glands) may not be feasible without extension of the periumbilical fasciotomy. Gill et al. described their initial experience with donor nephrectomy utilizing the E-NOTES approach with a periumbilical multiport [8]. They also described the use of a 2-mm needlescopic instrument to assist in retraction (placed through the subcostal Veress puncture site) and a suture placed transabdominally to help retract the ureter and gonadal vein anterolaterally (Fig. 4.1).

Alternatively, a small Pfannenstiel extraction incision is often utilized. While periumbilical LESS may be performed followed by extraction through an extended periumbilical or Pfannenstiel incision, we have described the utilization of the mini-Pfannenstiel incision (7–8 cm) for the port placement and performance of donor nephrectomies [9], obviating the need for additional fasciotomies at the navel (Fig. 4.2). This has resulted in decreased pain compared to conventional laparoscopic donor nephrectomy in a subsequent prospective, single-blinded, randomized controlled trial [10].

It is important to note that when utilizing Pfannenstiel incision as the LESS site, extra-long instruments, articulating instruments, and a deflectable tip videoscope may be necessary. Similarly, obese patients undergoing TUES may also require long instruments and a deflectable tip videoscope as lateralization of ports (a common practice in obese patients in conventional laparoscopic approach) is not possible. Such instruments and videoscopes will be described later in this chapter.

Often the use of a single needlescopic (3 mm) instrument or port has been utilized to facilitate

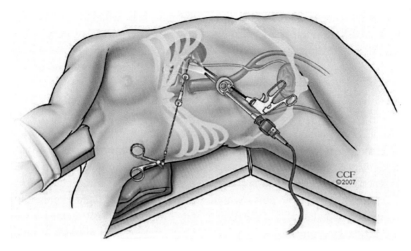

Fig. 4.1 LESS donor nephrectomy (transumbilical) with the use of a needlescopic instrument through Veress needle puncture site (From Gill et al. [8]. Reprinted with permission from Elsevier Limited)

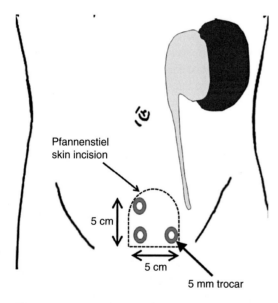

Fig. 4.2 LESS donor nephrectomy (via Pfannenstiel extraction incision) schematic diagram (From Andonian [9]. Reprinted with permission from Elsevier Limited)

LESS procedures. The placement of such a port can reestablish triangulation and facilitate in intracorporeal suturing or difficult retraction [11]. While not considered strictly LESS, such a puncture is rather small with minimal scar and may be necessary as the site of Veress needle insufflation or drain placement. One abstract at the 31st World Congress of Endourology revealed that the use of a single needlescopic accessory instrument may facilitate the adaptation of LESS into practice.

Another approach utilizing LESS is through the retroperitoneum (RP). Access is obtained in the standard fashion, with a small incision inferior to the twelfth rib at the mid-axillary line and dissection of the retroperitoneal space. Often a multiple -trocar port is utilized, and retroperitoneoscopy and surgery can be performed similar to the conventional multiple trocar approach. RP-LESS has been described for renal cyst decortications, ureterolithotomies [12], radical nephrectomies [13], renal ablations [14], pyeloplasties [15], and adrenalectomies in humans [16].

Most experience is noted with retroperitoneal LESS is with adrenalectomies. This approach offers the particular benefit of obviating the need for liver retraction, an issue encountered when performing a LESS right adrenalectomy from a single-site umbilical or transperitoneal subcostal approach. This benefit however is tempered by the obscurement of the adrenal vein, which is often furthest in the visual field and hidden by the adrenal tumor. In fact, one recent series comparing transumbilical, subcostal transperitoneal, and RP-LESS adrenalectomy, demonstrated a significant propensity to perform partial adrenalectomy when approaching from the

RP. Further, cosmetic benefit of RP-LESS was not superior to TUES, though RP-LESS did allow for shorter operative times [16].

Access: Ports

While access for LESS is obtained within a single site, it is not necessarily performed through a single incision. Access for LESS is obtained through either of two general approaches. One approach employs the placement of several ports within close proximity often within the folds of the umbilicus or the extraction incision. We refer to this approach as multiple trocar configuration. The other approach employs a single incision and fasciotomy through which a multiport device is placed (referred to as multiport approach) (Fig. 4.3) [17]. In their initial experience with TUES, Raman et al. favored three 5-mm ports placed in a periumbilical incision (multiple trocar configuration) over the then available 25-mm multiport [1]. The restriction in the range of motion associated with the multiport was cited as the reason why they favored the multiple trocar configuration.

Access: Ports: Multiple Trocar Configuration

There are many permutations of multiple trocar configuration. The premise however is the same. Three small ports (3 mm or 5 mm) are placed

through three separate periumbilical stab sites or within the extremes of exposed fascia within a single skin incision (Fig. 4.4) [1]. Most typically, the port utilized for the camera is both medial and in the middle for upper tract procedures and superior and in the middle for lower tract procedures approached from the umbilicus. This allows for a central view familiar to most surgeons from conventional laparoscopy.

While standard laparoscopic ports may be utilized, their most inner portions may crowd and restrict motion at the abdominal wall. One strategy often utilized is the staggering of port height above the incision in order to minimize external crowding. The use of low profile trocars such as the Curcillo very low profile trocar (Karl Storz, Tuttlingen, Germany) may help further minimize external crowding; however, these ports still contain rigid lumens which may interfere within the abdominal cavity. Novel trocars utilizing flexible silicone cannulas have been developed in order to better facilitate passage of pre-bent instruments and minimize internal crowding.

Many multichannel port devices will be reviewed in this chapter. Some have been featured in scholarly articles describing certain LESS cases, and information on others was obtained from commercial websites or personal experience. Xie et al. evaluated the performance of a multiport setup compared to the SILS Port and TriPort in a training simulator and discovered that multiports were associated with the least average load and the

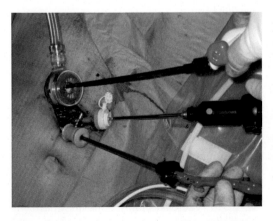

Fig. 4.3 LESS donor nephrectomy (via Pfannenstiel extraction incision)

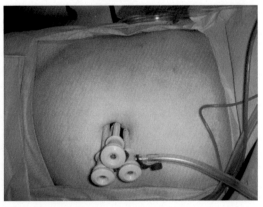

Fig. 4.4 Multiple trocars placed through a single site (From Raman et al. [1]. Reprinted with permission from Elsevier Limited)

shortest task performance times (Xie J Sur Res) [18]. While such multichannel port devices are well described commercially, comparisons of such devices are limited. A summary of multichannel port devices has been provided in Table 4.1.

AirSeal

The AirSeal trocar has been described for LESS [19] with the use of a non-FDA-approved 27-mm oval port. The AirSeal intelligent flow system creates a vortex of recycling carbon dioxide at the trocar site, obviating the need for a mechanical valve. This allows for decreased smudging of the camera and has been shown to be associated with shorter operative times and decreased CO2 consumption [20]. When adapted to a larger 27-mm oval port, which can accommodate several instruments without the loss of pneumoperitoneum, nine porcine single-port nephrectomies were performed at an average of 24 min.

AnchorPort

The AnchorPort (SurgiQuest, Milford, CT) is the "world's only self-adjusting, self-anchoring 5-mm port." Its elastomer construction and low profile external portion minimize crowding as its length is adjusted to fit the abdominal wall width – hence minimizing the crowding of the inner cannula noted with conventional ports. Further, as an extra safety measure, the AnchorPort comes with a bladeless optical port system in a handle that allows for visualization upon trocar placement (Fig. 4.5).

Access: Ports: Multichannel Port Devices

TriPort +/TriPort 15/QuadPort + (Olympus)

These represent the third generation of this line of single-port devices. Experience with the first-generation R-port in LESS has been sub-

stantial since its initial report in 2008 [2]. In principle these single-use devices utilize an inner diaphragm ring which is attached to a long clear plastic sleeve over which outer diaphragm containing three or four entry ports and an insufflation port is cinched over and secured when tight. Insertion is typically performed with an open (Hasson) technique. The inner ring is typically inserted with the aid of an injector introducer through a 2.5-cm fasciotomy (Fig. 4.6) [2].

SILS Port (Covidien)

The SILS Port is comprised of a single biconcave piece of foam with a valve for insufflation and three holes. These three holes can accommodate either three 5-mm low profile trocars (which come with the single-use device) or two 5-mm trocars and a 10–12-mm trocar (Fig. 4.7). It is inserted into a 2-cm skin and fascia incision (Hasson technique) with the aid of a Pean clamp (see Fig. 4.6).

GelPOINT (Applied)

The GelPOINT is similar to the GelPort used for hand-assisted laparoscopic surgery, save its smaller size, a valve for insufflation and smoke evacuation, and no pre-made incision in the gel. The device is comprised of an Alexis (Applied Medical, Rancho Santa Margarita, CA, USA) wound retractor, which can accommodate any facial incision between 1.5 and 7 cm, and the overlying gel. Sleeves are low profile trocars without any inner cannula made to be placed into the gel. The large surface area of the GelPOINT facilitates triangulation and minimizes external crowding. The GelPort has been described as a suitable access for robotic LESS (R-LESS), particularly as it provides excellent spacing and flexibility of port site placement [21]. Further, assistant port placement and specimen extraction were noted as additional benefits by Stein and colleagues (Fig. 4.8).

Table 4.1 Ports and platforms

Device	Company	Multiport?	Reusable?	Ports offered	Rotating?	Accessory valve	Size incision required	Removable top?	Features
AnchorPort	SurgiQuest (Orange, CT, USA)	No	No	Single 5-mm port	N/A	No	5 mm	N/A	Low profile, anchors abdominal wall, self-adjusting – minimizes internal crowding
AirSeal	SurgiQuest (Orange, CT, USA)	No (5 mm and 12 mm) and yes (27-mm oval port – not FDA approved)	No	5 mm, 12 mm, 27 mm	N/A	Tri-Lumen Filtered Tube Set – allows for airflow through side of trocar	5–27 mm	N/A (oval port – NO)	Valveless technology – decreased smudging, for the 27-mm oval port – positioning of instruments not fixed, facile placement of pre-bent instruments, continuous evacuation of smoke, reduction of CO_2 consumption, may lead to decreased OR times
TriPort +	Olympus (Southborough, MA, USA)	Yes	No	2 × 5-mm ports, 1 × 15-mm port (reducible)	No	2 valves (insufflation and smoke evacuation)	10–25 mm	Yes	Easy introduction and removal of instruments Accommodates a wide variety of laparoscopic instruments Easy insufflation and smoke evacuation Firmly grips incision to maintain pneumoperitoneum Reduces instrument clutter in operative field Controlled Hasson introduction Virtually eliminates scarring Full visibility upon entering abdominal cavity Removable top streamlines specimen removal

TriPort 15	Olympus (Southborough, MA, USA)	Yes	No	3×5-mm ports, 1×10-mm port (reducible)	No	2 valves (insufflation and smoke evacuation)	10–25 mm	Yes	
QuadPort +	Olympus (Southborough, MA, USA)	Yes	No	2×5-mm ports, 1×10-mm port (reducible), 1×12-mm port (reducible), 1×15-mm port (reducible)	No	2 valves (insufflation and smoke evacuation)	25–60 mm	Yes	
SILS port	Covidien (Dublin, Ireland)	Yes	No	3 slots, may accommodate 3×5-mm ports, or 2×5-mm and 1×10–12-mm port	No	1 valve with two-way stopcock	20 mm	Yes	
GelPOINT	Applied Medical (Rancho Santa Margarita, CA, USA)	Yes	No	May accommodate many various ports, either through sleeves or may utilize standard trocar	No	1 valve	15–70 mm	Yes	Placement of ports not prefixed, novel design allows for surgeon's desired placement of ports on a large surface area
Homemade Port – utilizing Alexis wound protector	Any surgical glove + Alexis wound protector (Applied Medical)	Yes	No	Up to 5 – any size	No	No	15 mm to 70 mm	Yes (but not replaceable)	Inexpensive (estimated $200 USD); however, construction and lack of trocar support may add to OR time
Octoport	Dalim SurgNET (Korea)	Yes	No	2×5 mm + 1×12 mm (reducible) ±1×10 mm	Yes	2 valves (insufflation and smoke evacuation)	15 mm to 50 mm	Yes	
SSL Access System	Ethicon Endo-Surgery (Cincinnati, OH, USA)	Yes	No	2×5 mm + 1×10/12 mm	Yes	1 valve	20–40 mm	Yes	Larger wound retractor allows for 7-cm abdominal wall thickness retraction. No profile trocar design – minimizes external crowding

(continued)

Table 4.1 (continued)

Device	Company	Multiport?	Reusable?	Ports offered	Rotating?	Accessory valve	Size incision required	Removable top?	Features
EndoCone (S-port EndoCone)	Karl Storz (Tuttlingen, Germany)	Yes	Yes	6×5-mm slots + 2×10/12-mm slots	No	1 valve		No	Low profile, compatible with S-Port Modular system which allows for placement of EndoCone or X-Cone type cap
X-Cone, Mini-X-Cone (S-Port X-Cone)	Karl Storz (Tuttlingen, Germany)	Yes	Yes	3×5-mm ports, 1×10-mm port (reducible)	Yes	2 valves (insufflation and smoke evacuation)	20–30 mm	Yes	Reusable up to 20 sterilizations, compatible with S-Port Modular system which allows for placement of EndoCone or X-Cone type cap
KeyPort	Richard Wolf (Knittlingen, Germany)	Yes	Yes	3 ports (typically 2×5 mm and 1×10/12 mm)	Yes	1 valve	30 mm and 36 mm	Yes	
Platforms									
SPIDER	TransEnterix (Durham, NC, USA)	Yes	Yes	Two flexible channels (instrument delivery tubes) and two rigid channels	No	3 valves		No	
Transport	USGI Medical (San Clemente, CA, USA)	Yes	Yes	4 large working channels	N/A	N/A	N/A	N/A	Platform for NOTES, may have application for LESS
Da Vinci Robot	Intuitive Surgical (Sunnyvale, CA, USA)	N/A	Yes	N/A	No	N/A	N/A	N/A	Da Vinci Si Robot allows for triangulation and allows surgeon's right hand to control right-sided instrument; second-generation instruments (VeSPA) available but lack EndoWrist

Homemade Port (Applied Wound Retractor Plus Glove)

Similar to the GelPOINT is the Homemade Port. This is classically comprised of a wound retractor and a sterile surgical glove that is secured to the wound retractor – utilizing suture or sterile rubber bands. This was initially described by a group in Korea that did not have access to commercial LESS single-port devices [22]. The glove (typically size 6.5–7.5) is sutured to the outer ring of the wound retractor. This configuration allows for the placement of five ports, essentially of any size (Fig. 4.9) [22]. In a report on 50 cases utilizing such access, both laparoscopic and robotic, Jeon et al. cited that there were no cases with leakage of pneumoperitoneum from the device, the devices offered wide range of motion, and the device was rather inexpensive (around $200) [23].

Octoport (Dalim SurgNET)

The Octoport is another single-port device that accommodates incisions from 15 to 50 cm with either of its two base sizes. This Korean product utilizes a wound retractor with various multiport attachments to allow for one, three, and four ports. A beneficial feature is this ports ability to rotate, minimizing the need to remove an instrument and place in another port (Fig. 4.10).

SSL Access System (Ethicon Endo-Surgery)

The SSL Access System is similar to the Octoport in that it utilizes a wound retractor and an attachment cap. This cap rotates as well, but it provides the additional advantage of a low profile cap – no trocar components protrude from the cap (both inside and outside the body). The wound retractors are fashioned for 2-cm or 4-cm fasciotomy, with the larger able to accommodate a 7-cm abdominal wall thickness. The cap accommodates two 5-mm instruments and a 10–12-mm instrument.

X-Cone (Karl Storz) and KeyPort (Richard Wolf)

Both of these single-port devices are relatively new and unlike all the previous ports are reusable. The Keyport has been described in a prospective evaluation of 31 LESS-radical prostatectomies, revealing a low positive margin rate, excellent aesthetic results, and very low postoperative pain levels [24]. The authors utilized an additional 3-mm incision for the placement of a port to facilitate intracorporeal suturing of the vesicourethral anastomosis and for drainage (Fig. 4.11).

SPIDER

The SPIDER surgical system (TransEnterix, Morrisville, NC, USA) is a novel platform created for LESS. It has been shown to be safe and effective in LESS cholecystectomy in an animal model and has recently gained FDA approval. An evaluation in the laboratory revealed that it was received well by experienced and inexperienced surgeons except for lack of strength required for retraction [25]. In the same report, the group from Cleveland Clinic demonstrated that it may not be ready for primetime as there were many issues associated with its first human use in the form of renal cyst decortications. The device was rather large and required the placement of a GelPort in order to provide enough room within the insufflated abdomen. In addition, prolonged operative time was partly attributed to the need for several repositioning attempts. Further, a straight lap instrument was added in order to facilitate with the decortications and subsequent suturing of a collecting system communication (Fig. 4.12).

Transport (USGI Medical, San Clemente, CA, USA)

Essentially, it is a flexible endoscope with four ports that allows for a flexible lens and three flexible instruments to be placed. While initially developed for NOTES, it has been attempted for E-NOTES.

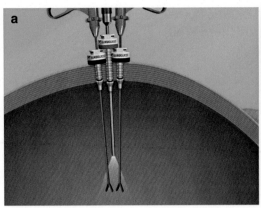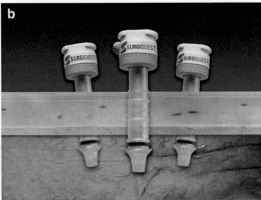

Fig. 4.5 The AnchorPort® Cannulas from SurgiQuest® (**a**)-Illustration of anchorports within insufflated abdomen, (**b**) Illustration of anchorports demonstrating low profile nature of port

Optics

Standard laparoscopes are typically straight, are relatively short, offer only one angle of view per lens, and are commonly attached to the camera and light source separately, often at 90° angle to one another. All of these features have been targeted for adaptation to LESS. By increasing length, incorporating the camera and light source in-line with the lens, and adding articulation, optical systems designed specifically for LESS offer the surgeon improvements in visualization with decreased internal and external crowding.

Karl Storz offers an extra-long lens in the Hopkins endoscope. This lens offers a working length of 50 cm which prevents the camera and light source, and assistant's hand, from being an additional contributor to external crowding associated with LESS.

Karl Storz also offers the ENDOCAMELEON endoscope. This lens offers the assistant control over the angle of visualization of the scope. A dial located near the insertion of the light cord allows the assistant to change the angle of visualization from 0 to 100°. This allows for the assistant to hold the scope more inferiorly minimizing external crowding and obviating the need for lens changes.

Another recent development has been the advent of flexible tip endoscopes. Both Olympus (EndoEyes) and Stryker (IDEAL EYES) offer a videoendoscope with assistant-controlled deflection. This deflection is particularly beneficial in LESS performed from an extraction site such as in Pfannenstiel donor nephrectomy [10]. In fact, the latest models of articulating videoscopes (such as the Endoeye Flex 3D LTF-190-10-3D, Olympus, Southborough, MA) offer not only angulated views of up to 100° in four directions (up, down, left, right), but also offer capability of either two-dimensional or three-dimensional viewing, focus-free viewing, and Narrow Band Imaging®. As highlighted by Olympus, based on laboratory studies, the benefit of three-dimensional viewing seems to help decrease the learning curve of specific surgical tasks and improves the speed and accuracy of grasping, suturing, and dissection independent of skill level [26]. Despite such claims, independent reports are critical in maintaining integrity with such claims. Though they are limited, one such evaluation by Goldsmith et al. reported that fixed rod lens system demonstrates the highest resolution and is not susceptible to significant attenuation of resolution noted in flexible videoscopes at flexion [27].

Several novel concepts in optics targeted for LESS surgery have been developed. Terry et al. described the use of a novel port camera system in a porcine model [28]. Their SPA Port Camera combines the camera, light source, and

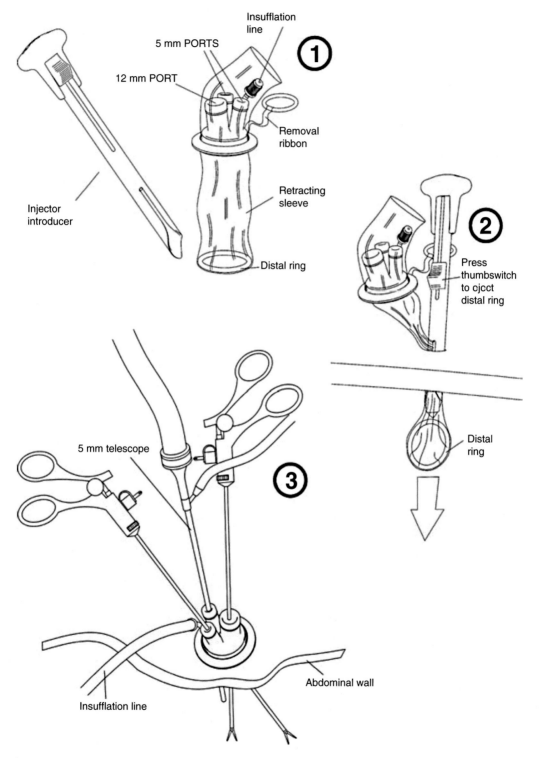

Fig. 4.6 Insertion and setup for R-Port (similar to any Olympus port – TriPort, QuadPort) (From Abhay et al. [2]. Reprinted with permission from Elsevier Limited)

monitor into an inexpensive cannula port. This obviated the need for a dedicated port for a camera and, consequentially, an assistant to hold such camera. Despite their low-cost model, several shortcomings were evident during the live surgery.

Another novel optic system is the well-described magnetically anchored guidance systems (MAGS) developed at University of Texas Southwestern. While not commercially available, such systems have been demonstrated in human cases with success [29], with equivalent or superior resolution and depth of focus compared to

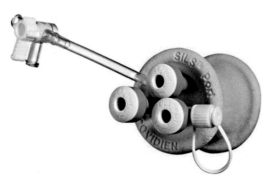

Fig. 4.7 SILS Port (Covidien) Insertion Copyright ©2014 Covidien. All rights reserved. Used with the Permission of Covidien

conventional laparoscope or flexible endoscope [30], and resultant decreased surgeon and camera driver work-load [31].

Instruments

LESS was originally performed with conventional laparoscopic instruments. Immediately apparent is that the use of straight instruments placed through a single site minimizes triangulation, often necessary for all but the simplest laparoscopic procedures. Further, in an effort to minimize external crowding, many have adopted crossing instruments. This effectively moved the triangulation point or fulcrum from the operative field to the point of insertion through the abdominal wall (through the point of single access). One strategy utilized to reestablish triangulation at the surgical field includes the utilization of pre-bent instruments. Another strategy employs the use of articulating instruments.

Pre-bent Instruments

Karl Storz and Peter Wolf have developed pre-bent instruments in the form of the S-portal and

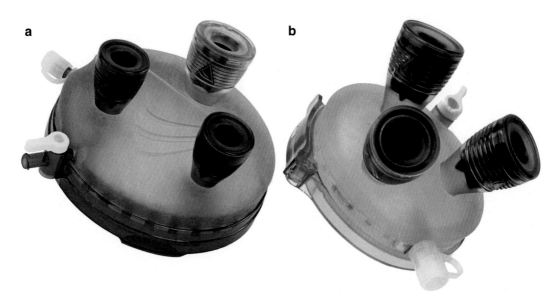

Fig. 4.8 GelPOINT (Applied Medical). (**a**) GelPOINT® Advanced Access Platform. (**b**) GelPOINT Mini Advanced Access Platform (Images courtesy of Applied Medical Resources Corporation)

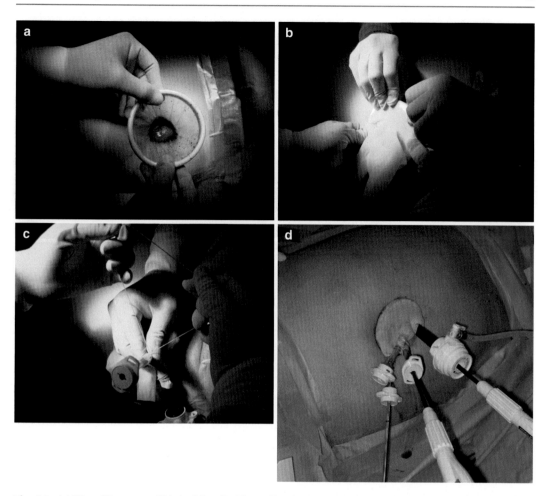

Fig. 4.9 (**a**) Wound Protector within incision (**b**) Glove affixed onto wound protector (**c**) Trocars placed into cut glove finger-tip and secured with suture tie (**d**) Final Setup of Homemade Port: made of wound retractor and glove (From Han et al. [22]. Reprinted with permission from Elsevier)

duo-rotate instruments, respectively. The benefit of such instruments is that they are often reusable, are boasting their economy, and are sturdy. Such pre-bent instruments require the use of flexible trocars or single-port systems. The duo-rotate instruments have been specifically utilized with some success in six consecutive LESS partial nephrectomies [32]. The authors contended that the ability to rotate the tip 360° allowed for improved maneuverability without loss of rigidity.

Clearly however, the use of such pre-bent instruments is not intuitive and may require a learning curve. Ninety medical students were evaluated on their ability to perform four typical laparoscopic tasks in the lab utilizing conventional laparoscopic instruments and port placement, LESS with one pre-bent and one straight laparoscopic instrument, or LESS with two pre-bent instruments [33]. As expected, the students performed significantly better on the conventional laparoscopic approach than the LESS approach. Their performance with the utilization of two pre-bent instruments was inferior to their performance with the use of a single pre-bent instrument, though this difference was not statistically significant. Despite their inferiority to conventional instruments, Stolzenberg identified pre-bent instruments as greater in maneuverability and less time-consuming compared to flexible instruments in another laboratory evaluation [34].

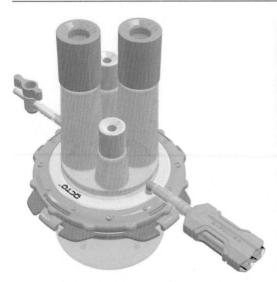

Fig. 4.10 Octoport (Dalim SurgNET) (Courtesy of Dalim SurgNET)

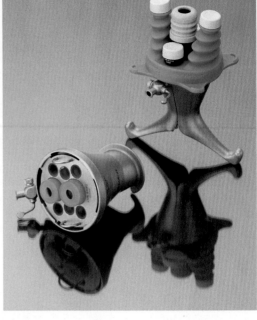

Fig. 4.11 X-Cone (Karl Storz) (©2013 Photo Courtesy of Karl Storz Endoscopy-America, Inc.)

Articulating Instruments

Articulating instruments may be another solution to overcome the limitation forced upon laparoscopy through a single access. Articulating instruments allow for the reestablishment of triangulation, however, with many additional steps. First, the surgeon must still be cognizant of potential crossing of instruments which will limit the motion of one instrument with respect to the other (internal clashing). Secondly, the surgeon must then operate in a mirror image fashion. In other words, the left hand controls the right-sided instrument which must be articulated toward the midline, with the opposite true for the opposite hand. Clearly, maneuvering such instrumentation requires much cognitive energy. Martinec et al. revealed that while expert laparoscopic surgeons were able to retain proficiency in a dry lab exercise when transitioning to flexible instruments, somewhat, novices had significantly greater difficulty [35]. Utilization of the da Vinci Si Robot may negate such difficult cognitive exercise by utilizing software that assigns control

to the instrument on one side of the screen to its ipsilateral hand.

Another limitation with the articulating instruments includes their loss of control and power at the point of articulation. Jeong et al. detailed the results of their mechanical experiments summarizing that first-generation articulating instruments do not provide sufficient forces necessary to meet the usual operative needs [36], though newer models may be improved in their mechanical properties [37].

Robotic Platform

The da Vinci Robotic platform was FDA approved in the USA for laparoscopic general and urologic surgery. Though it was not designed for LESS approach, its application to LESS has been ever-present. Over 55 studies have demonstrated the feasibility of the da Vinci Si Robot in LESS, with varying degrees of success. The initial hurdle that was cleared by R-LESS was the external and internal

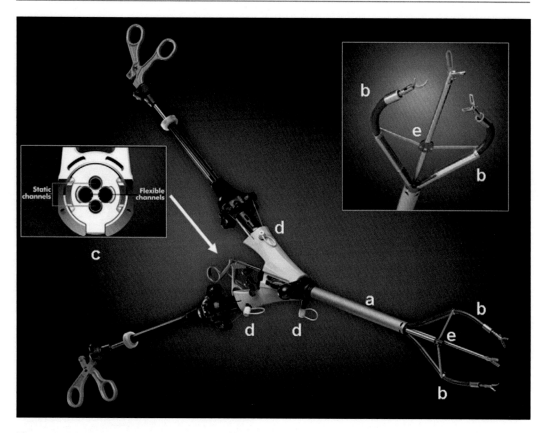

Fig. 4.12 SPIDER surgical system. (**a**) Main body port with cannula. (**b**) Extended-reach instrument delivery tubes (IDTs); being flexible, the IDTs allow for x, y, and z motion for a multidirectional approach into and throughout the surgical field. They are actuated by a gimbal system at the proximal end that provides 360 degrees of freedom at the distal end. (**c**) Four working channels, two flexible and two rigid. (**d**) Ports for insufflation/smoke evacuation. (**e**) Triangulation ratchet to adjust the width of the working area. (From Haber et al. [25]. Reprinted with permission from Elsevier Limited)

crowding associated with conventional placement of robotic arms through a single site. The "chopstick" technique has been demonstrated to decrease such sword-fighting, initially in the lab and subsequently in porcine models [38]. The chopstick technique is now the standard approach for R-LESS, particularly as the intuitive software allows for the surgeon's right hand control to control the instrument on the right side of the field and vice versa (limiting the mental strain associated with such technique in non-robotic LESS) [3].

R-LESS may be performed through multiple ports placed within a single incision, with a single-port device, or a combination of both. Figure 4.13 demonstrates robotic instruments placed through various ports [3]. Despite this,

Intuitive Surgical has developed a second-generation platform designed specifically for LESS for the use with the da Vinci Si, known as VeSPA (Fig. 4.14). Haber et al. demonstrated the feasibility of this platform in 16 R-LESS cases performed in the porcine model [39] with no complications, robotic system failures, or significant instrument clashing. However, their excitement was tempered by significant leakage of air, decreased optical resolution with the 8.5-mm videoscope (compared with the standard 12-mm videoscope), and the lack of an EndoWrist associated with the VeSPA instruments. Subsequent modifications including improvements in the multi-channel port and shorter curved trocars have allowed for improvements in air leakage and

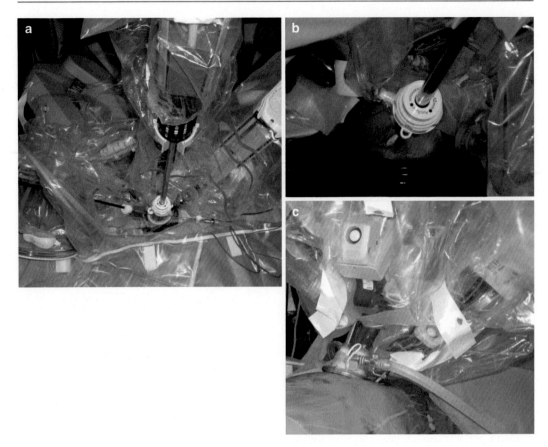

Fig. 4.13 Access devices to perform robotic laparoendoscopic single-site surgery: (**a**) SILS Port (Covidien), (**b**) GelPoint (Applied), and (**c**) TriPort (Olympus). Courtesy of Jihad Kaouk, Cleveland Clinic, Cleveland, OH, USA. (From Autorino et al. [3]. Reprinted with permission from Elsevier Limited)

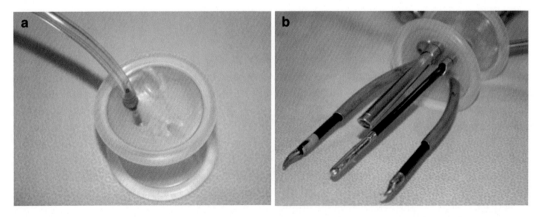

Fig. 4.14 VeSPA instruments (second-generation instruments purposely built for robotic LESS) (**a-c**) Multichannel port with trocars and instruments; (**d**) first- (longer) and second- (shorter) generation single-site trocars; (**e**) single-site instruments; (**f**) multichannel port inserted in the umbilicus. (From Kaouk et al. [40]. Reprinted with permission from Elsevier Limited)

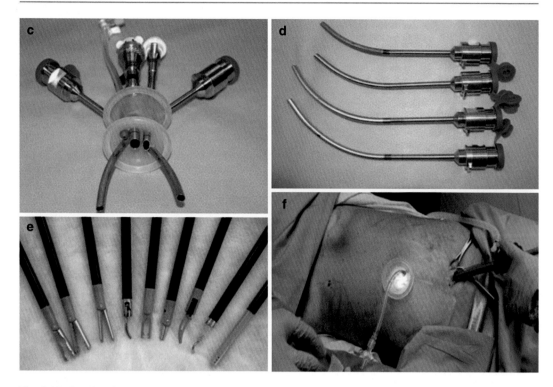

Fig. 4.14 (continued)

space issues in a subsequent evaluation in the cadaveric model [40]. Improvements are ever developing, and while Intuitive Surgical may eventually deliver EndoWrist technology to this new platform, many companies and collaborations are on the hunt for the next big advancement. Novel ideas and advances may allow us to offer patients nearly scarless surgery without increasing difficulty or decreasing safety. Perhaps, it is the next generation of robots that will herald LESS into widespread adaptation [3].

References

1. Raman JD, Bensalah K, Bagrodia A, Stern JM, Cadeddu JA. Laboratory and clinical development of single keyhole umbilical nephrectomy. Urology. 2007;70(6):1039–42. PubMed.
2. Rané A, Rao P, Rao P. Single-port-access nephrectomy and other laparoscopic urologic procedures using a novel laparoscopic port (R-Port). Urology. 2008;72:260–4.
3. Autorino R, Kaouk JH, Stolzenburg JU, et al. Current status and future directions of robotic single-site surgery: a systematic review. Eur Urol. 2013;63:266–80.
4. Kaouk JH, Autorino R, Kim FJ, et al. Laparoendoscopic single-site surgery in urology: worldwide multi-institutional analysis of 1076 cases. Eur Urol. 2011;60:998–1005.
5. Autorino R, White WM, Gettman MT, et al. Public perception of "Scarless" surgery: a critical analysis of the literature. Urology. 2012;80:495–502.
6. Song T, Cho J, Kim TJ, et al. Cosmetic outcomes of laparoendoscopic single-site hysterectomy compared with multi-port surgery: randomized controlled trial. J Minim Invasive Gynecol. 2013;20:460–7.
7. Kumar CVP. Different types of single incision laparoscopy surgery (SILS) ports. World J Laparosc Surg. 2011;4(1):47–51.
8. Gill IS, Canes D, Aron M, et al. Single port transumbilical (E-NOTES) donor nephrectomy. J Urol. 2008;180:637–41.
9. Andonian S, Herati AS, Atalla MA, et al. Laparoendoscopic single-site pfannenstiel donor nephrectomy. Urology. 2010;75:9–13.
10. Richstone L, Rais-Bahrami S, Waingankar N, et al. Pfannenstiel laparoendoscopic single-site (LESS) vs conventional multiport laparoscopic live donor nephrectomy: a prospective randomized controlled trial. BJU Int. 2013;112:616–22.

11. Liatsikos E, Kyriazis I, Kallidonis P, Do M, Dietel A, Stolzenburg JU. Pure single-port laparoscopic surgery or mix of techniques? World J Urol. 2012;30:581–7.

12. Tugcu V, Simsek A, Kargi T, Polat H, Aras B, Tasci AI. Retroperitoneal laparoendoscopic single-site ureterolithotomy versus conventional laparoscopic ureterolithotomy. Urology. 2013;81(3):567–72. doi:10.1016/j.urology.2012.11.033. Epub 2013 Jan 3. PubMed.

13. Dong J, Zu Q, Shi L, Gao J, Song T, Li H, Sun S, Zhang X, Cai W. Retroperitoneal laparoendoscopic single-site radical nephrectomy using a low-cost, self-made device: initial experience with 29 cases. Surg Innov. 2013;20(4):403–10. doi:10.1177/1553350612460768. Epub 2012 Dec 4. PubMed.

14. Nozaki T, Watanabe A, Fuse H. Laparoendoscopic single-site surgery for partial nephrectomy without ischemia using a microwave tissue coagulator. Surg Innov. 2013;20(5):439–43. doi:10.1177/1553350612459682. Epub 2012 Sep 10.

15. Chen Z, Chen X, Wu ZH, et al. Feasibility and safety of retroperitoneal laparoendoscopic single-site dismembered pyeloplasty: a clinical report of 10 cases. J Laparoendosc Adv Surg Tech A. 2012;22(7):685–90. doi:10.1089/lap.2012.0164. Epub 2012 Jul 30.

16. Wang L, Cai C, Liu B, Yang Q, Wu Z, Xiao L, Yang B, Chen W, Xu Z, Song S, Sun Y. Perioperative outcomes and cosmesis analysis of patients undergoing laparoendoscopic single-site adrenalectomy: a comparison of transumbilical, transperitoneal subcostal, and retroperitoneal subcostal approaches. Urology. 2013;82(2):358–64. doi:10.1016/j.urology.2013.03.060. PubMed.

17. Soroush Rais-Bahrami, Abhay Rane, Lee Richstone. Chapter 107. Smith's textbook of endourology, 3rd ed. West Sussex, UK. Wiley-Blackwell; 2012.

18. Xie XF, Zhu JF, Song CL, et al. Mechanical evaluation of three access devices for laparoendoscopic single-site surgery. J Surg Res 2013;185(2):638–44.

19. Leppert JT, Breda A, Harper JD, et al. Laparoendoscopic single-site porcine nephrectomy using a novel valveless trocar system. J Endourol. 2011;25(1):119–22. doi:10.1089/end.2010.0199. Epub 2010 Oct 26.

20. Herati AS, Andonian S, Rais-Bahrami S, et al. Use of the valveless trocar system reduces carbon dioxide absorption during laparoscopy when compared with standard trocars. Urology. 2011;77:1126–32.

21. Stein RJ, White WM, Goel RJ, et al. Robotic laparoendoscopic single-site surgery using GelPort as the access platform. Eur Urol. 2010;57:132–7.

22. Han WK, Park YH, Jeon HG, et al. The feasibility of laparoendoscopic single-site nephrectomy: initial experience using home-made single-port device. Urology. 2010;76:862–5.

23. Jeon HG, Jeong W, Oh CK, et al. Initial experience with 50 laparoendoscopic single site surgeries using a homemade, single port device at a single center. J Urol. 2010;183:1866–72.

24. Cáceres F, Cabrera PM, García-Tello A, et al. Safety study of umbilical single-port laparoscopic radical prostatectomy with a new DuoRotate system. Eur Urol. 2012;62(6):1143–9. doi:10.1016/j.eururo.2012.04.043. Epub 2012 May 5.

25. Haber GP, Autorino R, Laydner H, et al. SPIDER surgical system for urologic procedures with laparoendoscopic single-site surgery: from initial laboratory experience to first clinical application. Eur Urol. 2012;61:415–22.

26. Tanagho YS, Andriole GL, Paradis AG, et al. 2D versus 3D visualization: impact on laparoscopic proficiency using the fundamentals of laparoscopic surgery skill set. J Laparoendosc Adv Surg Tech A. 2012;22(9):865–70. doi: 10.1089/lap.2012.0220. Epub 2012 Oct 16.

27. Goldsmith ZG, Astroza GM, Wang AJ, et al. Optical performance comparison of deflectable laparoscopes for laparoendoscopic single-site surgery. J Endourol. 2012;26:10.

28. Terry BS, Schoen J, Mills Z, et al. Single port access surgery with a novel Port Camera system. Surg Innov. 2012;19(2):123–9. doi:10.1177/1553350611418988. Epub 2011 Sep 13.

29. Cadeddu J, Fernandez R, Desai M, et al. Novel magnetically guided intra-abdominal camera to facilitate laparoendoscopic single-site surgery: initial human experience. Surg Endosc. 2009;23(8):1894–9. doi:10.1007/s00464-009-0459-6. Epub 2009 May 9.

30. Arain NA, Cadeddu JA, Best SL, et al. A randomized comparison of laparoscopic, magnetically anchored, and flexible endoscopic cameras in performance and workload between laparoscopic and single-incision surgery. Surg Endosc. 2012;26:1170–80.

31. Han WK, Tan YK, Olweny EO, et al. Comparison between magnetic anchoring and guidance system camera-assisted laparoendoscopic single-site surgery nephrectomy and conventional laparoendoscopic single-site surgery nephrectomy in a porcine model: focus on ergonomics and workload profiles. J Endourol. 2013;27:4.

32. Cabrera PM, Caceres F, García-Tello A. Initial experience of umbilical laparoendoscopic single-site nephron-sparing surgery with KeyPort and DuoRotate system. J Endourol. 2013;27:5.

33. Miernik A, Schoenthaler M, Lilienthal K, et al. Prebent instruments used in single-port laparoscopic surgery versus conventional laparoscopic surgery: comparative study of performance in a dry lab. Surg Endosc. 2012;26:1924–30.

34. Stolzenburg JU, Kallidonis P, Oh MA, et al. Comparative assessment of laparoscopic single-site surgery instruments to conventional laparoscopic in laboratory setting. J Endourol. 2010;24:2.

35. Martinec DV, Gatta P, Zheng B, et al. The trade-off between flexibility and maneuverability: task performance with articulating laparoscopic instruments. Surg Endosc. 2009;23:2697–701.

36. Jeong CW, Kim SH, Kim HT, et al. Insufficient joint forces of first-generation articulating instruments for

laparoendoscopic single-site surgery. Surg Innov. 2013;20(5):466–70. doi: 10.1177/1553350612468961. Epub 2012 Dec 14.

37. Jung JW1, Cha WH, Lee BK, et al. Laparoendoscopic single-site surgery using innovative articulating instruments: preclinical evaluation of the prototype. J Endourol. 2014;28(3):281–5. doi: 10.1089/end.2013.0510. Epub 2013 Nov 22.

38. Joseph RA, Goh AC, Cuevas SP, et al. "Chopstick" surgery: a novel technique improves surgeon performance and eliminates arm collision in robotic single-incision laparoscopic surgery. Surg Endosc. 2010;24:1331–5.

39. Haber GP, White MA, Autorino R, et al. Novel Robotic da Vinci instruments for laparoendoscopic single-site surgery. Urology. 2010;76:1279–82.

40. Kaouk JH, Autorino R, Laydner H, et al. Robotic single-site kidney surgery: evaluation of second-generation instruments in a cadaver model. Urology. 2012;79:975–9.

5

Robotic Systems in Laparoendoscopic Single-Site Surgery

Riccardo Autorino and Jihad H. Kaouk

Introduction

Despite the increasing interest in LESS world-wide, the actual role of this novel approach in the field of minimally invasive urologic surgery remains to be determined [1].

One major technical disadvantage in LESS is the "sword fighting" among instruments. During standard LESS, as laparoscopic instruments are inserted into the abdominal cavity through a single incision, there can be a tendency to cross them just below the abdominal wall to obtain a separation between instrument tips without external collision of the handpieces. This crossing of the instruments allows a better range of motion, but the resultant reversal of handedness introduces a major mental challenge for the surgeon.

Novel non-robotic systems have been tested to offer intuitive instrument maneuverability and restored triangulation without external instrument

clashing, but their use remains experimental (Fig. 5.1) [2].

To overcome the current constraints of LESS, it has been postulated that robotic technology could be applied [3]. In 2009, Kaouk et al. reported the first successful series of single-site robotic procedures in humans, and the authors noted improved facility for intracorporeal dissecting and suturing because of robotic instrument articulation and stability [4]. Since then, there has been a growing interest from investigators in different surgical specialties.

In this chapter an overview of current and future robotic systems for application in urologic LESS is provided.

da Vinci® S and da Vinci® Si Platform

The da Vinci® surgical system was the first robotic system cleared by the Food and Drug Administration for use in general and urologic laparoscopic surgery. Some of its benefits over conventional laparoscopy include superior ergonomics, optical magnification of the operative field, enhanced dexterity, and greater precision.

It has been largely demonstrated by Kaouk and collaborators at the Cleveland Clinic that a variety of robotic LESS urologic procedures can be performed using different trocar configurations or purpose-built multichannel devices [5] (Fig. 5.2). In their initial experience, the da Vinci® S system

R. Autorino, MD, PhD, FEBU
Department of Urology, University Hospitals
Urology Institute, 27100 Chardon Rd,
Richmond Heights, OH 44143, USA
e-mail: riccardo.autorino@uhhospitals.org;
ricautor@gmail.com

J.H. Kaouk, MD, FACS
Professor of Surgery, Cleveland Clinic Lerner College of Medicine, Zagarek Pollock Chair in Robotic Surgery, Center for Robotic and Image guided Surgery, Glickman Urologic Institute, Cleveland, OH, USA
e-mail: kaoukj@ccf.org

© Springer Science+Business Media New York 2017
J.H. Kaouk et al. (eds.), *Atlas of Laparoscopic and Robotic Single Site Surgery*,
Current Clinical Urology, DOI 10.1007/978-1-4939-3575-8_5

Fig. 5.1 SPIDER™
Platform: this platform
features a main body
port/cannula, extended
flexible instrument
delivery tubes, four
working channels, and
ports for insufflation/
smoke evacuation
(Photo courtesy of
Transenterix Inc.)

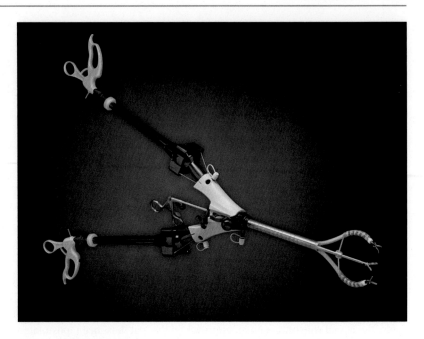

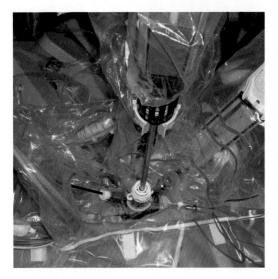

Fig. 5.2 Setup for robotic LESS prostatectomy using the da Vinci® Si platform and the SILS® multichannel port

was used. However, since the introduction of the Si system, this was preferred, given its enhanced visualization and ability to customize the console settings ergonomically. To reduce instrument clashing, instruments and, therefore, the robotic arms, were positioned parallel to the robotic camera. This subsequently required the camera lens and instruments to be moved in near unison to optimize range of motion.

To address limitations related to the coaxial arrangement of instruments, Joseph et al. [6] conceived a "chopstick" technique enabling the use of the robotic arms through a single incision without collision (Fig. 5.3). The robotic instruments cross at the abdominal wall to have the right instrument on the left side of the target and the left instrument on the right. To correct for the change in handedness, the robotic console is instructed to drive the left instrument with the right hand effector and the right instrument with the left hand effector. In this way, collision of the external robotic arms is prevented.

da Vinci Single-Site® Platform

Intuitive Surgical developed a novel set of single-site instruments and accessories specifically dedicated to LESS (Fig. 5.4). The set includes a multichannel access port with room for four cannulas and an insufflation valve. Two curved cannulas are for robotically controlled instruments, and the other two cannulas are straight; one cannula is 8.5 mm and accommodates the robotic endoscope, and the other cannula is a 5-mm bedside-assistant port. The curved cannulas are integral to the system, since their configuration allows

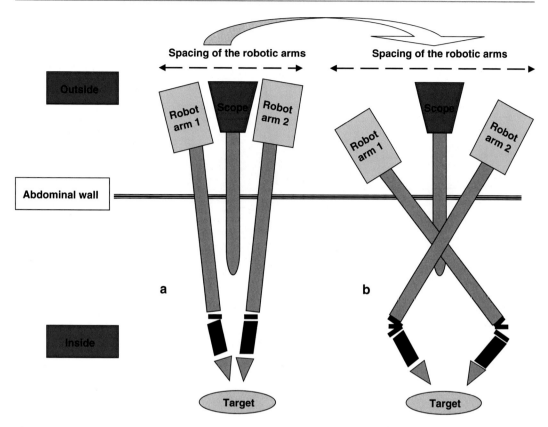

Fig. 5.3 Concept of "chopstick" surgery applied to robotic laparoendoscopic single-site surgery: (**a**) standard configuration and (**b**) chopstick configuration to minimize external clashing

the instruments to be positioned to achieve triangulation of the target anatomy. This triangulation is achieved by crossing the curved cannulas midway through the access port. Same-sided hand–eye control of the instruments is maintained through assignment of software of the Si system that enables the surgeon's right hand to control the screen right instrument even though the instrument is in the left robotic arm and, reciprocally, the left hand to control the screen left instrument even though the instrument is in the right robotic arm (Fig. 5.5). The second part of the platform is a set of semirigid, nonwristed instruments with standard da Vinci® instrument tips (Fig. 5.6).

The semirigid, flexible shaft allows for insertion down the curved cannula and triangulation of the anatomy. Robotic arm collisions are minimized externally because the curved cannulas angle the robotic arms away from each other. Internal collisions with the camera are avoided because the camera is designed to be placed into the middle of the curved cannula zone and is not in a parallel arrangement. The single-site instruments and accessories are intended to be used with the da Vinci® Si surgical system and are of similar construction to existing EndoWrist instruments, except they do not have a wrist at the distal end of the instrument.

Haber et al. described the first laboratory experience with VeSPA robotic instruments by assessing their feasibility and efficiency for urological applications [7]. Sixteen procedures (including four pyeloplasties, four partial nephrectomies, and eight nephrectomies) were performed without additional ports or need for conversions. During this feasibility evaluation, limitations of the platform were noted, including the lack of articulation at the tip of the instruments compared with the Endowrist™ instruments afforded by current da Vinci Si, making intracorporeal suturing more challenging.

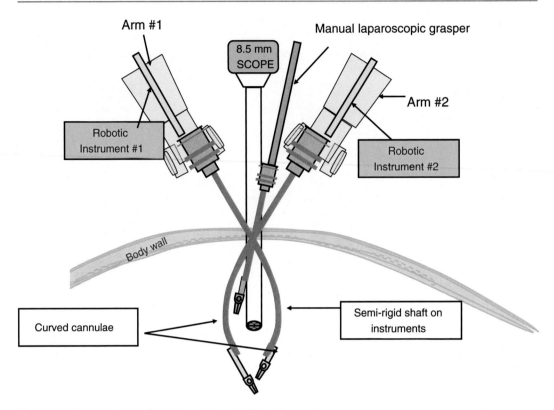

Fig. 5.4 da Vinci Single-Site® platform: schematic illustration

More recently, Kaouk et al. also reported the use of a second generation of da Vinci single-site instruments for robotic LESS to perform different kidney procedures in the cadaver model [8]. Three types of left side kidney procedures were successfully performed (one pyeloplasty, one partial nephrectomy, and one nephrectomy) in a female cadaver without the addition of extra ports.

Robotic Platforms for Single-Site Surgery: Open Issues

While the current da Vinci® system has shown to be a valuable ally in LESS, this is not what it was specifically designed for. The introduction of the da Vinci Single-Site® instrumentation has represented a step forward on one side, as it addresses some of the current drawbacks, mainly the clashing and lack of triangulation. However, the lack of EndoWrist® technology at the instrument tips, which probably has represented the main feature

of robotic surgery as compared with standard laparoscopy, remains a major limitation. The ideal robotic platform for LESS should have a low external profile, the possibility of being deployed through a single-access site, and the possibility of restoring intra-abdominal triangulation while maintaining the maximum degree of freedom for precise maneuvers and strength for reliable traction. A number of robotic prototypes are currently being developed and might be available in the near future for urologic LESS applications.

SPORT™ (Single-Port Orifice Robotic Technology) Surgical System

This novel prototype developed by Titan Medical works via a 25-mm single-access port which contains two snakelike robotic instruments and a 3D HD camera. Once inserted into the abdomen, the camera and instruments can then extend into the abdominal cavity. Similarly to the da Vinci®, the

SPORT™ is a master/slave system operated by the surgeon through a special nearby console (Fig. 5.7).

SPRINT (Single-Port lapaRoscopy bImaNual roboT)

It has been developed within the ARAKNES (Array of Robots Augmenting the Kinematics of Endoluminal Surgery) program coordinated by Dario and Cuschieri and funded by the EU

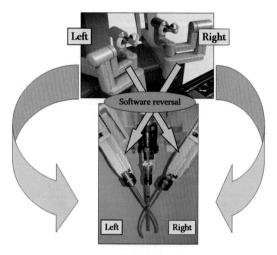

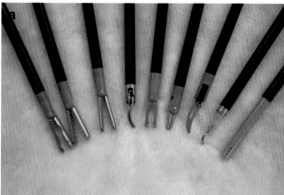

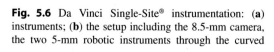

Fig. 5.5 Schematic explanation of the restored triangulation achieved through assignment of the Si system software that enables the surgeon's right hand to control the screen right instrument and, reciprocally, the left hand to control the screen left instrument

Framework 7 program [9]. This is a novel teleoperated bimanual robot specifically designed for single-access interventions. The system comprises two high-dexterity six DOF robotic arms, each one provided with a surgical tool, a stereoscopic camera, and a dedicated console for surgical tasks execution. The robotic arms may be placed inside the abdomen of the patient through a 30-mm access port (Fig. 5.8) [10].

At this stage of development, the SPRINT robot is less technically advanced than the da Vinci® system in terms of precision and easiness of surgical manipulation. However, it presents some unique features: it is intended to be assembled inside the patient and does not clutter the operating room to any extent; the surgeon operates closely to the patients within the sterile area and can intervene directly in the event of a major intraoperative complication, not relying on the assistant [11].

ALF-X (Advanced Laparoscopy Through Force-RefleCT(X)ion)

This system is the result of the research and development collaboration between the Italian pharmaceutical company SOFAR S.p.A. and the Joint Research Centre, the European Commission's in-house research body. The ALF-X is a four-armed surgical robotic system that uses eye tracking to control the endoscopic view and to enable activation

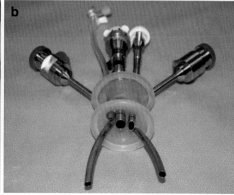

Fig. 5.6 Da Vinci Single-Site® instrumentation: (**a**) instruments; (**b**) the setup including the 8.5-mm camera, the two 5-mm robotic instruments through the curved cannulas, and the 5-mm assistant port, all inserted through the five-lumen port

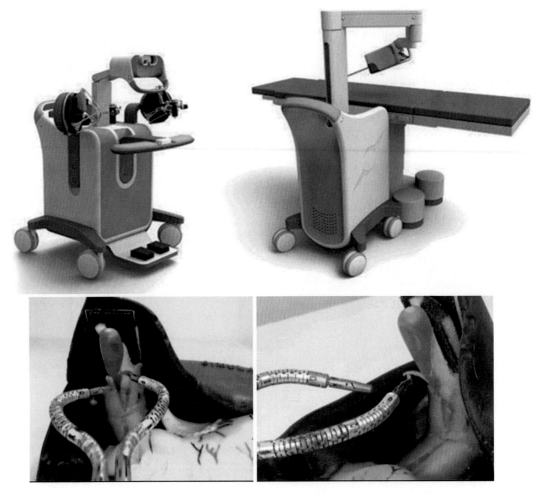

Fig. 5.7 SPORT™ (Single-Port Orifice Robotic Technology) Surgical System (Photos courtesy of Titan Medical Inc.)

of the various instruments. Compared to the da Vinci®, the system moves the base of the manipulators away from the bed (about 80 cm) and has a realistic tactile-sensing capability due to a patented approach to measure tip/tissue forces from outside the patient, with a sensitivity of 35 g (Fig. 5.9) [12].

HVSPS (Highly Versatile Single-Port System)

The concept of this platform is presented in Fig. 5.10. It features two hollow 12-mm manipulators that provide the introduction of flexible endoscopic instruments up to 4 mm and a double-bending

10-mm telescope [13]. Both manipulators and the telescope are inserted independently through an insert with three lumens. This ensemble is introduced gas tightly into the abdominal cavity using a 33-mm trocar and guided over a telemanipulator attached to the insert. The drive system is placed to the periphery, 2 m away from the patient.

IREP (Insertable Robotic End-Effectors Platform)

This platform can be inserted through a 15-mm trocar into the abdomen, and it uses 21 actuated joints for controlling two dexterous arms and a

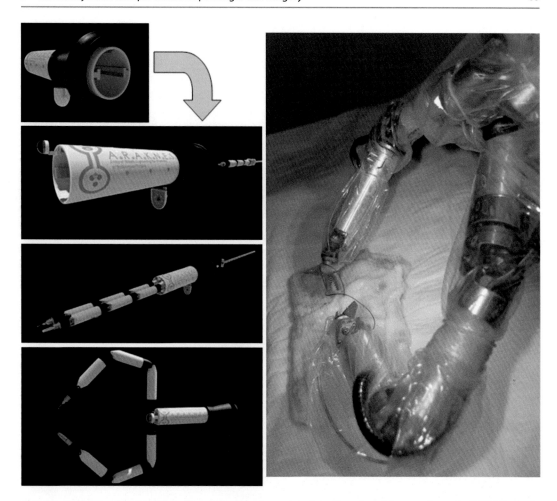

Fig. 5.8 SPRINT robot. (**a**) Illustration of the insertion sequence into the patient abdomen: umbilical access port with the introducer, insertion of the first arm through the introducer, insertion of the second arm, the SPRINT robot in the operative configuration (Courtesy of Prof. Paolo Dario, Scuola Superiore Sant'Anna, University of Pisa, Italy)

stereo-vision module. Each dexterous arm has a hybrid mechanical architecture comprised of a two-segment continuum robot, a parallelogram mechanism for improved dual-arm triangulation, and a distal wrist for improved dexterity during suturing (Fig. 5.11) [14].

Waseda University Robot

A new surgical prototype robot is being developed and tested by investigators from Japan. The robot consists of a manipulator for vision control, and dual tool tissue manipulators can be attached at the tip of a sheath manipulator (Fig. 5.12) [15]. The diameter of the insertable component is approximately 30 mm, and this part in its folded and straight configurations can be inserted into the abdomen through a 30-mm skin incision. The diameter of the flexible endoscope is 5 mm. The diameter of the tool manipulator for gripping is 8 mm; for cautery, its diameter is 6 mm. The length of the sheath manipulator, which is a two DOF snakelike continuum manipulator, is 50 mm.

Fig. 5.9 ALF-X
(Advanced
Laparoscopy through
Force-RefleCT(X)ion)
(Courtesy of SOFAR
spa)

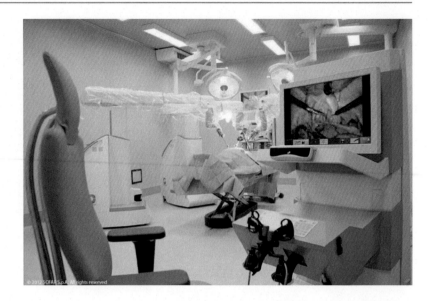

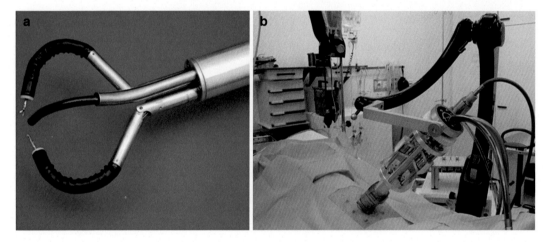

Fig. 5.10 (**a**) HVSPS (**b**) In vivo evaluation in an animal study (Courtesy of Research Group MITI, Klinikum r.d. Isar der TUM, Germany)

Nebraska University Robot

The group of Oleynikov is also developing a multidexterous miniature in vivo robotic platform that is completely inserted into the peritoneal cavity through a single incision (Fig. 5.13) [16, 17]. The platform consists of a multifunctional robot and a remote surgeon interface. The robot has two arms and specialized end effectors that can be interchanged to provide monopolar cautery, tissue manipulation, and intracorporeal suturing capabilities.

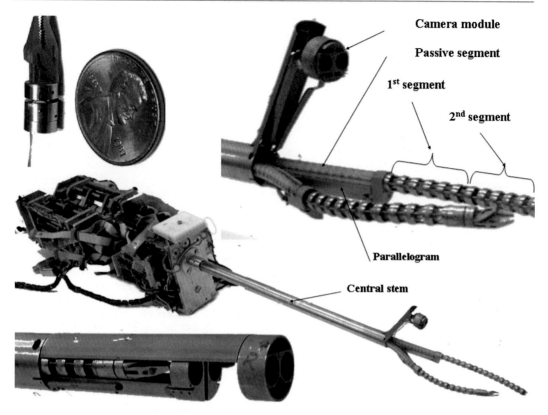

Fig. 5.11 The Insertable Robotic Effectors Platform (IREP) (Courtesy of Dr. Nabil Simaan)

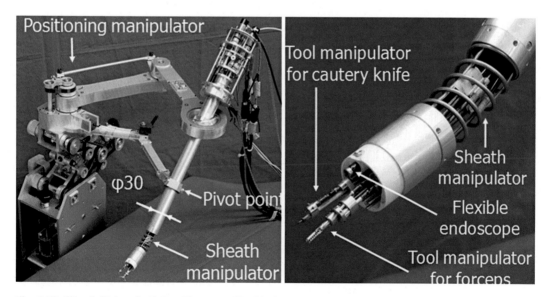

Fig. 5.12 Waseda University Robot (Courtesy of Dr. Yo Kobayashi, Waseda University, Japan)

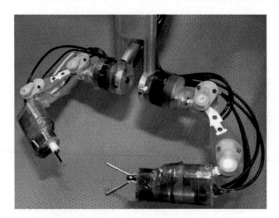

Fig. 5.13 Miniature robot for LESS (Courtesy of Drs Dmitry Oleynikov and Shane Farritor, University of Nebraska, Omaha, NE)

Conclusions

Significant advances have been achieved in the field of robotic LESS. The recent introduction of a purpose-built da Vinci® instrumentation represents a step forward. However, we are still far from the ideal robotic platform, as the currently available robot is bulky and not specific for what is necessary in single-site surgery. Further advances in the field of robotic technology are expected to overcome current limitations and provide the optimal interface to facilitate LESS.

References

1. Autorino R, Cadeddu JA, Desai MM, et al. Laparoendoscopic single site and natural orifice transluminal endoscopic surgery in urology: a critical analysis of the literature. Eur Urol. 2011;59:26–45.
2. Haber GP, Autorino R, Laydner H, et al. SPIDER surgical system for urologic procedures with laparoendoscopic single-site surgery: from initial laboratory experience to first clinical application. Eur Urol. 2012;61(2):415–22.
3. Autorino R, Kaouk JH, Stolzenburg JU, Gill IS, Mottrie A, Tewari A, Cadeddu JA. Current status and future directions of robotic single-site surgery: a systematic review. Eur Urol. 2013;63(2):266–80.
4. Kaouk JH, Goel RK, Haber GP, et al. Robotic single-port transumbilical surgery in humans: initial report. BJU Int. 2009;103:366–9.
5. White MA, Autorino R, Spana G, Hillyer S, Stein RJ, Kaouk JH. Robotic laparoendoscopic single site urological surgery: analysis of 50 consecutive cases. J Urol. 2012;187:1696–701.
6. Joseph RA, Goh AC, Cuevas SP, et al. "Chopstick" surgery: a novel technique improves surgeon performance and eliminates arm collision in robotic single-incision laparoscopic surgery. Surg Endosc. 2010; 24:1331–5.
7. Haber GP, White MA, Autorino R, et al. Novel robotic da Vinci instruments for laparoendoscopic single-site surgery. Urology. 2010;76(6):1279–82.
8. Kaouk JH, Autorino R, Laydner H, et al. Robotic single-site kidney surgery: evaluation of second-generation instruments in a cadaver model. Urology. 2012;79(5):975–9.
9. Tang B, Hou S, Cuschieri SA. Ergonomics of and technologies for single-port laparoscopic surgery. Minim Invasive Ther Allied Technol. 2012;21:46–54.
10. Petroni G, Niccolini M, Caccavaro S, et al. A novel robotic system for single-port laparoscopic surgery: preliminary experience. Surg Endosc. 2013;27(6): 1932–7.
11. Petroni G, Niccolini M, Menciassi A, Dario P, Cuschieri A. A novel intracorporeal assembling robotic system for single-port laparoscopic surgery. Surg Endosc. 2013;27(2):665–70.
12. Gidaro S, Buscarini M, Ruiz E, Stark M, Labruzzo A. Telelap Alf-X: a novel telesurgical system for the 21st century. Surg Technol Int. 2012;22:20–5.
13. Can S, Fiolka A, Mayer H, Knoll A, Schneider A, Wilhelm D, Meining A, Feussner H. The mechatronic support system "HVSPS" and the way to NOTES. Minim Invasive Ther Allied Technol. 2008;17(6):341–5.
14. Ding J, Goldman RE, Xu K, Allen PK, Fowler DL, Simaan N. Design and coordination kinematics of an insertable robotic effectors platform for single-port access surgery. IEEE ASME Trans Mechatron. 2013;18(5):1612–24.
15. Kobayashi Y, Tomono Y, Sekiguchi Y, et al. A surgical robot with vision field control for single port endoscopic surgery. Int J Med Robot. 2010;6:454–64.
16. Dolghi O, Strabala KW, Wortman TD, Goede MR, Farritor SM, Oleynikov D. Miniature in vivo robot for laparoendoscopic single- site surgery. Surg Endosc. 2011;5:3453–8.
17. Wortman TD, Strabala KW, Lehman AC, Farritor SM, Oleynikov D. Laparoendoscopic single-site surgery using a multi-functional miniature in vivo robot. Int J Med Robot. 2011;7:17–21.

Part III

Laparoscopic LESS Surgery

LESS Adrenal Surgery

6

Yinghao Sun, Wang Linhui, Liu Bing, and Wang Zhixiang

Introduction

Laparoscopic adrenalectomy has become the "gold standard" [1] of surgical treatment for adrenal tumors after two decades of extensive, worldwide clinical practice and verification. Over the last few years, there has been an increasing enthusiasm and growing interest in this novel minimally invasive surgical technique. Laparoendoscopic single-site (LESS) surgery has been conceived as a natural evolution to a further reduction of surgical trauma and has been steadily gaining momentum during the past 6 years. The population has a favorable perception of scarless surgery, even in the case of increased procedural risks of complications, in spite of cure and surgical safety being the main concerns. Proof by facts, the procedure of LESS adrenalectomy (LESS-AD) is one of the most performed LESS procedures in urologic surgery [2].

Anatomy

It is helpful to perform a successful adrenalectomy with a proper knowledge of the surgical anatomy of the adrenal gland and the vessels

associated with each gland. The adrenal glands lie immediately superior and slightly anterior to the upper pole of either kidney. Golden yellow in color, each gland possesses two functionally and structurally distinct areas, an outer cortex and an inner medulla. The glands are surrounded by connective tissue containing perinephric fat, enclosed within the renal fascia, and separated from the kidneys by a small amount of fibrous tissue.

Each gland is supplied by superior, middle, and inferior suprarenal arteries, whose main branches may be duplicated or even multiple. The superior suprarenal artery arises from the inferior phrenic artery. The middle suprarenal artery arises from the lateral aspect of the abdominal aorta at the level of the superior mesenteric artery. It ascends slightly and runs over the crura of the diaphragm to the suprarenal glands, where it anastomoses with the suprarenal branches of the inferior phrenic and renal arteries. The right middle suprarenal artery passes behind the inferior vena cava and near the right celiac ganglion and is frequently multiple. The left middle suprarenal artery passes close to the left celiac ganglion, splenic artery, and the superior border of the pancreas. The inferior suprarenal arteries arise from the renal arteries, usually from the main renal artery but occasionally from its upper pole branches. The right adrenal vein is very short, passing directly and horizontally into the posterior aspect of the inferior vena cava. The left

Y. Sun, MD, PhD (✉) • W. Linhui, MD, PhD
L. Bing, MD • W. Zhixiang
The Department of Urology, Changhai Hospital,
Second Military Medical University, Shanghai, China
e-mail: sunyh@medmail.com.cn; liubinglll@aliyun.com; wangzhixiangsmmu@hotmail.com

© Springer Science+Business Media New York 2017
J.H. Kaouk et al. (eds.), *Atlas of Laparoscopic and Robotic Single Site Surgery*,
Current Clinical Urology, DOI 10.1007/978-1-4939-3575-8_6

suprarenal vein descends medially, anterior and lateral to the left celiac ganglion.

There are three relatively bloodless planes around the adrenal. The first dissection plane between the perirenal fat and the anterior renal fascia is located at the superomedial side of the upper kidney pole, which is a potential anatomical plane. The second dissection plane is between the perirenal fat and the posterior renal fascia located on the lateral side of the upper kidney pole, and it meets upward in medial fashion with the first dissection plane. Third plane dissection progresses immediately adjacent to the parenchymal surface of the upper kidney pole.

Indications and Patient Selection

Masses of the adrenal gland can be categorized into two main groups, benign and malignant. Benign masses can be further subcategorized into functional and nonfunctional masses. Functional masses are those that secrete hormones, normally produced by the adrenal gland such as aldosterone (Conn's syndrome), cortisol (Cushing's syndrome), virilizing hormones, or sympathetic agents. Indications for adrenalectomy have been hyperaldosteronism, hypercortisolism, pheochromocytoma, incidentaloma, metastasis, lymphoma, and angiomyolipoma.

The roles of patient preparation and selection cannot be overemphasized in their ability to prevent and alter the outcomes of possible complications of surgery. This is especially true during the early learning curve of any newly developing surgical technique. The ideal patients for LESS adrenalectomy are relatively thin, have no surgical history of the abdominal cavity, and are otherwise physiologically healthy. A thorough cardiopulmonary evaluation is critical to avoid many possibly devastating complications. LESS adrenalectomy is more difficult than conventional laparoscopic adrenalectomy. These surgeries should be performed by skilled minimally invasive surgeons. Size is considered a relative contraindication to this approach for a malignant mass. Local invasion into adjacent structures is considered a contraindication to a minimally invasive approach. There are no absolute contraindications to a LESS adrenalectomy except for uncorrectable bleeding disorders. However, the risk is higher with larger tumors. As general principle, all eligible laparoscopic surgery patients may be considered for LESS depending on surgeons' own experience. As previously reported even with conventional laparoscopic surgery, in case of patients with tumor greater than 4 cm, the limited working space does represent a significant challenge, an issue that needs to be considered carefully. Although it was reported that tumors of more than 6 cm are generally associated with more bleeding in conventional adrenalectomy [3], based on recent reports, it is reasonable to consider laparoscopic adrenalectomy of large adrenal tumors greater than 6 cm when there is no evidence of local invasion or regional lymphadenopathy on preoperative imaging [4]. We suggest LESS adrenalectomy (laparoscopic or retroperitoneoscopic) is the surgical standard of care for small (<6 cm) and benign adrenal lesions requiring resection and especially for one during the early learning curve.

Preoperative Evaluation and Preparation

A thorough cardiopulmonary evaluation is critical to avoid many possibly devastating complications. The many physiologic changes associated with pneumoperitoneum are well documented. Pneumoperitoneum with the strict and exaggerated positions required for LESS adrenalectomy surgery places these patients at risk for potential cardiopulmonary compromise intraoperatively.

All functional masses are evaluated preoperatively and treated appropriately. Patients with pheochromocytoma are placed on several weeks of alpha blockade, followed by beta blockade prior to surgery. Calcium channel blockers can also be used to help control blood pressure and hypertensive episodes. Patients with cortisol producing masses are given preoperative steroids as the contralateral adrenal is severely suppressed by excessive production of cortisol by the mass.

To treat the patients with Cushing's syndrome from the glucocorticoid production of a primary tumor of the adrenal cortex, proper dose of glucocorticoids should be placed before surgery. The surgeon must determine and discuss the patient's expectations preoperatively. Informed consent, open communication, and presentation of realistic expectations are the hallmarks of patient satisfaction and the avoidance of malpractice suits. Anesthetic considerations related to pulmonary disease and the ability or inability to compensate for the hemodynamic, cardiovascular, and metabolic changes associated with laparoscopy may serve as relative contraindications.

Surgical Techniques

Patient Positioning and Port Site

Following standard laparoscopic principles, during adrenal surgical procedures, the patient is typically placed in full lateral position with gel pads used to support the operative side. After the induction of general anesthesia, the patient was placed in a standard lateral decubitus position. A 2–3-cm single longitudinal incision was made and extended down to the level of the peritoneum. In transperitoneal approach, the umbilicus or subcostal incision could be used as the port of entry. And in retroperitoneal approach, skin and fascial incisions (2–3 cm) were made along the lower margin of the 12th rib in the midaxillary line and entered the retroperitoneal space. The single-port device was inserted into the abdominal cavity with a specialized introducer, and insufflation began with a pressure of 14–15 mmHg [5].

Equipment

Surgical equipment and instruments. All the procedures were performed using a novel multichannel TriPort (Advanced Surgical Concepts, Wicklow, Ireland) and flexible and rigid laparoscopic instruments. The characteristics and technique of insertion were similar to those described by Gill et al. [6] and Rane and Rao [7]. Articulating instruments from Autonomy Laparo-Angle (Cambridge Endo, Framingham, MA) were selectively used to create triangulation. Using an extraumbilical skin incision, an ancillary 2-mm port was applied to facilitate retraction with a grasper during our first two procedures. A 5-mm, 30° rigid video laparoscope (Endo-EYE, Olympus Surgical, Orangeburg, NY) was used in all LESS procedures [5].

In LESS, the incision always hides inside the umbilicus in order to avoid a visible surgical "scar." A challenging and critical aspect of LESS is to establish a transumbilical access with a single small incision.

Many companies have developed innovative multichannel ports, and some surgeons have reported the use of homemade access devices for LESS [8]. And in our center, TriPort™ (Olympus) and QuaPort™ (Olympus) are used usually (Fig. 6.1).

SILS™ Hand Instruments (Covidien) and prebent laparoscopic instruments would be very useful during LESS adrenal surgery (Fig. 6.2). They provide a dynamic articulation allowing access to the surgical site from different angles by having handle moved off-axis. Main features include: locking system, increased shaft length, 360° tip rotation, and electrocautery connection. Their relative simple design ensures that the handles do not enter the operating range of the laparoscope and permit the surgeon to work in a comfortable, ergonomic position without the surgeon and camera assistant interfering with one another.

Chosen Approach

Laparoscopy requires insufflation of the peritoneal cavity with carbon dioxide gas to create a suitable working space for tissue visualization and dissection. Anterior laparoscopic access and exposure of the right adrenal gland typically entail mobilization of colon and liver, whereas left adrenal tumors often

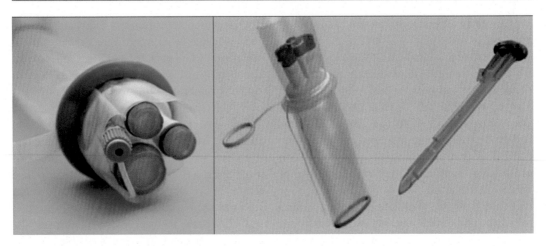

Fig. 6.1 TriPort access device (TriPort™ (Olympus) (With kind permission from Springer Science+Business Media: The Training Courses of Urological Laparoscopy, Chapter 6: The Laparoendoscopic Single-site Surgery (LESS) Training Module, 2012, pp 61–84, Sun et al.)

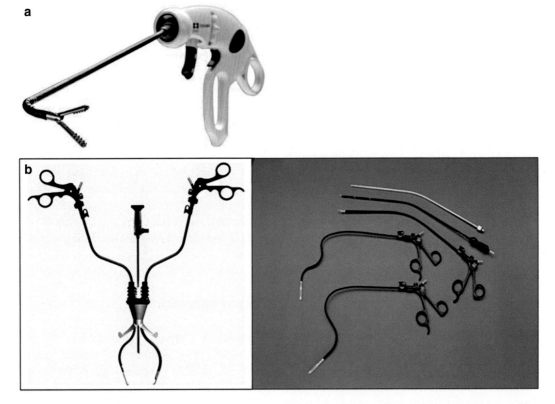

Fig. 6.2 (**a**, **b**) SILS™ Hand Instruments and pre-bent laparoscopic instruments: HiQ LS™ hand instruments (With kind permission from Springer Science+Business Media: The Training Courses of Urological Laparoscopy, Chapter 6: The Laparoendoscopic Single-site Surgery (LESS) Training Module, 2012, pp 61–84, Sun et al.)

require mobilization of the spleen, liver, stomach, and colon. In contrast, the retroperitoneoscopic approach provides more direct posterior access to the adrenals and avoids the peritoneal cavity. This is particularly advantageous for patients with a history of prior laparotomy, as intraperitoneal adhesions can preclude well-tolerated and timely laparoscopic surgery. The posterior approach is also favored for bilateral adrenalectomy, as it is performed in the prone position and does not require intraoperative patient repositioning. Lastly, insufflation with carbon dioxide can impair pulmonary and cardiovascular function, and many patients tolerate insufflation of the retroperitoneum better than the peritoneal cavity [4]. The relative contraindications for retroperitoneoscopic adrenalectomy include morbid obesity and caudally located tumors near the renal hilum. This procedure requires the placement of instrument port sites just under the costal margin posteriorly with cranial angulation; this often cannot be achieved in patients with a BMI exceeding 40 Kg/m^2. Furthermore, this posterior approach requires mobilization of the superior attachments of the kidney to expose the adrenal gland. Tumors located low near the renal hilum are difficult to expose [4]. And the retroperitoneal approach is more difficult than its transperitoneal counterpart due to the paucity of anatomic landmarks and abundance of retroperitoneal adipose tissue. Overall, retroperitoneoscopic adrenalectomy is a newer minimally invasive approach that utilizes the more direct posterior approach to access adrenal tumors. It is best suited for patients with a history of prior laparotomy and is most useful for small tumors located in the most cephalad portion of the adrenal glands. However, this approach is not ideal for large patients, large tumors, or in tumors located near the hilum of the kidney.

Superiority of LESS-AD compared with its conventional counterpart was demonstrated by authors [5]. Although maintaining the most cosmetic advantage, the transumbilical (TU) approach for LESS-AD appears to be more technically demanding because of the long distance and limited angle from the port site to

the operating field [9]. Alternatively, a subcostal portal site of entry, either transperitoneal or retroperitoneal, can be used to improve the ergonomics within the strict definition of LESS. LESS-AD is an effective procedure with a high level of cosmesis using a TU, TS, or RS approach. The surgeon's background, patient characteristics, and cosmetic perception must be carefully considered as a part of the entire clinical picture so that LESS-AD can be used for patients who will derive the most benefit [10].

Port Placement

As mentioned above, a 2–3-cm single longitudinal incision was made and extended down to the level of the peritoneum. In transperitoneal approach, the umbilicus or subcostal incision could be used as the port of entry. And in retroperitoneal approach, skin and fascial incisions (2–3 cm) were made along the lower margin of the 12th rib in the midaxillary line and entered the retroperitoneal space.

Tips and Tricks

The purported advantages of a single incision include improved cosmesis and decreased port-related morbidity. The clear disadvantages of this approach include instrument congestion around a single port and the inability to achieve adequate triangulation.

As mentioned above, in spite of a better cosmetic effect and better working space, during transumbilical LESS adrenalectomy, the distance between the umbilicus and the adrenal gland is longer, which usually makes the conventional laparoscopic instrument unable to reach the upper pole of the adrenal gland [11]. Moreover, in transperitoneal LESS adrenalectomy, liver or spleen retraction usually are inevitable [12].

Any additional instrument through the same incision in LESS increases the fighting of instruments, thus the difficulty performing LESS. In this respect, the use of 2- or 3-mm needlescopic instruments can represent an effective solution [12, 13]. Disadvantages related to the loss of the triangulation during LESS can be overcome by using special instruments. Several reports have described the use of fixed-shaft bent instruments to facilitate single-port surgery and several actively articulating instruments also have been developed [2]. Although the aforementioned instruments are helpful for attempting to resolve the problems of triangulation, the lack of sufficient strength to provide robust retraction and dissection persists.

The development of novel flexible/articulating instruments for LESS has addressed this key challenge of LESS. Many of these purpose-built instruments have been designed to restore triangulation, also using the crossing method (Fig. 6.3).

Step-by-Step Technique for LESS Adrenalectomy

Left Transperitoneal LESS Adrenalectomy

Step 1

Preparation of special instruments. TriPort and equipment used in left transperitoneal LESS adrenalectomy are shown in Fig. 6.4.

Step 2

Trocar placement. After the induction of general anesthesia, the patient was placed in a standard lateral decubitus position. A 2.5-cm single longitudinal incision was made and extended down to the level of the peritoneum. We then made a subsequent incision of the fascia and peritoneum, the length of which was identical to the skin incision. Then the

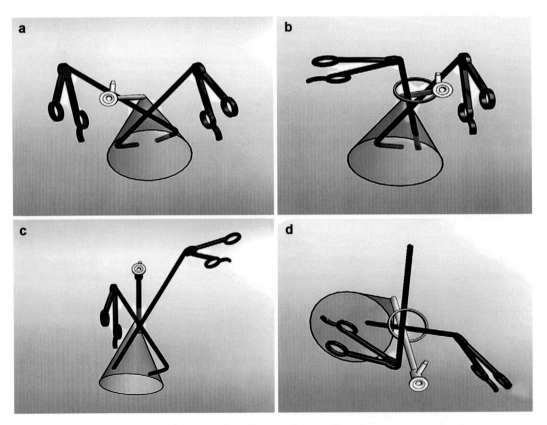

Fig. 6.3 The crossing method of instruments in LESS. (**a**) The crossing method of flexible instrument in LESS (**b**, **c**) The combination of the straight and articulating instruments in LESS (**d**) The crossing method of straight instruments in LESS

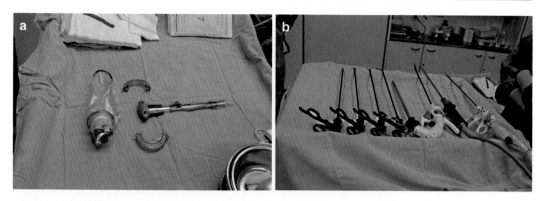

Fig. 6.4 (**a**, **b**) TriPort and equipment used in left transperitoneal LESS adrenalectomy

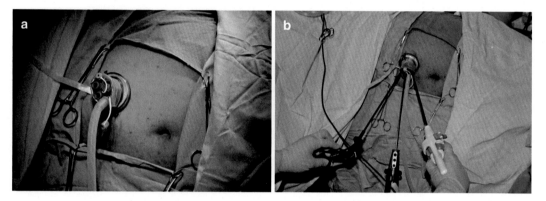

Fig. 6.5 (**a**, **b**) TriPort placement

TriPort was inserted to the peritoneal cavity. The single-port device was inserted into the abdominal cavity with a specialized introducer, and insufflation began with a pressure of 14–15 mmHg. A 5-mm, 30° rigid video laparoscope was inserted, and the initial exploration revealed no obvious abnormal findings. Standard laparoscopic instruments were used for the majority of the procedure and curved or bent instruments were used only selectively (Fig. 6.5).

Step 3

Peritoneal incision lateral to the descending colon and dissection between fusion fascia and Gerota's fascia. The peritoneum lateral to the descending colon (white line of Toldt) was incised caudally from the midportion of the left kidney. Recognition of this plane is important, as inadvertent entry into the mesentery can lead to bleeding as well as mesenteric

defects with potential for internal herniation. The articulated grasper held a portion of the peritoneum just lateral to the white line and retracted it in a lower right direction on the monitor, when the peritoneum was incised. Dissection of the plane between the fusion fascia and the anterior renal fascia (so-called Gerota fascia) was also performed at this level. Premature entry into Gerota's fascia can create bleeding and limit visualization of the renal hilum. The dissection is carried cephalad toward the upper pole of the kidney (Fig. 6.6).

Step 4

Next, the peritoneal incision was lengthened in a cephalad direction around the spleen. Dissection of the plane was subsequently performed. The portion of the peritoneum that was grasped by the articulated instrument, with the right hand of the surgeon, was retracted in a lower left direction on the monitor. The spleen

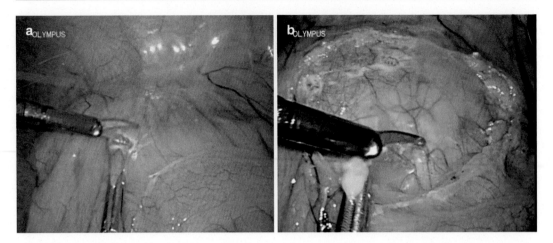

Fig. 6.6 (**a**, **b**) On the *left side* (**a**), the *line* of Toldt was incised with an articulating scissor. The junction of the colonic mesentery and Gerota's fascia was identified and dissected. The descending colon was mobilized medially

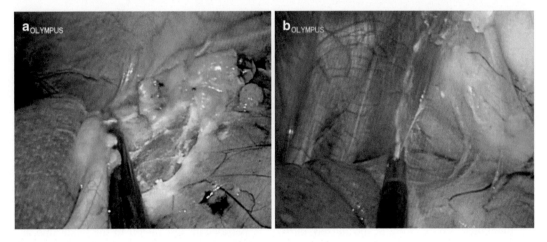

Fig. 6.7 (**a**, **b**) The lienorenal and splenocolic ligaments were divided

and pancreatic tail were carefully separated. In most cases, the spleen fell away sufficiently by gravity without having to extend the dissection above the spleen (Fig. 6.7).

Step 5

Incision of anterior renal fascia, exposure of left renal vein, and transection of left adrenal vein. After opening the anterior renal fascia, hold the fascia that contained the lymphatics. The fascia was retracted in an upper left direction on the monitor (Fig. 6.8).

Step 6

The left renal vein was fully exposed, and the left adrenal vein was identified. Adequate tension to the adrenal vein was necessary to clip and transect it. Once the adrenal vein is divided, the adrenal gland is gently retracted medially, and meticulous dissection between the adrenal gland and the upper pole of the kidney is carried out. The use of clips or a thermal energy device is beneficial in this area due to the highly vascular nature of the adrenal gland. If bleeding is encountered in this area, the application of gentle pressure is usually effective in obtaining hemostasis. If inferior phrenic arterial branches are encountered, they are clipped and divided. In addition, renal arterial branches between the upper pole of the kidney

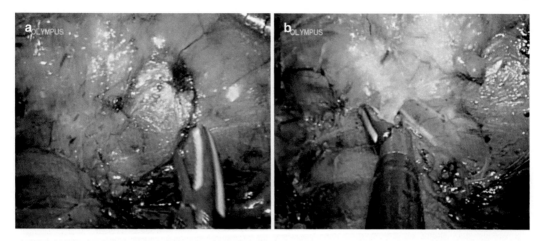

Fig. 6.8 (**a, b**) The plane of the colonic mesentery and Gerota's fascia was dissected to the renal vein

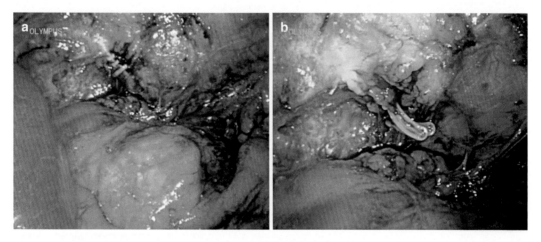

Fig. 6.9 (**a, b**) The adrenal vein was dissected free, doubly clipped on the body side, singly on the specimen side, with 5-mm Hem-o-Lok clips (Weck, Research Triangle Park, NC) and titanium clips (Olympus, Tokyo, Japan), and divided

and adrenal gland are not uncommonly encountered during this portion of the dissection, and one must exercise caution to avoid inadvertent vascular injury (Fig. 6.9).

Step 7

Division of the tissue surrounding the adrenal gland. After transection of the left adrenal vein, the avascular space caudal and dorsal to the adrenal gland was opened to expose the fascia of quadratus lumborum muscle. Further elevation of the adrenal gland could be obtained by a support instrument, according to the laterality of the tissue being treated. Extensive splenic mobilization is required to provide adequate exposure of the upper pole

of the kidney and adrenal gland, if necessary. With adequate mobilization, the spleen should fall medially without requiring active retraction (Fig. 6.10).

Step 8

Medial and lateral wings that contained small vessels were divided using Hem-o-lok clips, and the gland was completely freed (Fig. 6.11).

Step 9

Removal of specimen and insertion of drain. The specimen was enclosed in an endoscopic pouch and removed. After the absence of active bleeding and organ injury was confirmed, a suction drain was placed. And bleeding from the adrenal arteries was controlled

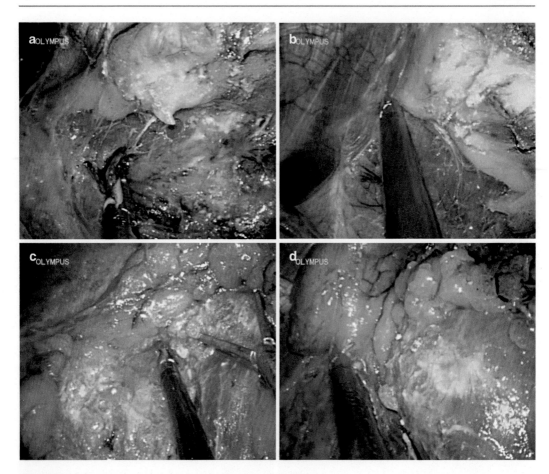

Fig. 6.10 (**a–d**) Division of the tissue surrounding the adrenal gland

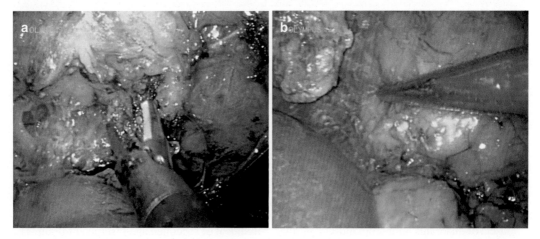

Fig. 6.11 (**a, b**) The adrenal vein was used to lift the gland up and develop the plane along the posterior abdominal wall

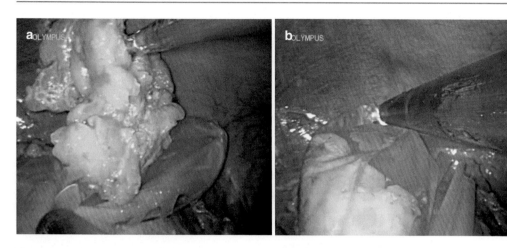

Fig. 6.12 (**a, b**) The adrenal gland was fully mobilized using the 5-mm ultrasonic surgical system Sonosurg (Olympus, Tokyo, Japan)

with Hem-o-Lok clips when they were encountered (Fig. 6.12).

Follow-Up

Follow-up after operation. Wound closure. After removal of the TriPort, the peritoneum, the rectus fascia, and the skin were closed with 3-0 polyglactin sutures. Representative healed skin incision scars of patients who underwent laparoendoscopic single-site surgery adrenalectomy. Transperitoneal subcostal scar, 2 cm, 18 months after surgery (Fig. 6.13).

Right Transperitoneal LESS Adrenalectomy

During right transperitoneal LESS adrenalectomy, the right triangular ligament is divided in order to mobilize the liver adequately for exposure of the adrenal gland. The posterior peritoneum is divided close to the liver edge and this incision is carried from the inferior vena cava to the abdominal side wall. Extensive liver mobilization is required such that the superior aspect of the adrenal gland is visible (Fig. 6.14).

The right middle suprarenal artery passes behind the inferior vena cava and near the right celiac ganglion and is frequently multiple. If inferior phrenic arterial branches are encountered, they are clipped and divided or can be controlled using a bipolar vessel-sealing device. The

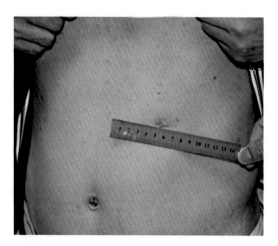

Fig. 6.13 Transperitoneal subcostal scar, 2 cm, 18 months after surgery

right adrenal vein is identified, dissected from surrounding tissues, ligated with clips, and divided. Care must be taken when manipulating the right adrenal vein due to its short length and insertion into the inferior vena cava. Dissection continues circumferentially around the adrenal gland. As bleeding is easily encountered, this dissection is best accomplished using clips or a thermal energy device.

With adequate mobilization, the spleen or liver should fall medially without requiring active retraction. Diamond retract would be very useful in retracting spleen or liver in LESS adrenalectomy (Fig. 6.15).

Fig. 6.14 (**a**, **b**) Position of patient and port placement

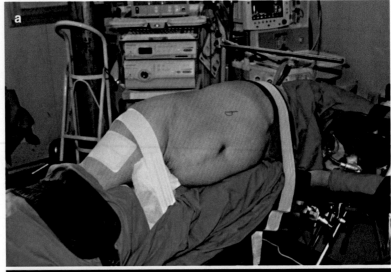

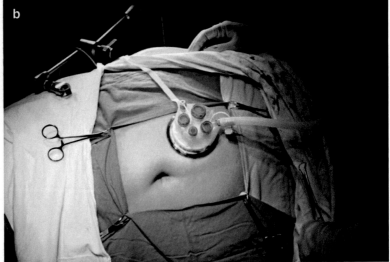

Right Retroperitoneal LESS Adrenalectomy

Step 1

Port placement: anesthesia and patient position.

The patients were secured on an operating table in the lateral decubitus position under general anesthesia. A 2.5-cm transverse skin incision is made along the lower margin of the 12th rib in the midaxillary line. The underlying musculature is spared by blunt splitting of the obliques and transversalis. The thoracolumbar fascia is next exposed and penetrated for entrance to the retroperi-

toneum. The retroperitoneal space is initially developed using blunt finger dissection to push the peritoneum forward. A balloon dilator (Chenhe Inc., Zhejiang Province, China) then is placed into the retroperitoneal space and inflated with 800 ml of air. The balloon is subsequently deflated, and the introducer of the TriPort aids in the facile introduction of the internal ring into the retroperitoneal space. The TriPort then is fixed as described previously. Carbon dioxide is instilled through the insufflation channel of the TriPort to a maximum pressure of 15 mmHg.

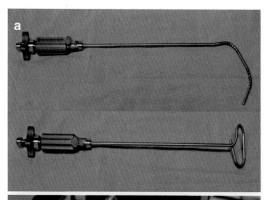

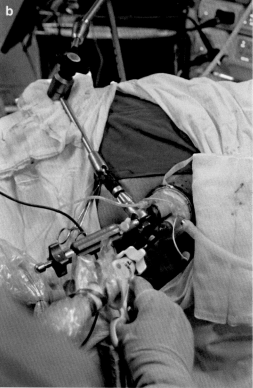

Fig. 6.15 (**a**, **b**) Diamond retract and its application during LESS adrenalectomy

Step 2

Clearance of retroperitoneal fat tissue outside Gerota's fascia. The retroperitoneal fat was sharply resected en bloc outside the posterior renal fascia, from immediately inferior of the diaphragm and downward to the iliac fossa (Fig. 6.16).

Step 3

Open the Gerota's fascia. After the Gerota's fascia is incised, the first dissection plane between the perirenal fat and the anterior renal fascia located at the superomedial side of the kidney is explored (Fig. 6.17). The adrenal can be identified at the initial stage of the operation.

Identification of anatomic markers in retroperitoneoscopy. Clearance and retrieval of the retroperitoneal fat were routinely performed to provide a greater retroperitoneal working space and for easier identification of the following anatomic structures: retroperitoneum fold, psoas, diaphragm, and posterior renal fascia.

Step 4

Orderly entry into the three relatively bloodless fascial planes (mentioned above) for dissection of adrenal tumors [14–16]. After Gerota's fascia was longitudinally incised near the diaphragm, dissection of the adrenal tumor proceeded into the following three relatively bloodless fascial planes. The first plane is between the perirenal fat and the anterior renal fascia under the diaphragm, where we can find the adrenal tumor at the first stage of the operation and expose its anterior surface. Loose areolar tissue and some vertical septa are identified as the landmarks indicating the correct dissection plane. The second plane is between the perirenal fat and posterior renal fascia located on the lateral side of the upper kidney pole, where we can expose the adrenal tumor's lateral and posterior surfaces. The upper adrenal arteries from the diaphragmatic muscle should be kept to facilitate the subsequent separation. The adrenal arteries were controlled with Hem-o-Lok clips when they were encountered (Fig. 6.18).

Step 5

Subsequently, the adrenal gland can be sharply dissected in the third plane between the adrenal and parenchymal surface of the upper pole of the kidney. For patients with an abundant perinephric fat, clearance and retrieval of the perinephric fat at the upper pole of the kidney were performed before dissection of the third bloodless fascial plane. To prevent these potential sources of bleeding, we treated the adrenal arteries using a Weck clip or coagulated them using a harmonic scalpel.

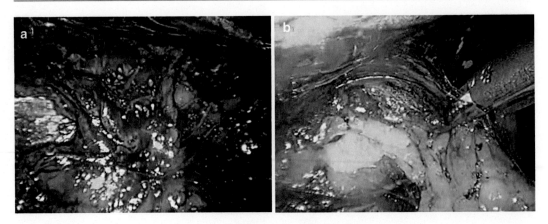

Fig. 6.16 (**a**, **b**) Clearance of retroperitoneal fat tissue outside Gerota's fascia

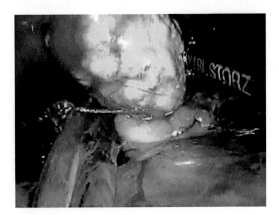

Fig. 6.17 Open the renal fascia

After the dissection of the third bloodless fascial plane, the inferior and middle suprarenal artery were usually bluntly dissected at the lower or middle gland border of the adrenal tumor and then treated with a Weck clip or using a harmonic scalpel. The superior suprarenal arteries should not be cut until the adrenal gland has been totally separated and the central vein has been divided. It will be similar to a retractor hanging the adrenal gland. Anomalous vessels that are encountered must be controlled and divided. The medial and inferior surfaces of the adrenal gland are dissected off the renal vein and the vena cava. If inferior phrenic vessels are encountered, they are clipped and divided. The inferior surface of the adrenal gland is dissected off the upper pole of the kidney (Fig. 6.19).

Step 6

Control of adrenal vein. The adrenal vein of a large adrenal tumor is more difficult to control than that of a small one, especially in right-sided cases. After dissection of the three planes, the working space will be larger for easier treatment of the adrenal vein. For right-sided cases, the inferior vena cava can be exposed fully after deep dissection along the dissected anterior surface of the adrenal tumor. Next, the lower gland border of the adrenal tumor is lifted. Blunt dissection of the posterolateral aspect of the vena cava leads to identification of the main adrenal vein which is meticulously isolated, ligated, and divided. For left-sided cases, after the lower gland border of the adrenal tumor has been lifted, blunt dissection can be done between the lower pole of the adrenal tumor and the upper pole of the left kidney. The adrenal vein can then be finally exposed at the inferior margin of the left adrenal gland. The adrenal vein should be securely ligated with one or two Hem-o-lok clips and disconnected (Fig. 6.20).

Step 7

Specimen retrieval and drainage tube insertion. The lateral surface is the final portion that is dissected. After the adrenal tumor has been completely isolated, it should be placed in an entrapment sack and retrieved through the posterior-axillary trocar port site. The

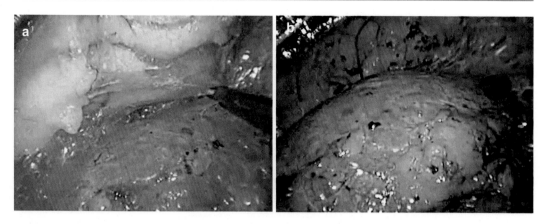

Fig. 6.18 (**a**, **b**) Dissect perirenal fat and expose the anterior posterior surface of the right kidney

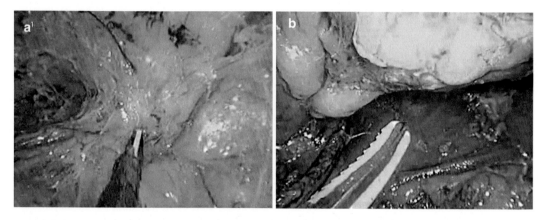

Fig. 6.19 (**a**, **b**) The plane between kidney and adrenal is dissected

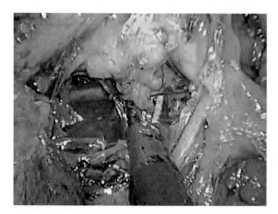

Fig. 6.20 Control of adrenal vein

skin incision can be suitably lengthened, if necessary. Next, a rubber drainage tube is usually inserted at the suprarenal bed, exit-

ing from the trocar port above the iliac crest (Fig. 6.21).

Step 8

Finally, after bleeding from the adrenal arteries controlled with Hem-o-Lok clips when encountered, then all the skin incisions are closed.

Left Retroperitoneal LESS Adrenalectomy

Removal of the left adrenal gland begins with the identification of the renal hilum. Blunt dissection and caudal retraction of the left renal artery leads to identification of the left adrenal vein, which is meticulously isolated, ligated, and divided. The superior aspect of the adrenal gland is dissected

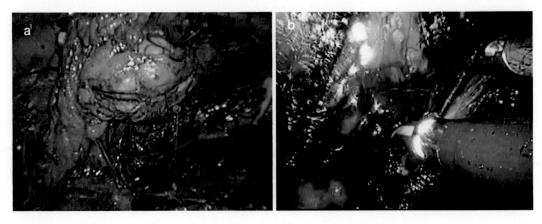

Fig. 6.21 (**a, b**) The adrenal gland was fully mobilized using the 5-mm ultrasonic surgical system Sonosurg

from the diaphragm. Inferior phrenic vessels, if encountered, require vascular control. The lateral surface of the adrenal gland is then dissected off the kidney. Cephalad retraction allows dissection of the inferior surface. The medial surface of the adrenal gland is the final portion that is dissected.

LESS Partial Adrenalectomy

The first report of LESS-PA was reported by Yuge and his colleagues [17]. The indications for partial adrenalectomy for benign tumors in adrenal gland are still controversial. For example, oral medications, such as an anti-aldosterone drug, are also indicated for the treatment of bilateral primary aldosteronism. Following standard laparoscopic principles, the steps to dissect adrenal in LESS-PA are the same as LESS adrenalectomy. In LESS-PA, there is a risk of bleeding on the cut surface of the adrenal gland, and hemostasis of the remnant adrenal gland is very important. In the previous reports, the procedure was performed safely by using, for example, electrocautery and an ultrasonic scalpel to resect the adrenal tumors from normal adrenal parenchyma [18]. Fibrin glue was also used to prevent late hemorrhage from the cut surface.

> **Conclusion**
>
> LESS adrenal surgery appears to be a safe and feasible alternative to its conventional laparoscopic counterpart, with decreased postoperative pain noted, albeit with a longer operative

time. As a promising and emerging minimally invasive technique, however, the current evidence has not verified other potential advantages (i.e., cosmesis, recovery time, convalescence, port-related complications, etc.) of LESS adrenal surgery.

References

1. Smith CD, Weber CJ, Amerson JR. Laparoscopic adrenalectomy: new gold standard. World J Surg. 1999;23(4):389–96.
2. Autorino R, Cadeddu JA, Desai MM, Gettman M, Gill IS, Kavoussi LR, et al. Laparoendoscopic single-site and natural orifice transluminal endoscopic surgery in urology: a critical analysis of the literature. Eur Urol. 2011;59(1):26–45.
3. Hall DW, Raman JD. Has laparoscopy impacted the indications for adrenalectomy? Curr Urol Rep. 2010;11(2):132–7.
4. Nehs MA, Ruan DT. Minimally invasive adrenal surgery: an update. Curr Opin Endocrinol Diabetes Obes. 2011;18(3):193–7.
5. Wang L, Liu B, Wu Z, Yang Q, Chen W, Sheng H, et al. Comparison of single-surgeon series of transperitoneal laparoendoscopic single-site surgery and standard laparoscopic adrenalectomy. Urology. 2012;79(3):577–83.
6. Gill IS, Canes D, Aron M, Haber GP, Goldfarb DA, Flechner S, et al. Single port transumbilical (E-NOTES) donor nephrectomy. J Urol. 2008;180(2):637–41; discussion 641.
7. Rane A, Rao P, Rao P. Single-port-access nephrectomy and other laparoscopic urologic procedures using a novel laparoscopic port (R-port). Urology. 2008;72(2):260–3; discussion 263–4.

8. Khanna R, White MA, Autorino R, Laydner HK, Isac W, Yang B, et al. Selection of a port for use in laparoendoscopic single-site surgery. Curr Urol Rep. 2011;12(2):94–9.

9. Ishida M, Miyajima A, Takeda T, Hasegawa M, Kikuchi E, Oya M. Technical difficulties of transumbilical laparoendoscopic single-site adrenalectomy: comparison with conventional laparoscopic adrenalectomy. World J Urol. 2013;31(1):199–203.

10. Wang L, Cai C, Liu B, Yang Q, Wu Z, Xiao L, et al. Perioperative outcomes and cosmesis analysis of patients undergoing laparoendoscopic single-site adrenalectomy: a comparison of transumbilical, transperitoneal subcostal, and retroperitoneal subcostal approaches. Urology. 2013;82(2):358–64.

11. Rane A, Cindolo L, Schips L, De Sio M, Autorino R. Laparoendoscopic single site (LESS) adrenalectomy: technique and outcomes. World J Urol. 2012;30(5):597–604.

12. Chung SD, Huang CY, Wang SM, Tai HC, Tsai YC, Chuch SC. Laparoendoscopic single-site (LESS) retroperitoneal adrenalectomy using a homemade single-access platform and standard laparoscopic instruments. Surg Endosc. 2011;25(4):1251–6.

13. Cindolo L, Gidaro S, Neri F, Tamburro FR, Schips L. Assessing feasibility and safety of laparoendoscopic single-site surgery adrenalectomy: initial experience. J Endourol. 2010;24(6):977–80.

14. Zhang X, Fu B, Lang B, Zhang J, Xu K, Li HZ, et al. Technique of anatomical retroperitoneoscopic adrenalectomy with report of 800 cases. J Urol. 2007;177(4):1254–7.

15. Wang B, Ma X, Li H, Shi T, Hu D, Fu B, et al. Anatomic retroperitoneoscopic adrenalectomy for selected adrenal tumors >5 cm: our technique and experience. Urology. 2011;78(2):348–52.

16. Shi TP, Zhang X, Ma X, Li HZ, Zhu J, Wang BJ, et al. Laparoendoscopic single-site retroperitoneoscopic adrenalectomy: a matched-pair comparison with the gold standard. Surg Endosc. 2011;25(7):2117–24.

17. Yuge K, Miyajima A, Hasegawa M, Miyazaki Y, Maeda T, Takeda T, et al. Initial experience of transumbilical laparoendoscopic single-site surgery of partial adrenalectomy in patient with aldosterone-producing adenoma. BMC Urol. 2010;10:19.

18. Liao CH, Chueh SC, Wu KD, Hsieh MH, Chen J. Laparoscopic partial adrenalectomy for aldosterone-producing adenomas with needlescopic instruments. Urology. 2006;68(3):663–7.

Laparoscopic Single-Site Radical Nephrectomy

Rodrigo Donalisio da Silva, Diedra Gustafson, and Fernando J. Kim

Introduction

Laparoendoscopic single-site surgery (LESS) is now accepted as a general term for all new surgical procedures using one skin incision to provide access for camera and instruments, with or without an additional port of maximum 5 mm [1].

Since the introduction of laparoscopic technique in urology, laparoscopic radical nephrectomy (LRN) has been refined and adopted as a standard of care for appropriate renal masses, reporting advantages including decreased blood loss, lower narcotic requirements, shorter hospital stays, and more rapid return to normal activities with same oncologic efficacy when compared with open radical nephrectomy [2, 3]. With improvements in laparoscopic surgical instrumentation and technique, laparoscopic partial nephrectomy (LPN) emerged as an alternative to open partial nephrectomy with comparable oncological outcomes for select patients.

Combining working trocar sites and the extraction site into a single location, LESS limits the invasiveness of laparoscopic surgery and may enhance advantages associated with traditional laparoscopy. Due to interest in reducing incisional morbidity and improving cosmesis, there has been an increased interest in applying this technique to treat renal tumors.

Since first described by Raman et al. in 2007, many standard laparoscopic operations in urology have been successfully performed using LESS. Also, increasingly complex procedures have been successfully performed using LESS platform including partial nephrectomies, cytoreductive nephrectomy, large renal masses, and renal vein thrombectomy [4, 5, 7, 8].

A recent meta-analysis of LESS nephrectomy cases related a longer operative time and higher conversion rate when compared to conventional laparoscopy nephrectomy. However, LESS radical nephrectomy was associated with less postoperative pain, lower analgesic requirement, short hospital stay, short recovery time, and a better cosmetic outcome. Furthermore, no significant differences were found in perioperative complications or estimated blood loss [6].

There are intrinsic challenges for LESS radical nephrectomy compared to other modalities, i.e., mini-laparoscopy [9].

R. Donalisio da Silva, MD • D. Gustafson, BS
Department of Urology, Denver Health Hospital and Authority, Denver, CO, USA
e-mail: Rodrigo.DonalisiodaSilva@DHHA.org; Diedra.Gustafson@DHHA.org

F.J. Kim, MD, MBA/MHA, FACS (✉)
Surgery/Urology, Denver Health Medical Center, Denver, CO, USA

Minimally Invasive Urological Oncology, University of Colorado Denver, Denver, CO, USA
e-mail: Fernando.kim@dhha.org

© Springer Science+Business Media New York 2017
J.H. Kaouk et al. (eds.), *Atlas of Laparoscopic and Robotic Single Site Surgery*,
Current Clinical Urology, DOI 10.1007/978-1-4939-3575-8_7

Indications

LESS technique is indicated in those patients where radical nephrectomy is required to treat their renal tumors. Depending on surgeon's experience, more challenging cases can be performed safely, but large renal masses and renal venous thrombus into vena cava must be considered as relative contraindication.

The general rule is LESS radical nephrectomy must be considered for any patient that is a candidate for laparoscopic radial nephrectomy to optimize cosmesis since benefits regarding social recovery have not been well established and only experienced laparoscopic surgeons should consider applying this technique [6, 10, 11].

Surgical Technique

Preoperative Care

In general, the only recommendations are for large renal masses that may involve the colon or the gastrointestinal tract. Bowel preparation can be accomplished by consuming one bottle of magnesium citrate 1 day before the surgery, with or without the addition of erythromycin and neomycin base antibiotics. It is essential to discuss the expectation of the surgery and possible conversion to laparoscopic with more port sites and even a conversion to open procedure with the patient.

Single-Site Devices

LESS access devices have different configurations concerning numbers of ports, port dimensions, and adaptation to abdominal wall (Table 7.1). Different types of articulating instruments (Table 7.2) and cameras with different diameters, degree of angulation, and view were developed and have been used to facilitate triangulation and ergonomic position for the procedure (Table 7.3).

Conventional laparoscopic instruments and cameras can be used, but ergonomics and view of the surgical field can be limited.

Materials

- Veress needle
- LESS access device
- Laparoscopic suction irrigator
- Flexible digital laparoscope (Endoeye™)

Table 7.1 LESS access devices

Access device	Company	Characteristics	Comments
Triport	Olympus	Three instruments, 1×12 mm; 2×5 mm	Adapts to size of incision and abdominal wall
Quadraport	Olympus	4 instruments: 1×15 mm; 1×10 mm; 2×5 mm	Adapts to size of incision and abdominal wall
GelPOINT	Applied Medical	Pseudo abdomen platform; self-retaining trocars	Adapts to size of incision and abdominal wall. Enhanced triangulation
X-Cone	Karl Storz	Three instruments, 5 or 12 mm	Reusable, rigid
SILS port	Covidien	Three individual ports	Possible to exchange different sized ports
Endocone	Karl Storz	Multiple	Rigid seal cap, reusable
Single-site laparoscopy access system	Ethicon Endo-Surgery	1×15 mm and 2×5 mm	360° seal cap rotation to allow reorientation of instruments
OCTO-port	Dalim SurgNet	Three or four channels	Inferior base plate under skin edge in the peritoneum and a external transparent silicone disk
SPIDER surgical system	TransEnterix	Four channels	Platform access device and stabilizer with a bed clamp

Table 7.2 LESS articulating instruments

Instrument	Company	Comments
Real hand high dexterity	HD	5 mm hand instrument allowing 360° reticulation mimicking hands movement. Significant learning curve
Autonomy laparo-angle instruments	Cambridge Endoscopic	360° movements and can be locked into position
Roticulator	Covidien	Articulating in one plane only, limiting degree of freedom
SILS stitch instrument	Covidien	Distal shaft articulation, needle jaw tip rotation, and additional shaft length

Table 7.3 Optics

Optic	Company	Comments
Endoeye	Olympus	High definition, 5 mm, 30°, control section can be bent by as much as 90°, integrated light and camera
Endoeye LS	Olympus	High definition, 5–10 mm, 0° with a deflectable tip in all directions (100° angulation)
IDEAL EYES	Striker	10 mm, friction-assist brake, over 100° of flexion in all directions
endoCAMeleon	Karl Storz	10 mm, variable direction (0–120°)

- Laparoscopic bipolar instrument or other energy-based laparoscopic instrumentation (Ultrasonic, Plasmakinetic)
- Laparoscopic deBakey and other graspers
- Laparoscopic vascular clips (Titanium or Weck clips)
- Laparoscopic vascular stapler
- Laparoscopic organ removal bag
- Camera holder (optional)

Anesthesia and Patients' and Surgeon's Position

Patients should undergo general anesthesia with placement of an orogastric tube at the beginning of the case to decompress the stomach and gastrointestinal content to minimize possible perforation of bowel during Veress needle and ports placement.

Patients will be in supine modified flank position with a "chest roll" placed under the ipsilateral flank side of the patient. A Foley catheter is placed using the standard sterile technique, and then the patient is padded in all pressure points and taped to the table using the shoulder, hip, and thigh levels to prevent the patient from sliding off the operating table while the patient is at a 70° rotation (Fig. 7.1).

The lower extremities should be slightly flexed and well padded. Special attention must be taken to prevent neurological injuries to brachial and perineal plexus. Patient must be secured, preferably with a 3 in. cloth tape.

A camera holder is positioned at the level of the patient's shoulder, and auxiliary surgeon can be seated, allowing the surgeon to operate freely (Fig. 7.2).

Pneumoperitoneum and Trocar Placement

Pneumoperitoneum is accomplished by placing Veress needle in the umbilicus region or the subcostal upper quadrant area if previous abdominal surgery has been performed. The optimal CO_2 insufflation pressure ranges from 15 to 20 mmHg (Fig. 7.3).

The skin incision site must be well planned for an optimal final cosmetic result and also for the operation of the camera. The periumbilical site is usually elected for the LESS port placement and removal of the specimen, and the length of the incision must be at least 2.5 cm depending on the LESS port elected (Fig. 7.4).

Left-Side LESS Radical Nephrectomy

The Endoeye™ laparoscope is inserted in the abdomen through the LESS port. The avascular line of Toldt is incised to mobilize the

Fig. 7.1 Patient
positioned in supine
modified flank position
with pads under all
pressure points and
taped at the shoulder,
hip, and thigh to prevent
patient from sliding
during the procedure

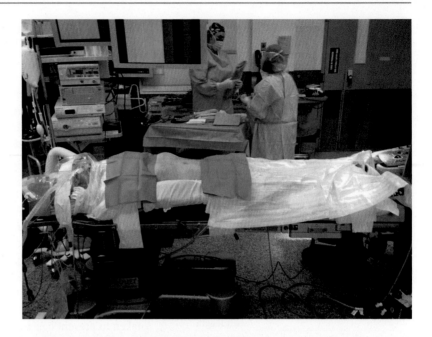

Fig. 7.2 Camera holder
is positioned at the level
of patients shoulder,
permitting auxiliary
surgeon to be seated,
allowing surgeon to
operate freely

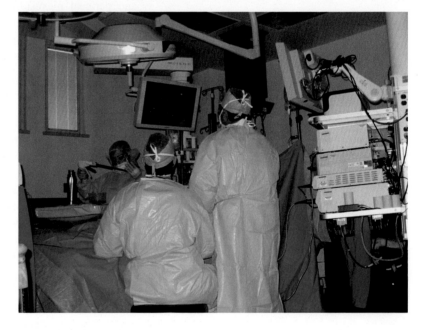

colon medially and allow access to the retro-peritoneum. The incision of the peritoneum must be taken down to the level of iliac vessels and up to the splenic junction to expose the kidney and ureter (Fig. 7.5). A bipolar laparoscopic device may be used to dissect and perform hemostasis in conjunction with laparoscopic vascular clips.

Identification of the psoas muscle, left ureter, and renal hilum is mandatory. The distal pancreas can be injured during this dissection, and patient must be rotated to 70° with the operating table in full rotation to allow optimal visualization.

To facilitate access to renal hilum, retraction of the ureter and gonadal vein must be performed upward, separating them from psoas muscle and

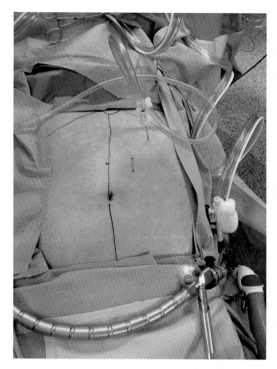

Fig. 7.3 Veress needle placement at the subcostal upper quadrant and CO2 insufflation

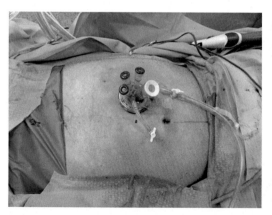

Fig. 7.4 Single-port placement at the periumbilical site

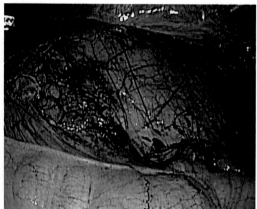

Fig. 7.5 Avascular line of Toldt incision and colon mobilization medially to allow access to the retroperitoneum

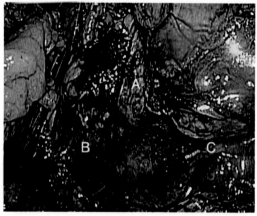

Fig. 7.6 Left-side renal hilum dissection. (*A*) Renal vein, (*B*) adrenal vein, (*C*) gonadal vein

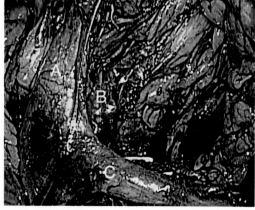

Fig. 7.7 Left renal hilum with individualized structures. (*A*) Renal vein, (*B*) renal artery, (*C*) gonadal vein

preserving the superficial fascia layer of the muscle and ligating possible lymphatic channels as the dissection continues toward the renal hilum. The renal vein and artery must be identified and carefully dissected and adrenal vein individualized (Fig. 7.6).

The renal vein and artery must be dissected carefully to allow proper ligation with the stapler or vascular clips (Figs. 7.6, 7.7, and 7.8).

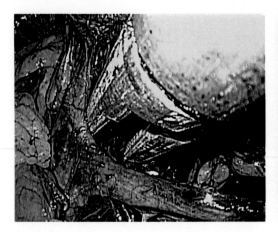

Fig. 7.8 Vascular stapler placed in the left renal artery

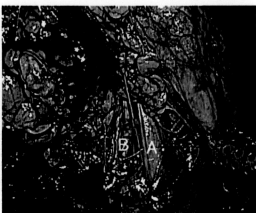

Fig. 7.10 Right renal hilum. (*A*) Renal vein, (*B*) renal artery

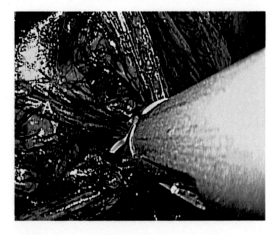

Fig. 7.9 Vascular clip placed in the distal ureter

The distal ureter is clipped with vascular clips and divided (Fig. 7.9). Lastly, the kidney is released from its posterior and lateral attachments, and a laparoscopic organ removal bag is used to extract the specimen.

A careful review of the hemostasis with low insufflation pressure (<8 mmHg) must be performed.

Ports are closed with absorbable sutures under direct vision using a fascia closure device. The specimen is taken out by extension of skin and fascia incision, and the fascia closure is made with absorbable sutures. Alternatively, the skin incision and specimen extraction can be performed by a separate site with Pfannenstiel technique at the bikini line. The skin is closed with absorbable sutures and dressing is applied.

Right-Side LESS Radical Nephrectomy

The same steps of the procedure performed on the left can be followed for the right side. Few differences are noted. The peritoneum can be incised closer to the medial side of the right kidney to identify the ureter and gonadal vein and access the retroperitoneum by mobilizing the colon medially (Fig. 7.10). Special care must be taken to avoid injury to the duodenum when dissecting the renal hilum, particularly when using laparoscopic energy-based devices since thermal injury may occur with lateral energy spread.

For the right-side LESS radical nephrectomy, an additional 5 mm port may be necessary to retract the liver, but when the tumor is large, it pushes the right lobe of the liver anteriorly allowing access to the medial side of the kidney and vessels.

Often, the coronary ligament is divided with a bipolar device to better expose the upper border of the adrenal gland and inferior vena cava. The inferior phrenic vessels can be identified and divided with a bipolar device and the adrenal vein clipped with vascular clips and divided.

Careful dissection of the renal hilum can be effectively performed with the laparoscopic suction irrigator and blunt dissection. The right renal artery and vein can be divided with vascular staplers. Finally, the gonadal vein can be preserved or ligated depending on the length of the renal vein and its relationship with the adrenal vein.

The ureter can be clipped with vascular clips and be divided.

Finally, the kidney is released from posterior and lateral attachments, and if adrenal gland preservation is going to be performed, it is gently separated from the upper pole of the kidney with a bipolar device; otherwise, the adrenal gland is removed in bloc when indicated. The specimen pouch is used to collect the specimen.

A careful review of the hemostasis is performed. The specimen is taken out by fascia incision and the fascia closure is made with absorbable sutures. Ports are closed with absorbable stitches under direct vision and dressing is applied.

Complications

Intraoperative Complications

During LESS radical nephrectomy, the most challenging complications are related to bleeding (vascular injury). Surgeon's experience and accurate surgical technique are mandatory to prevent this complication [12]. According to Irwin et al., most conversion from LESS to conventional laparoscopy is performed to facilitate dissection and/or bleeding control, needing additional ports [12]. Patient selection can play an important role in preventing complications during LESS radical nephrectomy [12, 13].

Postoperative Complications

After LESS upper urinary tract surgery, patients can experience postoperative complications, but most of them are minor complications. Minor complications (Clavien grade 1 and 2) can be estimated about 7 %, and major complications (Clavien grade 3 and 4) occur in about 2 % of procedure [13].

LESS radical nephrectomy can be performed with a low complication rate, low morbidity, and good cosmetic results [6].

Postoperative Care

Pain control is better achieved with a combination of analgesics and low-dose opioids. Patients should be encouraged to start early ambulation to prevent pulmonary complications and venous thrombosis. Serum creatinine and blood count should be evaluated if indicated. The postoperative follow-up can be scheduled within 2 weeks.

Conclusion

In conclusion, the LESS radical nephrectomy must be safely performed with good clinical outcomes when patients are well selected for this procedure and it is performed by experienced laparoscopic surgeons.

The most common complication seen with LESS radial nephrectomy is vascular that can be managed by conversion to a laparoscopic procedure with additional port placement.

Lastly, one must have required instrumentation to perform a successful procedure since the triangulation of instrumentations is challenging during LESS.

References

1. Gill IS, Advincula AP, Aron M, Caddedu J, Canes D, Curcillo 2nd PG, Desai MM, Evanko JC, Falcone T, Fazio V, Gettman M, Gumbs AA, Haber GP, Kaouk JH, Kim F, King SA, Ponsky J, Remzi F, Rivas H, Rosemurgy A, Ross S, Schauer P, Sotelo R, Speranza J, Sweeney J, Teixeira J. Consensus statement of the consortium for laparoendoscopic single-site surgery. Surg Endosc. 2010;24(4):762–8.
2. Clayman RV, Kavoussi LR, Soper NJ, Dierks SM, Merety KS, Darcy MD, Long SR, Roemer FD, Pingleton ED, Thomson PG. Laparoscopic nephrectomy. N Engl J Med. 1991;324(19):1370–1.
3. Dunn MD, Portis AJ, Shalhav AL, Elbahnasy AM, Heidorn C, McDougall EM, Clayman RV. Laparoscopic versus open radical nephrectomy: a 9-year experience. J Urol. 2000;164(4):1153–9.
4. Autorino R, Cadeddu JA, Desai MM, Gettman M, Gill IS, Kavoussi LR, Lima E, Montorsi F, Richstone L, Stolzenburg JU, et al. Laparoendoscopic single-site and natural orifice transluminal endoscopic surgery in urology: a critical analysis of the literature. Eur Urol. 2011;59(1):26–45.
5. Greco F, Veneziano D, Wagner S, Kawan F, Mohammed N, Hoda MR, Fornara P. Laparoendoscopic single-site radical nephrectomy for renal cancer: technique and surgical outcomes. Eur Urol. 2012;62(1):168–74.
6. Merseburger AS, Herrmann TR, Shariat SF, Kyriazis I, Nagele U, Traxer O, Liatsikos EN. EAU guidelines on robotic and single-site surgery in urology. Eur Urol. 2013;64(2):277–91.

7. Kaouk JH, Autorino R, Kim FJ, Han DH, Lee SW, Yinghao S, Cadeddu JA, Derweesh IH, Richstone L, Cindolo L, et al. Laparoendoscopic single-site surgery in urology: worldwide multi-institutional analysis of 1076 cases. Eur Urol. 2011;60(5):998–1005.

8. Rosoff JS, Fine RG, Velez MC, Del Pizzo JJ. Laparoendoscopic single-site radical nephrectomy for large renal masses. J Endourol Endourol Soc. 2013;27(1):34–9.

9. Autorino R, Kim FJ, Rassweiler J, De Sio M, Ribal MJ, Liatsikos E, Damiano R, Cindolo L, Bove P, Schips L, et al. Mini-laparoscopy, laparoendoscopic single-site surgery and natural orifice transluminal endoscopic surgery-assisted laparoscopy: novice surgeons' performance and perception in a porcine nephrectomy model. BJU Int. 2012;110(11 Pt C):E991–6.

10. Fan X, Lin T, Xu K, Yin Z, Huang H, Dong W, Huang J. Laparoendoscopic single-site nephrectomy compared with conventional laparoscopic nephrectomy: a systematic review and meta-analysis of comparative studies. Eur Urol. 2012;62(4):601–12.

11. Kim J, Yu HS, Cho KS, Han WK, Ham WS. A comparative study of laparoendoscopic single-site surgery versus conventional laparoscopy for upper urinary tract malignancies. Korean J Urol. 2013;54(4):244–8.

12. Irwin BH, Cadeddu JA, Tracy CR, Kim FJ, Molina WR, Rane A, Sundaram CP, Raybourn 3rd JH, Stein RJ, Gill IS, et al. Complications and conversions of upper tract urological laparoendoscopic single-site surgery (LESS): multicentre experience: results from the NOTES Working Group. BJU Int. 2011;107(8):1284–9.

13. Autorino R, Kaouk JH, Yakoubi R, Rha KH, Stein RJ, White WM, Stolzenburg JU, Cindolo L, Liatsikos E, Rais-Bahrami S, et al. Urological laparoendoscopic single site surgery: multi-institutional analysis of risk factors for conversion and postoperative complications. J Urol. 2012;187(6):1989–94.

LESS Partial Nephrectomy

8

Hak J. Lee and Ithaar H. Derweesh

Introduction/Historical Background

Laparoendoscopic single-site surgery has demonstrated advantages with respect to reduction of narcotic requirements and hospital stay as well as cosmesis [1]. Partial nephrectomy is a high-risk and technically demanding operation regardless of approach with significant risk for intraoperative hemorrhage and morbid procedure-specific complications such as urinary fistulae and pseudoaneurysm. Indeed, these concerns have hindered adoption of nephron-sparing surgery despite demonstrated oncological equivalence to radical nephrectomy for small renal mass and the benefits of nephron preservation [2].

While initially described for ablative procedures such as cyst decortication, cryoablation, and nephrectomy, refinement of technique and increasing experience with single-site platforms led to investigation of utility of the single-site platform for partial nephrectomy. Indeed, since 2009, there have been several single-center and multicenter studies demonstrating

feasibility and safety of LESS partial nephrectomy for select tumors, with both transperitoneal and retroperitoneoscopic approaches being described. A common theme running through these reports has been careful patient selection as well as the challenges posed by instrument clashing during the complex technical tasks such as tumor resection and renorrhaphy [3, 4].

More recent reports demonstrating application of the da Vinci robotic platform have shown promise with respect to improvement in easy of suturing and dissection; however, significant technical hurdles with respect to instrument clashing have remained, and while the most recent iteration of the robotic platform can ameliorate clashing and improve visibility and safety, wider adoption of this high-risk procedure has eluded its enthusiasts, and application of LESS or robotic LESS approaches beyond experienced minimally invasive surgeons means that the current status of LESS partial nephrectomy is that of a niche procedure on well-selected patients by experienced and high-volume minimally invasive urologic surgeons [5, 6].

Perioperative Work-Up

Patient Selection

Patient selection for LESS-PN is critical. Thinner patients with small/exophytic tumors are potential candidates for LESS-PN. Initial selection cri-

H.J. Lee, MD
Robotics/Minimally Invasive Surgery and Urologic Oncology, Gordon Urology, Gordon Hospital, Calhoun, GA, USA
e-mail: hak.j.lee15@gmail.com

I.H. Derweesh, MD (✉)
Urology, UCSD Medical Center,
San Diego, CA, USA
e-mail: iderweesh@ucsd.edu

© Springer Science+Business Media New York 2017
J.H. Kaouk et al. (eds.), *Atlas of Laparoscopic and Robotic Single Site Surgery*,
Current Clinical Urology, DOI 10.1007/978-1-4939-3575-8_8

teria for LESS-PN included BMI <30 Kg/m², tumor size <7 cm, and anterior exophytic tumor at interpolar or lower pole location and no prior abdominal surgery [7]. Evolving experience has demonstrated feasibility with retroperitoneoscopic approaches and endophytic polar location enabling a heminephrectomy approach.

Contraindications

The absolute and relative contraindications for LESS-PN are the same to conventional laparoscopic nephrectomy and partial nephrectomy with the further caveat that transperitoneal approaches that are periumbilical are inherently problematic in patients with significant obesity (BMI >35 kg/m²); furthermore, careful consideration should be given to patient indication for partial nephrectomy independent of tumor size/location.

Operative Technique

Patient Positioning

For a transperitoneal approach, the patient is placed in modified flank position (45° angle relative to bed, table in flex close to 110°l Fig. 8.1a). For a retroperitoneoscopic approach, the patient is placed in a pure flank position (90° angle relative to bed, table in flex close to 110°;

Fig. 8.1b). For both approaches, the dependent leg is flexed, and in order to prevent postoperative neuromuscular injury, foam padding is required for all pressure points, especially the knee and ankle in contact with the bed. The upper leg is straight and three pillows are used in between the legs. An axillary roll using an intravenous bag or towel roll is also required for supporting the axilla to prevent injury of the brachial plexus. In addition, for the arms, multiple pillows, a mayo stand, or arm rest can be used to support the upper arm, also bending close to 90° at the elbow. The support for the arm should be close to the level of the shoulder for neutral positioning and padding to prevent neuromuscular strain. Patient's ASIS should be at the level of the kidney to allow maximal opening of the flank when the bed is flexed.

Instruments and Access

Transperitoneal

There are multiple devices that have been developed and are in the market for LESS technique. Different investigators have used single-port devices that are commercially available or that are homemade. However, no randomized controlled trials have been performed to demonstrate the benefit of one device over another (Table 8.1), and the authors' preference is to proceed with a single-site approach and to place staggered ports of

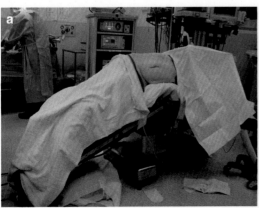 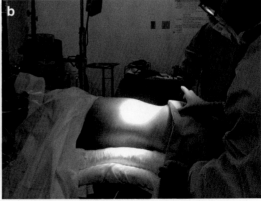

Fig. 8.1 (a) Patient positioning for transperitoneal LESS-PN and for (b) retroperitoneal LESS-PN

Table 8.1 Different types of commercially available single-port devices with size of incision and port description of device

Device	Manufacturer	Incision	Description	
R-Port (Tri/QuadPort)	Olympus	TriPort: 12–25 mm QuadPort: 25–65 mm	TriPort: 2×5 mm (ports) TriPort:+ 1×5–15 mm 3×5 mm 1×5–10 mm	QuadPort+: 2×5 mm (ports) 1×5–10 mm 1×5–12 mm 1×5–15 mm
SILS port	Covidien	15×20 mm	SILSPT12: 3×5 mm 1×5–12 mm	
SSLAS (single-site laparoscopic access system)	Ethicon	20–40 mm	SSLAS: 2×5 mm 1×5–15 mm	
X/Endocone	Storz	X-Cone: 20–25 mm Endocone: 35 mm	X-Cone: 2×5 mm 1×10–12 mm	Endocone: 6×5 mm 2×10–12 mm
Uni-X	P-Navel	15 mm	Uni-X: 3×5 mm	
GelPoint/Port:	Applied medical	GelPoint: 156–70 mm Mini: 15–30 mm	GelPoint: 3×10 mm 1×12 mm	GelPoint Mini: 3×5–10 mm
AirSeal	SurgiQuest	AirSeal: 18 mm AnchorPath: 5 mm	AirSeal: 1×18 mm	AnchorPort: 3×5 mm
SITRACC (Single Trocar Access)	Edlo	20–30 mm	SITRACC: 3×5 mm 1×10 mm	
Octo-Port	Dalim SurgNet	Octo-V2: 15–30 mm 35–50 mm	Octo-V2: 2×5 mm 1×5–12 mm	Octo-V2 A/B: 2×5 mm 1×5–10 mm 1×5–12 mm

different sizes to create a "Manhattan effect" to minimize instrument clashing and to create a zone of external triangulation (Fig. 8.2).

Retroperitoneal

The authors prefer a single-site approach for this also and utilize conventional retroperitoneoscopic (balloon dilator and cuffed trocar by Covidien, Inc.) and transperitoneal instruments (corkscrew low-profile 5-mm trocar, Xcel extra-long trocar).

Surgical Instruments

Tissue dissection is largely performed with standard extra-long laparoscopic instruments (non-locking laparoscopic deBakey bowel forceps, right-angle dissector, Maryland dissector, Endo Shears), laparoscopic Kittner dissector and 5-mm harmonic ACE 36-cm curved shears (Ethicon Endo-Surgery). Flexible, reticulating, bent, and

otherwise modified instrumentation is available, but not used. Utilization of extra-long instruments creates extracorporeal triangulation, which compensates for the intracorporeal triangulation afforded by spaced trocars in multisite laparoscopy. Furthermore, utilizing ports placed in a horizontal plane and performing tissue dissection in a vertical plane and observing traction/countertraction surgical principles allow for minimal instrument clashing.

Transperitoneal Access (Fig. 8.3)

A 4-cm periumbilical incision is made, and dissection is carried up to Scarpa's fascia. In our early experience, we cleared tissue overlying the fascia prior to trocar placement; to reduce air leaks, we eventually took to placing trocars once we got to Scarpa's. Pneumoperitoneum is obtained by placement of a Veress needle, and the abdomen is insufflated to 15 mmHg or alternatively by introducing a 5-mm extra-long (150-

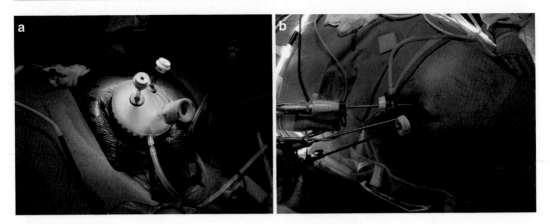

Fig. 8.2 (**a**) GelPoint transperitoneal access (Applied Medical, Rancho Santa Margarita, CA); (**b**) single-site transperitoneal access with staggered instrument lengths to minimize clashing

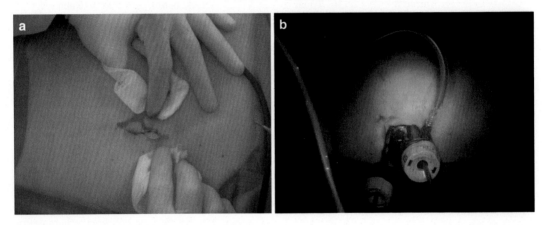

Fig. 8.3 (**a**) Transperitoneal periumbilical incision for single-site approach and (**b**) placement of trocars of different lengths

mm length) Endopath Xcel trocar with Visiport (Ethicon Endo-Surgery, Cincinnati, OH) in the cranial-most aspect of the incision (with a 5-mm zero-degree 35-cm-long laparoscope, Stryker, Kalamazoo, MI) which is inserted through the obturator of the 5-mm Endopath port to visualize the abdominal layers as the port is inserted. Once abdominal visualization has been established, then under direct vision, a 5-mm non-shielded low-profile trocar (65-mm length, Ethicon) is placed 1–1.5 cm caudal and at the 4 o'clock position to the extra-long trocar, eventually functioning as the camera port. A 12-mm standard length (100 mm) Xcel trocar (Ethicon) is inserted 1.5 cm caudal to the 5-mm low-profile port. The resulting configuration has a triangular arrangement (Fig. 8.3). If the 12-mm lens is desired for better

visualization, then a 12-mm Xcel trocar can be placed in between the extra-long 5-mm Xcel trocar and 5-mm low-profile trocar.

The variety of trocar lengths allows staggering of the external profiles of the trocars in order to minimize instrument clashing. Trocars are adjusted to minimize intracorporeal length and vary extracorporeal profile, allowing greater degree of freedom and less restriction of motion by adjacent instruments (Fig. 8.3).

Retroperitoneal Access (Fig. 8.4)

A 4-cm incision is made caudal to the tip of the twelfth rib – though more anterior and lateral than a conventional multiport retroperitoneoscopic

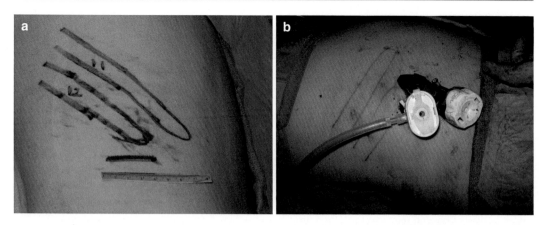

Fig. 8.4 (**a**) 4-cm incision for retroperitoneal LESS-PN; (**b**) port placement for right-sided retroperitoneal LESS-PN

approach so as to facilitate a wider working space from the incision (Fig. 8.4a). The incision is taken down to the transverse abdominis, which is then entered along a 1-cm portion in the median aspect of the incision; after blunt dissection to create a space between the posterior aspect of Gerota's fascia and the intercostals muscles, a balloon-dilating trocar (Covidien) is placed and the retro-peritoneal space is dissected under direct vision utilizing a zero-degree 10-mm laparoscope (Stryker). This is then exchanged for a 10/12-mm cuffed retroperitoneal trocar (Covidien), and then (from left to right for a right-sided operation and opposite for a left-sided operation) a corkscrew 5-mm low-profile trocar (Ethicon) and 5-mm Xcel extra-long 5-mm trocar are placed adjacent to the balloon-cuffed trocar, with the 5-mm cork-screw serving as the camera port (Fig. 8.4b).

Initial Dissection

Transperitoneal LESS-PN: Following takedown of the white line of Toldt, the 0° laparoscope is exchanged for a 5-mm, 45-cm, 30° laparoscope with a right-angle adaptor and inline camera head (Stryker) further minimizing instrument and camera clashing. On the right side, the hepatocolic ligament was incised, and on the left side, the splenocolic and splenorenal ligaments are also taken down to facilitate medial rotation of the large bowel and exposure of the kidney, followed by ureteral identification. Dissection of the ureter is mini-

mized; however, a packet of periureteral tissue is utilized as a fulcrum from which vertical traction is obtained to facilitate a cephalad march to the lower pole and then the renal hilum. For transperitoneal approach, we dissect which facilitates renal arterial dissection. Occasionally for upper pole anterior tumors on the left or the right, we have placed an Endo Paddle retractor to assist in splenic or hepatic retraction placed through a cephalad 12-mm Xcel trocar inserted through the single-site incision.

Retroperitoneal LESS-PN: The peritoneal reflection is medially mobilized to facilitate access to the posterolateral aspect of Gerota's fascia, though this dissection can be minimized in more posteromedial tumors. Following peritoneal mobilization, the outer lamella of Gerota's fascia is incised along it's attachment to the psoas medially to facilitate exposure of the renal hilum. While upward traction is placed on the lower pole, dissection and skeletalization of renal artery can take place.

Mass Isolation and Hilar Control

Following renal hilar dissection, steps of trans-peritoneal and retroperitoneal are identical. Once sufficient hilar dissection has been obtained to facilitate placement of vascular bulldog clamps (Aesculap or Scanlon), Gerota's fascia is incised in the peritumoral area to facilitate tumor identification. For endophytic tumors or tumors in which hostile retroperitoneal fat impedes tumor visualization and identification, we utilize a renal ultrasound with a laparoscopic probe to identify the mass and delineate margins (BK Diagnostics or Aloka, Inc.). The lesion is circumscribed and margins are marked by utilizing electrocautery.

We routinely only clamp the renal artery for hilar control. For small exophytic tumors, vascular clamping may not be necessary. However, for centrally located tumors or if there is significant bleeding from the renal bed with the renal artery clamped, then we elect to clamp the renal vein for better visualization. It is critical, when dissecting the renal hilum to dissect beyond the vessel to allow proper and safe placement of the vascular clamp.

Mass Excision and Renorrhaphy

Mass excision is carried out with cold laparoscopic scissors. Reconstruction is then carried out: For the deep layer, a running 12–15-cm-long, 3-0 Monocryl on a SH needle is used to obtain hemostasis of the renal bed. At the end of this running suture, we place a 10-mm Hem-o-lok clip (Teleflex Medical, Research Triangle Park, NC) and a Lapra-Ty clip (Ethicon, Endo-Surgery, Blue Ash, OH) just distal to the clip to prevent slippage of the suture. This running stitch is anchored from the outside of the renal bed and incorporates the renal capsule for back tension. After the sewing is completed in the renal bed and hemostasis is maintained, the needle is

brought to the renal capsule on the opposite side of the initial anchoring stitch. If there are other areas of bleeding on the renal bed, we place interrupted figure-of-eight sutures with 3-0 Monocryl for hemostasis to those specific areas. These stitches do not have a Hem-o-lok or Lapra-Ty placed at the end of the suture. If hemostasis is deemed to be sufficient at this point, arterial clamp is removed. Renorrhaphy is further continued by utilizing multiple 4-in. interrupted 0 Vicryl sutures on a CT-1 needle to help compress and apposition the cut edges of the kidney together. Again, a Hem-o-lok and Lapra-Ty clips are secured in the distal ends of the suture to maintain tension, and alternatively, the arterial clamps are removed at this point. Application of hemostatic agents (thrombin-gelatin matrix, oxidized cellulose) is optional and may be utilized to assure hemostasis following clamp removal.

Specimen Retrieval and Closure (Fig. 8.5)

The resected specimen is placed in a 10-mm Endo Catch (Covidien, Mansfield, Massachusetts) specimen extraction bag, and extraction for most lesions can be carried out through the 12-mm port, or by slight extension of the incision through this. We also deploy a ten flat Jackson-Pratt drain prior to closure. The drain is placed through the caudal-most port (transperitoneal) or the medial

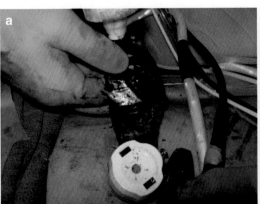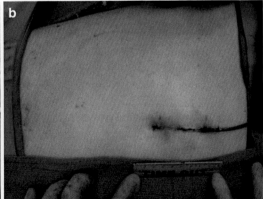

Fig. 8.5 (**a**) Specimen extraction through 12-mm trocar for retroperitoneal LESS-PN; (**b**) drain placement through single-site incision (transperitoneal)

port (retroperitoneal). We obtain intraoperative pathology consultation to verify negative.

Once the renal mass is extracted through the 12- or 15-mm port, then the 12-mm port site/extraction site is closed using interrupted 0-PDS on a UR-6 needle for the fascia and a running subcuticular suture with a 4 Monocryl on a RB-1 needle for the skin incision.

Robotic Application

Robotic LESS (R-LESS) is more suitable for a partial nephrectomy due to the meticulous intracorporeal suturing which is required for a partial nephrectomy [6, 7]. Where conventional LESS does not allow for easy suturing and movements due to clashing, the da Vinci robot (Intuitive, Sunnyvale, CA) has been utilized to improve the movements to overcome these technical difficulties. However, because LESS sets a limit for port triangulation and more coaxial port placement, clashing is inevitable with the robotic arms and camera. Moreover, since the current robot arms are externally bulky and do not allow for curved or flexible articulating instrumentation, it enhances the clashing. In order to minimize the clashing, a 30°-up camera position can be used to move the camera out of the way of the robotic arms and instruments. In addition, a chopstick technique, where the instruments crosses at the abdominal wall so that the right instrument is crossed to the left side and the left instrument is crossed to the right side to minimize external collision of the robotic arms. In order to correct for the change in handedness and work with the correct arm with the correct position of the instrument, changes can be made on the robotic console to adjust for this change. On the console, the position of the left instrument can be aligned for the right arm and the right instrument aligned for the left arm. These techniques overall enhance the movements of the arms and increase the functionality of the robot for LESS. However, even with these changes, the current system is not perfect for LESS partial nephrectomy. There are still limitations compared to a multiport partial nephrectomy. Therefore, as with conventional LESS, surgeons with significant robotic and LESS experience should attempt these cases. Once a surgeon is more comfortable with the limitations in movement with the robotic technique, they can expand the indications for R-LESS partial nephrectomy to patients with endophytic and upper pole lesions.

Perioperative Care

All LESS-PN patients are managed postoperatively by a common clinical care pathway. Patients are given standing dose intravenous acetaminophen starting in the operating room and standing dose tramadol postoperatively. Patients are started on clear liquids after leaving the recovery room and ambulated. Diet is advanced to regular on postoperative day 1, and in patients with exophytic lesions without major collecting system repair, the Foley catheter and Jackson-Pratt drain are removed on postoperative day 1 and the patient is discharged home. Patients with more endophytic lesions or those with significant collecting system repair are usually observed closely to 48 h, with Foley and Jackson-Pratt removal occurring on postoperative day 2 [4].

References

1. Derweesh IH. Whither the long march of LESS. J Urol. 2012;187(5):1531–2.
2. Hollenbeck BK, Taub DA, Miller DC, Dunn RL, Wei JT. National utilization trends of partial nephrectomy for renal cell carcinoma: a case of underutilization? Urology. 2006;67(2):254–9.
3. Greco F, Autorino R, Rha KH, et al. Laparoendoscopic single-site partial nephrectomy: a multi-institutional outcome analysis. Eur Urol. 2013;64(2):314–22.
4. Bazzi WM, Stroup SP, Kopp RP, Cohen SA, Sakamoto K, Derweesh IH. Comparison of laparoendoscopic single-site and multiport laparoscopic radical and partial nephrectomy: a prospective, nonrandomized study. Urology. 2012;80(5):1039–45.
5. Khanna R, Stein RJ, White MA, et al. Single institution experience with robot-assisted laparoendoscopic single-site renal procedures. J Endourol. 2012;26(3):230–4.
6. Tiu A, Shin TY, Kim KH, Lim SK, Han WK, Rha KH. Robotic laparoendoscopic single-site transumbilical partial nephrectomy: functional and oncologic outcomes at 2 years. Urology. 2013;82(3):595–9.
7. Aron M, Canes D, Desai MM, Haber GP, Kaouk JH, Gill IS. Transumbilical single-port laparoscopic partial nephrectomy. BJU Int. 2009;103(4):516–21.

Laparoendoscopic Single-Site Nephroureterectomy

9

Sung Yul Park

Abbreviations

LESS   Laparoendoscopic single-site surgery
NU   Nephroureterectomy
TCC   Transitional cell carcinoma

Introduction

The standard treatment for patients with upper urinary tract transitional cell carcinoma (TCC) is surgical removal of the kidney and ureter with bladder cuff excision. Because of reasonable outcome compared with open surgery, laparoscopic nephroureterectomy (NU) became alternative treatment option for upper urinary tract TCC with minimal invasiveness. Recently, laparoendoscopic single-site surgery (LESS) has been gradually evolving in urologic fields. A few studies of LESS NU have been reported with early experiences [1–4]. In these studies, perioperative outcomes seem to be similar with those of conventional laparoscopic NU. LESS NU is more difficult than other LESS urologic surgeries because of the extreme range of surgical field. LESS NU has two broad objectives. First is nephrectomy in cephalic field, and second is distal ureterectomy in caudal field. These extremities make some limitations with LESS technique. Same as laparoscopic NU, LESS NU also have some debate about optimal management of the distal ureter and surrounding bladder cuff. In an attempt to adhere to the oncologic principles, various techniques have been used when performing distal ureterectomy and bladder cuff excision, including standard extravesical open excision of bladder cuff technique [5], cystoscopic resection of the ureteral orifice (modified pluck technique) [6, 7], and laparoscopic stapling of the bladder cuff [8].

This chapter describes the procedure of LESS NU and management technique for distal ureter and bladder cuff.

Indications and Contraindications

The indications and contraindications for LESS NU are the same as those for laparoscopic and open NU. In case such as advanced tumor, previous renal surgery, and concomitant severe inflammatory conditions, LESS NU may be more challenging.

S.Y. Park, MD
Department of Urology, Hanyang
University College of Medicine,
17 Haengdang-dong, Seongdong-gu,
Seoul 133-792, South Korea
e-mail: syparkuro@hanyang.ac.kr

© Springer Science+Business Media New York 2017
J.H. Kaouk et al. (eds.), *Atlas of Laparoscopic and Robotic Single Site Surgery*,
Current Clinical Urology, DOI 10.1007/978-1-4939-3575-8_9

Operative Technique

Positioning

Sometimes, intraoperative repositioning for supine or Trendelenburg position can be needed for distal ureterectomy. So, tiltable operation table is helpful for intraoperative repositioning. A modified flank position allows repositioning of patient from flank position to supine or Trendelenburg position.

Port Placement

Several designs of ports are now available. Most of commercial LESS port is needed just for 2–2.5-cm skin incision. If you use a homemade single port during the procedure, umbilical skin incision can afford to about 4 cm because of relatively big specimen size of NU. For the placement of homemade single port, a medium-sized Alexis wound retractor (Applied Medical, Rancho Santa Margarita, CA) was inserted through the incision. A single-port device was made by attaching a surgical glove to the wound retractor and then securing three or four trocars to the fingers of the glove using rubber bands [3]. The glove was fixed to the outer ring of the wound retractor by silk ties (Fig. 9.1).

Mobilization of the Colon

For LESS nephrectomy, complete colon mobilization is essential procedure. During the LESS, traction of adjacent organs such as liver and colon is more difficult than conventional laparoscopic surgery. Complete colon mobilization can make reflection of the colon medially by using gravity without additional traction. Make an incision at the white line of Toldt lateral to the colon in the lateral to the liver or the spleen cranially and the caudal direction of the bifurcation of the common iliac vessels with laparoscopic scissors or hook (Fig. 9.2). For right side, hepatocolic ligaments must be divided as possible for further mobilizing the colon medially.

For left side, removal of the attachments lateral to the spleen is important. It makes that the spleen will fall medially along with the pancreas and colon.

Dissection and Ligation of the Ureter

Identify the ureter medial to psoas muscle and gonadal vein. During the dissection of the ureter, keep a wide margin of tissue surrounding the ureter for oncologic principle. Ligate the ureter at the distal portion of tumor to prevent spillage of tumor cells to the bladder in the subsequent part of surgery. Make a space between perirenal fat and psoas muscle using a blunt dissection. Extend this space cranially by placing anterior traction on the perirenal fat and lower pole of the kidney until the renal hilum is identified (Fig. 9.3).

Control the Renal Hilum

The ureter is a useful landmark for identification of renal hilum. Identify the renal vein and make an incision in Gerota's fascia. For right side, atraumatic blunt dissection of the duodenum from the kidney is essential for approach to renal vein. For left side, dissect the renal vein carefully with identifying and control its branches such as adrenal, gonadal, and lumbar vein. Usually, renal artery is found posterior to renal vein. Dissect the renal artery from surrounding tissues such as dense lymphatic tissue or lymph nodes using dissector or electrocautery device. Ligate and divide renal artery and vein with an endovascular stapler or multiple clips (Fig. 9.4). Dissect the superior pole attachment of the kidney to complete freeing of the kidney.

Dissection of Distal Ureter

During this procedure, change of patient position to Trendelenburg position is helpful for reflection of bowels cranially by using gravity without additional traction. Continue the peritoneal incision caudally to completely expose the distal

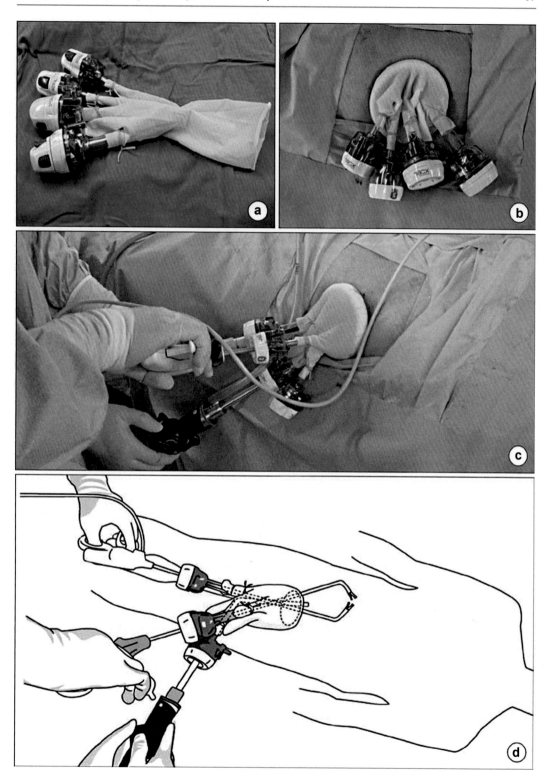

Fig. 9.1 Homemade single-port device (except wound retractor) (**a**). Applied homemade single-port device on umbilical incision (**b**). Instruments and laparoscope posi- tioning with homemade single-port device (**c**). Schematic illustration showing intraperitoneal positioning of instru- ments and laparoscope through the port device (**d**)

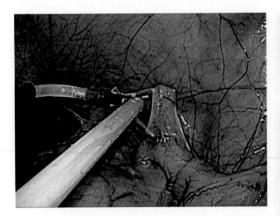

Fig. 9.2 The lateral attachments of the descending colon are divided along the white line of Toldt

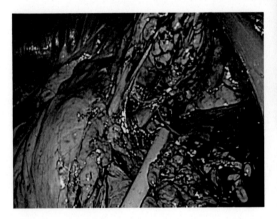

Fig. 9.3 After dissection of the ureter, a space between perirenal fat and psoas muscle is made using a blunt dissection by placing anterior traction on the perirenal fat and lower pole of the kidney

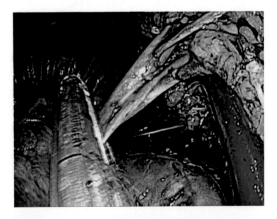

Fig. 9.4 The renal vein is divided with an endovascular stapler

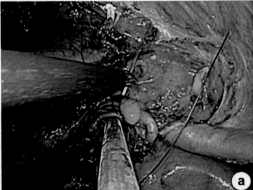

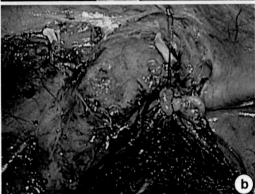

Fig. 9.5 A suture on a straight needle through the abdominal wall and through tissues or structures around the bladder cuff (**a**). A suture on a straight needle elevated around bladder cuff tissues for dissection of ureterovesical junction (**b**)

ureter. Dissect the ureter completely until identifying the insertion site of the ureter into the bladder. If the space around the bladder cuff is too narrow, pass a suture on a straight needle through the abdominal wall and penetrate tissues or structures around the bladder cuff to be elevated or retracted, and pass the needle back out through the anterior abdominal wall for the comfortable management of distal ureter and bladder cuff (Fig. 9.5).

Management of the Distal Ureter and Bladder Cuff

Standard oncologic protocol necessitates resection of a 1-cm bladder cuff around the ipsilateral ureteral orifice to excise and completely remove the distal intravesical ureter. There are still debates regarding the optimal management of bladder cuff excision. Various techniques have been used when performing distal ureterectomy and bladder cuff excision.

Standard Extravesical Open Excision of Bladder Cuff Technique

This technique remains one of the most reliable procedures based on oncologic principle. In conventional laparoscopic NU, the results using this technique for distal ureter management showed that the procedure was as oncologically effective as open surgery [5]. After identifying the ureterovesical junction, two stay stitches are placed on the bladder cuff just at the edges of the dissected detrusor muscle using 2-0 Vicryl suture (Fig. 9.6). The bladder mucosa is opened including a 1-cm bladder cuff (Fig. 9.7). The cystostomies are exposed by elevating the stay stitches and closed with one-layer continuous suture by pre-applied two stay stitches using a conventional rigid needle driver and dissector (Fig. 9.8).

Cystoscopic Resection of the Ureteral Orifice (Modified Pluck Technique)

After nephrectomy, dissect the ureter as distally as possible. Ligate and divide the ureter on ureterovesical junction. Following this, move the patient to the lithotomy position and carry out an aggressive transurethral resection of the ipsilateral ureter [6, 7].

Laparoscopic Stapling of the Bladder Cuff

After dissection of the distal and intramural ureter, the ureter is retracted superiorly while the endovascular stapler is placed as distally as possible to remove the en bloc excision distal ureter and bladder cuff [8].

Conclusion

LESS NU may be an alternative minimal invasive treatment option for all eligible laparoscopic surgery patients with upper urinary tract urothelial carcinoma, but it is still challenging for advanced cases [4]. In operative technique, the principle of surgical treatment

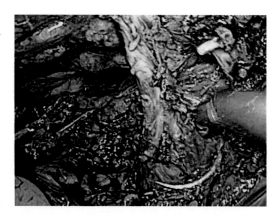

Fig. 9.6 Two stay stitches are placed on the bladder cuff just at the edges of the dissected detrusor muscle

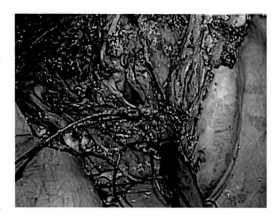

Fig. 9.7 The bladder mucosa is opened including a 1-cm bladder cuff

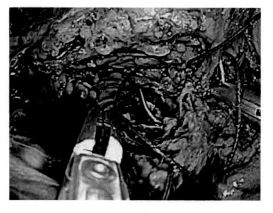

Fig. 9.8 The cystostomy is closed in one layer with a continuous suture using a conventional rigid needle driver

for upper urinary tract urothelial carcinoma is NU with en bloc excision of bladder cuff without tumor spillage. Excision of bladder cuff is much debated point in NU related with oncologic principle.

References

1. Rais-Bahrami S, Kavoussi LR, Richstone L. Laparoendoscopic single site (LESS) nephroureterectomy: an overview of techniques & outcomes. Arch Esp Urol. 2012;65:311–7.
2. Seo IY, Hong HM, Kang IS, Lee JW, Rim JS. Early experience of laparoendoscopic single-site nephroureterectomy for upper urinary tract tumors. Korean J Urol. 2010;51:472–6.
3. Lee JY, Kim SJ, Moon HS, Kim YT, Lee TY, Park SY. Initial experience of laparoendoscopic single-site nephroureterectomy with bladder cuff excision for upper urinary tract urothelial carcinoma performed by a single surgeon. J Endourol. 2011;25:1763–8.
4. Park SY, Rha KH, Autorino R, Derweesh I, Liastikos E, Tsai YC, et al. Laparoendoscopic single-site nephroureterectomy for upper urinary tract urothelial carcinoma: outcomes of an international multi-institutional study of 101 patients. BJU Int. 2013;112(5):610–5.
5. Waldert M, Remzi M, Klingler HC, Mueller L, Marberger M. The oncological results of laparoscopic nephroureterectomy for upper urinary tract transitional cell cancer are equal to those of open nephroureterectomy. BJU Int. 2009;103:66–70.
6. Kural AR, Demirkesen O, Arar O, Onder AU, Yalçin V, Solok V. Modified "pluck" nephroureterectomy for upper urinary tract disorders: combined endourologic and open approach. J Endourol. 1997;11(2):131–4.
7. Hayashi M, Tanaka G, Okutani T. Modified pluck method in en bloc nephroureterectomy with bladder cuff for upper urothelial cancer. Int J Urol. 2005;12(6):539–43.
8. Shalhav AL, Dunn MD, Portis AJ, Elbahnasy AM, McDougall EM, Clayman RV. Laparoscopic nephroureterectomy for upper tract transitional cell cancer: the Washington University experience. J Urol. 2000;163(4):1100–4.

Laparoendoscopic Single-Site Donor Nephrectomy

Matthew J. Maurice, Önder Kara, and Jihad H. Kaouk

Introduction

From a recipient and societal standpoint, kidney transplantation is the optimal treatment for end-stage renal disease, improving recipient survival and quality of life and decreasing cost compared to dialysis [1, 2]. In particular, living donor kidney transplantation offers unique advantages to the recipient, namely, decreased time to transplantation, decreased risk of rejection, and improved allograft and overall survival, compared to deceased-donor transplantation [3]. Despite the proven safety of kidney donation, one of the greatest barriers to donation is donor burden, including pain, convalescence, and cosmetic concerns [3, 4]. In fact, while the waiting list for kidney transplantation continues to grow, donation has been decreasing, especially among young donors [1]. While the reasons for this decline are unclear, donor burden may be a contributing factor.

M.J. Maurice, MD (✉) • Ö. Kara, MD
Department of Urology, Laparoscopic and Robotic Surgery, Glickman Urological and Kidney Institute, Cleveland Clinic, 9500 Euclid Ave Q10-1, Cleveland, OH 44195, USA
e-mail: mauricm2@ccf.org; karao@ccf.org; onerkara@yahoo.com

J.H. Kaouk, MD, FACS
Professor of Surgery, Cleveland Clinic Lerner College of Medicine, Zagarek Pollock Chair in Robotic Surgery, Center for Robotic and Image guided Surgery, Glickman Urologic Institute, Cleveland, OH, USA
e-mail: kaoukj@ccf.org

Over the last 20 years, advancements in minimally invasive surgery have improved the morbidity of living donor kidney procurement. By decreasing blood loss, minimizing surgical pain, shortening convalescence, and improving quality of life for the donor, laparoscopic donor nephrectomy (LDN) helped mitigate the disincentives to live donation without compromising transplant quality [5–8]. Since the first laparoscopic donor nephrectomy reported in 1995, over 90 % of donor nephrectomies are now performed laparoscopically [4, 9]. With the goal of further expediting recovery and improving cosmesis, surgical techniques have continued to evolve, from pure transperitoneal laparoscopy to hand-assisted and retroperitoneal approaches, and most recently to laparoendoscopic single-site surgery (LESS), natural orifice transluminal endoscopic surgery (NOTES)-assisted laparoscopy, mini-laparoscopy, and robotic-assisted laparoscopy [9–15].

LESS nephrectomy offers unique benefits compared to conventional laparoscopy, including decreased postoperative pain, faster recovery, and better cosmesis [16]. In a recent meta-analysis of 1,467 cases, specifically looking at the outcomes of LESS LDN, Autorino et al. showed that LESS patients had lower analgesic requirements and similar surgical and functional outcomes compared to standard LDN [17]. However, LESS was associated with longer operative times (without a significant difference in the duration of warm ischemia) and higher rates of open conversion, highlighting the increased technical difficulty of the operation [16, 17]. Importantly, the safety of LESS LDN appears to be comparable to standard LDN [17].

Just as the technical difficulty of advanced laparoscopy initially limited its application, there are intrinsic challenges for LESS LDN. Nevertheless, improving pain control and cosmesis through LESS is a worthwhile endeavor that may foster kidney donation, especially among young, healthy donors. By enhancing optics, reducing instrument clashing, and improving ergonomics, new robotic platforms may allow for the more general application of LESS to LDN in the future [18].

Indications

There are no absolute indications for LESS LDN. LESS technique may be considered in kidney donors who desire optimization of cosmesis. However, due to the absence of high-quality data, the exact role for LESS LDN remains to be defined [17]. Based on the available literature, candidates for LESS LDN appear to be similar to those undergoing standard LDN, i.e., younger, nonobese, female patients [17]. LESS has been used preferentially for left-sided LDN, but this is likely due to the longer length of the graft renal vein. Pending the availability of high-level evidence to guide utilization, as a general rule, LESS LDN should be applied conservatively to uncomplicated cases, i.e., in nonobese patients without history of prior surgery.

In living donor kidney procurement, the safety of the donor is of utmost importance, and there is little to no margin for error. Given the technical difficulty of LESS, it is generally accepted that only advanced laparoscopic surgeons should apply this approach in clinical practice [19]. More so for LDN, only experienced LESS surgeons with expertise in standard LDN should consider attempting this technique. At this time, widespread use of LESS LDN is not advised [17].

Surgical Technique

Preoperative Evaluation

Presently, there are no randomized controlled trials that have studied the optimal testing for evaluation of a living kidney donor. Due to significant variation in the preoperative evaluation of kidney donors, the Organ Procurement and Transplantation Network (OPTN) implemented a policy in 2013 to standardize this process at transplant centers throughout the United States [20–22]. The OPTN recommends that the preoperative evaluation of potential donors include a thorough psychosocial and medical evaluation to assess general health, surgical risk, and individual risks of living with a solitary kidney; immunologic compatibility; transmissible diseases; and renal anatomy. Absolute contraindications to living donation as defined by the OPTN include age <18 years, inability to provide informed consent, active malignancy, acute symptomatic infection, untreated psychiatric illness, HIV infection, donor coercion, illegal donor compensation, or any condition making the donor unsuitable for organ donation. Although there is significant variation in the criteria used to evaluate donor suitability, other possible contraindications to live donation beyond the OPTN requirements include uncontrolled hypertension, diabetes mellitus, abnormal GFR for age, proteinuria >300 mg/24 h, hematuria, history of bilateral kidney stones, significant risk factors for thromboembolic disease, significant medical disease (coronary artery disease, chronic lung disease), active chronic infection, obesity, and certain psychiatric disorders [23].

Aside from understanding the usual risks of laparoscopic nephrectomy, all patients who elect LESS LDN should be well informed of an approximately 8.5 % risk of conversion to a standard laparoscopic approach with additional port site incisions and a 0.2 % risk of conversion to an open approach [17].

LESS Devices

Multiple devices have been adapted specifically for LESS applications, including multichannel access ports, small-diameter high-definition rigid and deflecting laparoscopes with built-in cameras, and articulating instruments. While conventional laparoscopic devices may be used for LESS, specialized devices optimize visualization, triangulation, and ergonomic positioning for the procedure.

Materials

Multichannel Port
- GelPOINT® device containing three to four preplaced trocars (Applied Medical, Rancho Santa Margarita, CA), or
- TriPort/QuadPort R-port (Advanced Surgical Concepts, Dublin, Ireland)

Laparoscopic camera
- 5-mm 30° rigid laparoscope (a bariatric laparoscope may be needed for additional length during a Pfannenstiel approach), or
- 5-mm deflectable-tip laparoscope with integrated camera head (ENDOEYE™ or ENDOEYE FLEX 3D™, respectively, Olympus, Orangeburg, NY)

Standard laparoscopic instruments

Specialized articulating instruments
- EndoLink™ (Novare Surgical Systems, Cupertino, CA), or
- Autonomy™ Laparo-Angle™ (Cambridge Endo, Framingham, MA)

Laparoscopic suction irrigator

Laparoscopic bipolar energy device

Laparoscopic vascular staplers

Laparoscopic extraction bag (optional depending on the approach)

Anesthesia and Surgical Positioning

Once the patient arrives in the operating room, intermittent pneumatic compression stockings are applied to the bilateral lower extremities for deep vein thrombosis prophylaxis. After the placement of intravenous lines and external monitors, general endotracheal anesthesia is induced. Placement of an orogastric tube is used for bowel decompression. A Foley catheter is inserted in the usual sterile fashion.

The patient is then repositioned in a modified flank position (Fig. 10.1). All pressure points are padded appropriately, and the extremities are maintained in neutral positions to avoid neurological injuries. Lastly, the patient is secured to the table with wide cloth tape.

Pneumoperitoneum and Port Placement

Intraperitoneal access is achieved using either transumbilical Veress needle entry or an open Hasson technique (Fig. 10.2). A 2–2.5-cm intraumbilical incision is made in the skin, and dissection is carried down to the anterior rectus fascia. A 2–3-cm longitudinal fasciotomy is made, and the abdominal cavity is entered. Alternatively, intraperitoneal access is obtained through a Pfannenstiel incision. A multichannel access port is inserted and secured. The peritoneal cavity is insufflated to 15 mmHg.

Left-Sided LESS LDN

LESS LDN reproduces the standard LDN technique. The white line of Toldt is incised from the level of the pelvic brim to the splenic flexure, and the colon is reflected medially, exposing the retroperitoneum. Hemostasis is maintained with electrocautery.

At the level of the lower pole of the kidney, the ureter and gonadal vein are identified and elevated off the psoas muscle. The gonadal vein is traced cephalad to the renal hilum. In order to maintain upward retraction on the kidney, stay sutures may be placed affixing Gerota's fascia to the lateral abdominal side wall. Once the renal hilum is identified, the renal vein and artery are carefully

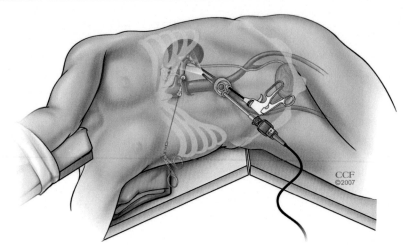

Fig. 10.1 Patient positioning and port placement demonstrating a multichannel port site at the umbilicus and an accessory 2-mm Veress needle port site at the hypochondrium (Reprinted with permission, Cleveland Clinic Center for Medical Art & Photography © 2007–2015. All Rights Reserved)

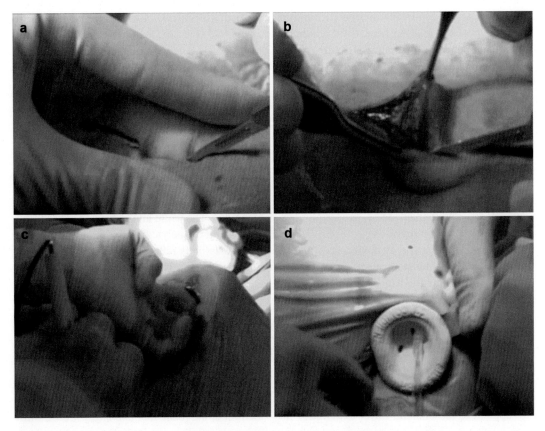

Fig. 10.2 (**a–c**) Intraumbilical incision, subcutaneous dissection, and intraperitoneal entry with finger sweep confirming the absence of adhesions. (**d**) Multichannel port insertion with the aid of curved forceps and retractor

skeletonized. The renal vein is dissected as far medial as the interaortocaval region, and the renal artery is dissected to its ostium at the aorta. The adrenal vein is ligated and divided between metal clips. If needed, the lumbar vein is divided between metal clips. After completing the hilar dissection, attention is turned to fully mobilizing the kidney. The adrenal gland is dissected off the upper pole of the kidney and spared. Finally, the remaining lateral and posterior renal attachments are divided, leaving the perirenal fat intact.

Once the recipient team is ready, the ureter and gonadal vein are divided at the level of the pelvic brim. A dose of intravenous mannitol is administered, and a brisk outflow of urine is confirmed from the divided ureter prior to proceeding with ligation of the vessels (Fig. 10.3).

The renal artery and vein are sequentially ligated with a non-cutting vascular stapling device. The vessels are then divided with laparoscopic scissors, leaving all staples on the stay side. Alternatively, a cutting vascular stapler may be used. When a Pfannenstiel incision is chosen as the site of the multichannel access port, the specimen may be extracted through this site. After removing the multichannel port, a gloved hand is inserted into the abdomen. The kidney is extracted via the Pfannenstiel incision and placed on ice.

Alternatively, the specimen may be retrieved through the same umbilical incision used for the multichannel access port. In this case, prior to ligating the vessels, a specimen retrieval bag is inserted, placed around the kidney, and loosely cinched at the hilum. The vessels are ligated and divided as above. The multichannel port is removed; the fascial incision is opened cranially and caudally; and if needed, the umbilical skin incision is extended. The pre-bagged kidney is then extracted and iced.

The multichannel port is replaced, which may require partial closure of the rectus fascia, and the abdomen is re-insufflated. The surgical bed is inspected with low insufflation pressure, and hemostasis is confirmed. The fascia and skin are closed in the standard fashion. The skin incision is infiltrated with local anesthesia prior to closure, and sterile dressings are applied.

Right-Sided LESS LDN

In general, the left kidney is preferred for LDN because of the renal vein's longer length, but right-sided LESS LDN is accomplished through essentially the same steps [24]. A few exceptions are worth noting. The liver may impede dissection of the upper pole of the kidney, requiring placement of an additional trocar through the multichannel port for liver retraction. A laparoscopic articulating retractor may be used for this purpose. After reflecting the colon, the duodenum is kocherized to expose the inferior vena cava. The ureter is identified and traced

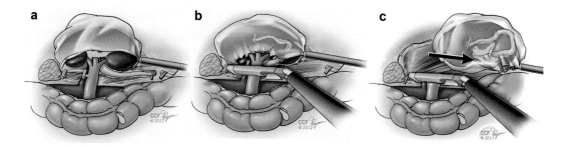

Fig. 10.3 (**a**) Kidney mobilized and partially encircled in a specimen retrieval bag (which was detached from its introducer, rolled, and inserted through the 12-mm inlet of the multichannel port) with the renal hilum skeletonized and ready for harvesting. (**b**) Vascular stapler introduced through the same 12-mm inlet and positioned for ligation of the hilum. (**c**) Renal artery and vein sequentially ligated and divided, leaving staple lines on the stay side, and retrieval bag closed around the graft for extraction (Reprinted with permission, Cleveland Clinic Center for Medical Art & Photography © 2007–2015. All Rights Reserved)

cranially to the hilum, maintaining the gonadal vein medially, which is spared. The adrenal vein is also spared. Otherwise, the procedure is similar to a left-sided LESS LDN.

Complications

Intraoperative

The primary risks of LESS LDN are bleeding, warm ischemia, longer operative duration, and conversion. The estimated blood loss and duration of warm ischemia for LESS LDN are comparable to standard LDN; however, the LESS technique is associated with significantly longer operative times and a higher rate of conversion [16, 18, 25]. In a recent meta-analysis, LESS LDN was actually associated with lower intraoperative blood loss than standard LDN [17]. As with any surgery, the bleeding risk may be lessened by attention to meticulous surgical technique and prudent intraoperative decision-making. Conversion most frequently involves placement of additional ports, with open conversion occurring infrequently (8.5 % vs. 0.2 % of cases, respectively) [17]. The main reasons for conversion during LESS nephrectomy (in order of most to least common) are difficult retraction, bleeding, difficult dissection, failure to progress, and difficult access [16].

Postoperative

The overall postoperative complication rate for LESS LDN is estimated at 8.0 %, which is not significantly different from that of standard LDN [17, 26]. Most postoperative complications (79.8 %) are minor (Clavien grade I or II) [17]. The rate of major complications (Clavien III-V) is less than 1 % [26].

In well-selected patients, LESS LDN is a safe procedure, comparable to standard LDN, when performed by experienced surgeons at specialized centers [16, 17, 26].

Postoperative Care

Postoperative pain control is achieved with acetaminophen and low-dose opioids. Stool softeners are administered to prevent constipation. Clear liquids are allowed on the first postoperative evening as tolerated, and a regular diet is usually initiated on postoperative day 1. Deep vein thrombosis prophylaxis is accomplished with early ambulation, as most patients are young with low risk for thromboembolic disease, but subcutaneous chemoprophylaxis is used if warranted. An initial serum creatinine and complete blood count are checked on postoperative day 1 and thereafter if indicated. Patients are usually discharged on the first or second postoperative day pending adequate pain control, toleration of a regular diet, and ambulation. Patients are seen in clinic for follow-up in 1–2 weeks.

Challenges and Future Directions

At present, LESS LDN is cumbersome due to its high level of technical difficulty and poor ergonomics, limiting its widespread use. Even with the most experienced LESS surgeons using specialized single-site laparoscopic instruments, LESS LDN is more technically challenging than standard LDN, causing longer operating times and a higher likelihood of conversion [17]. The greatest challenge of the LESS technique is the clashing of instruments and restricted field of view that occurs from attempting to triangulate multiple instruments and a camera through a single small incision. Recently, the application of robotic technology to LESS has shown great promise in overcoming many of the constraints of traditional LESS [27]. In robotic LESS (R-LESS), the articulation of robotic instruments and the use of novel port placement have minimized the importance of and dependence on port triangulation, thus allowing for improved intracorporeal dissecting and suturing within the confines of a single surgical site [27, 28]. New single-site robotic instruments have been developed for R-LESS, which facilitate the application of R-LESS using the current robotic platform [29]. While the feasibility of R-LESS using novel single-site instruments has been demonstrated, significant limitations still exist due to impaired wrist articulation, external collisions, and limited working space for the bedside assistant [13, 30, 31]. To date, the only report of R-LESS LDN was achieved using a hybrid LESS-NOTES approach with one robotic instrument placed transvaginally [13].

Multiple new robotic platforms for single-site surgery are currently being developed [18]. Recently, the da Vinci® Sp™ surgical system, a new robotic platform specifically designed for LESS, has been tested with promising results for a wide variety of urologic applications, including nephrectomy [32].

Conclusion

In highly skilled hands, LESS LDN has been shown to improve cosmesis and minimize morbidity for the donor without compromising graft function for the recipient. By providing potential donors with a more favorable outcome, LESS LDN may help increase the donor pool. Unfortunately, the technical limitations of current LESS technology have prevented its widespread use. Therefore, the current role of LESS LDN in clinical practice is limited. Emerging purpose-built robotic platforms may overcome these challenges and permit the mainstream application of R-LESS to LDN and a wide variety of other urological surgeries.

References

1. Matas AJ, Smith JM, Skeans MA, et al. OPTN/SRTR 2012 annual data report: kidney. Am J Transplant. 2014;14 Suppl 1:11.
2. Eggers P. Comparison of treatment costs between dialysis and transplantation. Semin Nephrol. 1992;12:284.
3. Weitz J, Koch M, Mehrabi A, et al. Living-donor kidney transplantation: risks of the donor – benefits of the recipient. Clin Transplant. 2006;20 Suppl 17:13.
4. Axelrod DA, McCullough KP, Brewer ED, et al. Kidney and pancreas transplantation in the United States, 1999–2008: the changing face of living donation. Am J Transplant. 2010;10:987.
5. Greco F, Hoda MR, Alcaraz A, et al. Laparoscopic living-donor nephrectomy: analysis of the existing literature. Eur Urol. 2010;58:498.
6. Andersen MH, Mathisen L, Oyen O, et al. Postoperative pain and convalescence in living kidney donors-laparoscopic versus open donor nephrectomy: a randomized study. Am J Transplant. 2006;6:1438.
7. Nicholson ML, Elwell R, Kaushik M, et al. Health-related quality of life after living donor nephrectomy: a randomized controlled trial of laparoscopic versus open nephrectomy. Transplantation. 2011;91:457.
8. Wilson CH, Sanni A, Rix DA, et al. Laparoscopic versus open nephrectomy for live kidney donors. Cochrane Database Syst Rev. 2011;(11):CD006124.
9. Ratner LE, Ciseck LJ, Moore RG, et al. Laparoscopic live donor nephrectomy. Transplantation. 1995;60:1047.
10. Velidedeoglu E, Williams N, Brayman KL, et al. Comparison of open, laparoscopic, and hand-assisted approaches to live-donor nephrectomy. Transplantation. 2002;74:169.
11. Bachmann A, Wolff T, Ruszat R, et al. Retroperitoneoscopic donor nephrectomy: a retrospective, non-randomized comparison of early complications, donor and recipient outcome with the standard open approach. Eur Urol. 2005;48:90.
12. Gill IS, Canes D, Aron M, et al. Single port transumbilical (E-NOTES) donor nephrectomy. J Urol. 2008;180:637.
13. Kaouk JH, Khalifeh A, Laydner H, et al. Transvaginal hybrid natural orifice transluminal surgery robotic donor nephrectomy: first clinical application. Urology. 2012;80:1171.
14. Breda A, Schwartzmann I, Emiliani E, et al. Mini-laparoscopic live donor nephrectomy with the use of 3-mm instruments and laparoscope. World J Urol. 2015;33:707.
15. Hubert J, Renoult E, Mourey E, et al. Complete robotic-assistance during laparoscopic living donor nephrectomies: an evaluation of 38 procedures at a single site. Int J Urol. 2007;14:986.
16. Fan X, Lin T, Xu K, et al. Laparoendoscopic single-site nephrectomy compared with conventional laparoscopic nephrectomy: a systematic review and meta-analysis of comparative studies. Eur Urol. 2012;62:601.
17. Autorino R, Brandao LF, Sankari B, et al. Laparoendoscopic single-site (LESS) vs laparoscopic living-donor nephrectomy: a systematic review and meta-analysis. BJU Int. 2015;115:206.
18. Autorino R, Kaouk JH, Stolzenburg JU, et al. Current status and future directions of robotic single-site surgery: a systematic review. Eur Urol. 2013;63:266.
19. Merseburger AS, Herrmann TR, Shariat SF, et al. EAU guidelines on robotic and single-site surgery in urology. Eur Urol. 2013;64:277.

20. Rodrigue JR, Pavlakis M, Danovitch GM, et al. Evaluating living kidney donors: relationship types, psychosocial criteria, and consent processes at US transplant programs. Am J Transplant. 2007;7:2326.
21. Brar A, Jindal RM, Abbott KC, et al. Practice patterns in evaluation of living kidney donors in United Network for Organ Sharing-approved kidney transplant centers. Am J Nephrol. 2012;35:466.
22. Organ Procurement and Transplantation Network: OPTN. New OPTN requirements and resources for the living donor kidney transplant programs. Prog Transplant. 2013;23:117.
23. European Association of Urology: Guidelines on Renal Transplantation. 2014. http://uroweb.org/wp-content/uploads/27-Renal-Transplant_LRV2-May-13th-2014.pdf. Accessed 31 Aug 2015.
24. Ruszat R, Wyler SF, Wolff T, et al. Reluctance over right-sided retroperitoneoscopic living donor nephrectomy: justified or not? Transplant Proc. 2007;39:1381.
25. Aull MJ, Afaneh C, Charlton M, et al. A randomized, prospective, parallel group study of laparoscopic versus laparoendoscopic single site donor nephrectomy for kidney donation. Am J Transplant. 2014;14:1630.
26. Ramasamy R, Afaneh C, Katz M, et al. Comparison of complications of laparoscopic versus laparoendo-scopic single site donor nephrectomy using the modified Clavien grading system. J Urol. 2011;186:1386.
27. Kaouk JH, Goel RK, Haber GP, et al. Robotic single-port transumbilical surgery in humans: initial report. BJU Int. 2009;103:366.
28. Joseph RA, Salas NA, Johnson C, et al. Video Chopstick surgery: a novel technique enables use of the Da Vinci Robot to perform single-incision laparoscopic surgery. Surg Endosc. 2010;24:3224.
29. Haber GP, White MA, Autorino R, et al. Novel robotic da Vinci instruments for laparoendoscopic single-site surgery. Urology. 2010;76:1279.
30. Cestari A, Buffi NM, Lista G, et al. Feasibility and preliminary clinical outcomes of robotic laparoendo-scopic single-site (R-LESS) pyeloplasty using a new single-port platform. Eur Urol. 2012;62:175.
31. Komninos C, Tuliao P, Kim DK, et al. Robot-assisted laparoendoscopic single-site partial nephrectomy with the novel da vinci single-site platform: initial experience. Korean J Urol. 2014;55:380.
32. Kaouk JH, Haber GP, Autorino R, et al. A novel robotic system for single-port urologic surgery: first clinical investigation. Eur Urol. 2014;66:1033.

Transvaginal NOTES Nephrectomy

Antonio Alcaraz, Luís Peri, and Mireia Musquera

Introduction

Over the last 20 years, surgery has changed dramatically, from open to laparoscopic and more recently to new minimally invasive techniques like laparoscopic single-site surgery (LESS) and natural transluminal endoscopic surgery (NOTES). The current goal with these techniques is to reduce morbidity and improve cosmetic results while maintaining functional and oncological results. Natural orifice transluminal endoscopic surgery uses natural orifices to enter the abdominal cavity avoiding abdominal incisions becoming a scarless surgery technique. NOTES was performed for the first time in animal models at the beginning of the 2000s and posteriorly has been applied in different experimental procedures and in some surgeries in humans, but it has not experimented the same acceptance than laparoscopy. NOTES, especially pure NOTES, increases complexity in comparison to laparoscopic approach and even over LESS (Fig. 11.1).

Specifically, the application of NOTES in urology is complex because the current technology does not allow an easy performance of a complete pure NOTES procedure. The current surgical tools are not designed for retracting large organs like a kidney; bleeding control and clashing of instruments are also other surgeon's obstacles. For this reason the hybrid and assisted approach have been developed and used by the groups with experience in these techniques. These variations of NOTES are feasible in urological surgery, obtaining good cosmetic results and reducing morbidity.

Among possible approaches, the vagina offers a good surgical channel and specimen removal orifice. Many published series have confirmed the feasibility and reproducibility of hybrid and assisted NOTES simple, radical and living donor nephrectomy.

In this chapter we proceed to summarize the NOTES nephrectomy history review with an actualization of all published data, an overview of all instruments and optics available to perform this technique and finally a surgical description of radical and living donor nephrectomy.

History

Surgery has changed dramatically over the last 20 years towards minimally invasiveness, and urology can be considered a pioneer speciality in that sense, as endoscopic surgeries have been done for many years. Since the first laparoscopic nephrectomy performed by Clayman et al. [1] in

A. Alcaraz, MD, PhD (✉) • L. Peri, MD
M. Musquera, MD, PhD
Department of Urology, Hospital Clinic,
Barcelona, Spain
e-mail: aalcaraz@clinic.ub.es; lperi@clinic.ub.es

© Springer Science+Business Media New York 2017
J.H. Kaouk et al. (eds.), *Atlas of Laparoscopic and Robotic Single Site Surgery*,
Current Clinical Urology, DOI 10.1007/978-1-4939-3575-8_11

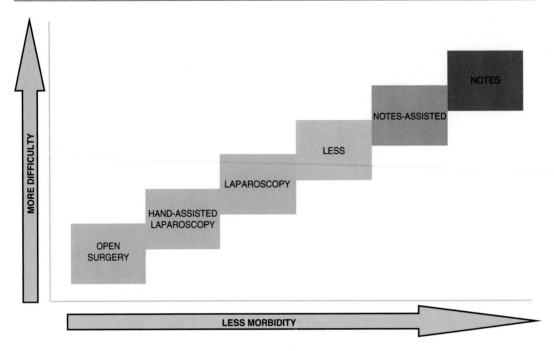

Fig. 11.1 Scheme of surgery evolution

1991, this surgical technique has been adapted worldwide because of its great advantages in front of the open approach. Currently, open nephrectomies are an example of surgical evolution. As many other open surgeries, they are nearly extinguished because laparoscopy offers advantages. Some of these advantages are small incisions (avoiding lumbotomy in nephrectomies cases), less needs of analgesia, less bleeding, faster recovery and lower risk of herniation.

The next step, after laparoscopy, in the minimal invasive surgery evolution is towards the concept of scarless surgery: entering the peritoneal cavity of a patient without injuring the abdominal wall, which might result in a complete absence of visible scars. The absence of these incisions would offer an obvious improvement in cosmetic results, but it also might improve postoperative pain while maintaining the same functional and oncologic results. Furthermore, it would decrease postoperative complications like hernias.

In that way, natural orifice transluminal endoscopic surgery (NOTES) has been recently developed [2, 3]. NOTES uses natural orifices (the mouth, anus, nares, vagina and urethra) of

the body with the intention to puncture hollow viscera (the bladder, vagina, colon, stomach and oesophagus) in order to enter an otherwise inaccessible body cavity.

To date, NOTES has been successfully completed experimentally in different fields and many surgeries. In 2002, Gettman et al. described the first experimental NOTES transvaginal nephrectomy in a porcine model [4]. Kalloo et al. later reported the first NOTES using a transgastric port also in a porcine model [5], while at the same time Pai et al. described a transcolonic approach with important limitations (lack of sterility and difficulties on an effective closure method) [6]. In addition, Lima et al. designed the transluminal vesical (transvesical) port for NOTES applications [7], and Bazzi et al. developed and demonstrated the feasibility of transrectal NOTES nephrectomy in a cadaveric and porcine model [8, 9].

As we mentioned before, pure NOTES in urology is really difficult to perform because the current type of instruments available is not designed to retract large organs. These instruments have an excess of flexibility that difficult large organ retraction such as the kidney; another difficulty is the limited space through the port access and this implies clashing of instruments inside the abdominal cavity and clashing hands outside; to obtain a good haemostasis with the existent devices is another limitation of NOTES. Ureteroscopes and gastroscopes were designed primarily as diagnostic tools, and they are far from being ideal for being used in NOTES. Finally, an important disadvantage is the viscera closure after the surgery that has not been resolved yet. Some devices are currently being developed with promising results, but no definitive evidence of its safety is available.

In order to overcome current technical limitations inherent in pure NOTES, variations on that with conventional laparoscopic combination have been described leading to the concept of hybrid or assisted NOTES [10]. Following the Nomenclature Consortium definition, a hybrid NOTES procedure is any surgery that uses transabdominal instruments or ports, but the majority (>75 %) of the procedure is carried out by the instrumentation inserted through the natural orifice. A hybrid NOTES surgery allows perforation of the organ under direct vision, minimizing the risk of injuring adjacent tissues. It also improves the spatial orientation as laparoscopic cameras can be used while maintaining triangulation, which also facilitates tissue retraction with the assistance of one or two transabdominal ports. Hybrid NOTES technique improves the safety of the pure NOTES procedure while minimizing the invasiveness of the laparoscopic approach. The use of a natural orifice as an additional port for insertion of an instrument or an endoscope for visualization during laparoscopic surgery should be designated as NOTES-assisted surgery, following the Nomenclature Consortium definitions [10].

In our opinion, the most important advantage of hybrid or assisted NOTES is to avoid an abdominal incision for the specimen removal, which might result in a better cosmetic result and probably an improved postoperative recovery. The benefit is equally obtained regardless of the use that surgeons do of the transvaginal port or the percentage of the surgical procedure performed through it. This is the main reason why hybrid or assisted NOTES is obsolete terms that made sense when LESS was being developed in order to clarify terminology. Nowadays, only NOTES-assisted surgery is extensively used by few groups.

NOTES in Renal Surgery

Twenty years ago, when laparoscopy was introduced in urology, the vagina was considered an excellent route for kidney retrieval after laparoscopic nephrectomy. In that way Breda et al. reported the first case [11]. A decade later Gill et al. reported an initial series using the vagina for intact specimen extraction [12]. Six years later, in 2008 appears the first publication in hybrid NOTES nephrectomy for an atrophic kidney in humans described by Branco et al. [13]. In this case two abdominal 5-mm trocars were used and a transvaginal access to entrance the endoscope. Some months later, Alcaraz et al. performed the first hybrid NOTES nephrectomy for a kidney tumour [14]. Since then, some surgeons have reported their clinical experience in the so-called hybrid or assisted transvaginal NOTES nephrectomy.

After our first experience in hybrid NOTES transvaginal radical nephrectomy [14], we performed and described a series of NOTES-assisted laparoscopic simple and radical nephrectomies, becoming pioneers in this approach. Concretely, we reported a total of 14 transvaginal NOTES-assisted laparoscopic nephrectomy for T1–T3a N0M0 renal cancer. The mean age of the women was 53.9 years (range 34–78 years). The mean operative time was 122 min (range 80–270 min) and the mean estimated blood loss was 167.5 mL (range 30–400 mL). One patient required a blood transfusion after surgery. The mean hospital stay was 4.1 days. In this first series, a major complication occurred in one patient. This woman had had previous abdominal and pelvic surgery and a colon injury occurred. This patient underwent surgery and a temporary colostomy was carried out [15].

After this experience in NOTES-assisted laparoscopic nephrectomies, we adapted the surgical technique to living donor nephrectomy. So far, we have performed more than 80 cases by adding one more abdominal port. Females represent around two-thirds of all living donors. In a group of people who will be submitted to a mutilating surgery being completely healthy, it is of the utmost importance to avoid morbidity. The potential advantages the transvaginal approach might offer are reducing and hiding abdominal scars (with an obvious improvement in the cosmetic result) and decreasing postoperative pain while maintaining the graft outcomes.

Sotelo et al. [16] described a NOTES hybrid transvaginal radical nephrectomy technique without extra-umbilical trocar. They described four cases using two multichannel devices, one in the umbilicus and the other one through the vagina; of those, just one case could be completed. The surgery took 3.7 h and no complications were seen.

Kaouk et al. in 2010 successfully carried out the first unique transvaginal "pure" NOTES nephrectomy in a 58-year-old woman using a multichannel device through the vagina [17]. Although this experience must be considered a complete success, the procedure took more than 7 h, and several changes of the access port in the vagina were required because of air leakage and instrument collision, so the authors themselves considered this was not a reproducible technique and

important improvements in armamentarium were needed before trying to repeat the procedure.

One year later Porpiglia et al. published a first case of transvaginal NOTES-assisted nephrectomy using mini-laparoscopic instruments through the abdominal wall with good results, being easier than a pure NOTES while obtaining excellent cosmetic results [18].

Apart from being an excellent route for big specimen retrieval, the vagina can be easily closed from the outside. This fact resolves the problem of wound closure that appears in other NOTES routes as the stomach or the rectum, where no appropriate closure methods have been validated. Besides, we count on the uro-gynaecological experience where countless patients have undergone transvaginal access to the peritoneal cavity for a wide variety of procedures with a low complication rate (infections, incisional hernias).

Allaf et al. described a successful laparoscopic living donor nephrectomy with vaginal extraction in March 2009 [19]. We performed the first NOTES-assisted radical nephrectomy for kidney tumour in 2009. Afterwards, we adapted NOTES-assisted laparoscopic nephrectomies to living donation, and in 2011 we published the first and largest series of NOTES-assisted living donor nephrectomy [20]. We compared the results of 20 transvaginal with a matched pair of 40 conventional laparoscopic ones. The transvaginal

Table 11.1 Summary of different transvaginal nephrectomy series published by different authors

Author	Year	Terminology	Surgery	N trocars
Branco et al.	2008	Hybrid NOTES	One simple neph	5-mm umbilical
				5-mm extraumbilical
Alcaraz et al.	2009	Hybrid NOTES	Four simple neph and ten radical	10-mm umbilical
				5-mm extraumbilical
				10-mm vaginal
Kaouk et al.	2009	Hybrid NOTES	One simple neph	TriPort vaginal
				5-mm umbilical
Sotelo et al.	2010	Hybrid NOTES	One radical neph	TriPort vaginal
				TriPort umbilical
Kaouk et al.	2010	Pure NOTES	One simple neph	GelPort vaginal
Porpiglia et al.	2011	Hybrid NOTES	One simple neph	10-mm vaginal
				3 of 3.5-mm abdominal
Alcaraz et al.	2011	Assisted NOTES	20 living donor nephrectomies	10-mm vaginal
				Two 10-mm/5-mm abd

approach offered an improvement in cosmetics, less needs of analgesia with same graft results [20]. Despite the longer warm ischemia time (which was under 5 min) in comparison with conventional laparoscopic nephrectomy, there was no effect on graft function, so it might be considered a good alternative procedure that might increase the living donor rate in the female population. To date we have done more than 80 transvaginal living donor nephrectomies and in our centre this procedure represents the first choice when feasible for females (Table 11.1).

Instruments and Optics

Although for a pure transvaginal NOTES nephrectomy no appropriate instruments are currently available, to start performing a transvaginal hybrid or assisted NOTES nephrectomy in a laparoscopic centre, very few specific instruments are required.

Trocars

A 12-mm trocar for bariatric surgery is required as common trocars are not long enough to reach the Douglas pouch. The trocar will be inserted under direct vision at the beginning of the surgery and it should maintain the same position without needing an exterior pressure.

Optics

The optics required depend on the surgical technique. If the camera is inserted through an abdominal trocar (see surgical approach), a regular 30° optic will be the only requirement. On the contrary, if we want to place the camera through the vaginal port, we will need a 0° camera with a deflectable-tip laparoscope (with or without 3D). A second 0° camera will be used after creation of the pneumoperitoneum, to assess the entrance of the transvaginal trocar and when removing the specimen. The deflectable laparoscope placed through the vagina trocar will be used during the rest of the surgical procedure, offering a conventional laparoscopic view.

Currently in the market, there are different laparoscopes. The only deflectable-tip laparoendoscope that is essential for a mixed NOTES transvaginal nephrectomy is the Endoeye® by Olympus™ (Figs. 11.2 and 11.3).

During the recent years, the 3D technology has been entering in the laparoscopic world as an improvement in vision. Surgeons that have used 3D feel much more comfortable when performing fine and difficult dissections, and they refer a

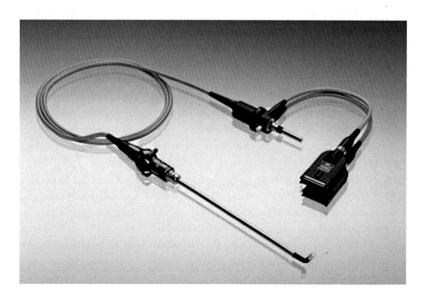

Fig. 11.2 Optics

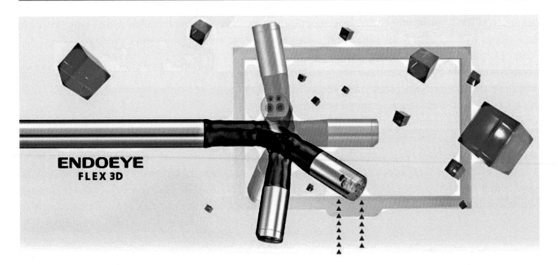

Fig. 11.3 Optics mobility

Surgical Technique

better view of the operating field. Although it is not mandatory, 3D technology can be helpful if available.

Before starting any surgical procedure, it is essential to have an appropriate surgical strategy. Basically, two items are required: physical exam and image evaluation. The great advances in image technologies that have taken place during the recent years (CT scan, MRI, etc.) are very helpful at this point, as we can see the peculiarities of each case in detail: tumour size, extra capsular invasion, existence of tumour vein thrombus and number and disposition of the pedicle vessels. The multidetector computed tomography with a 64-row scanner is the technique of choice for preoperative evaluation of living renal donors, as it offers an accuracy of nearly 100 % in vascular pedicle evaluation [21]. With axial reconstructions of 0.8 mm, this technology allows the detection of arteries smaller than 2 mm, which is what is required for an appropriate living donor assessment [22] (Fig. 11.4). Apart from that, the radiological exam offers information about pelvic varicosities that might contraindicate the transvaginal approach.

Patient and Donor Selection

All women suitable for the transvaginal approach need a vaginal exploration. It is important to assess the characteristics of the skin (atrophy, lesions, etc.) and existence of pelvic organ prolapses and, most important, assess the distensibility of the vagina and the introit to anticipate for any trouble during specimen extraction. The presence of vaginal sclero-atrophy or a non-distensible introitus might preclude the transvaginal extraction. This assessment is especially important in living donation. Although the specimens obtained in radical nephrectomies are normally larger and the tumour size might be a contraindication for transvaginal removal, in these cases there is no time limit due to warm ischaemia, and the specimen could be handled with "less" care. On the contrary, in living donor surgery, the specimen size tends to be smaller, but it must be handled with optimal care to obtain a good graft quality, so it is not desirable to push the future graft through a small canal.

It is better to avoid patients/donors with pelvic varicosities. Although this is not an absolute contraindication, when tearing the vagina aperture with the fingers, we can injure those vessels and get an important bleeding (Fig. 11.5).

One relative contraindication for NOTES surgery is overweight, as it depends on the

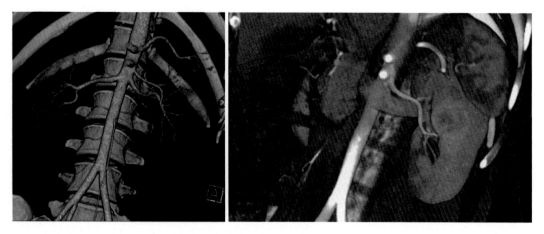

Fig. 11.4 CT scan of living donor. Vessels and parenchyma anatomy

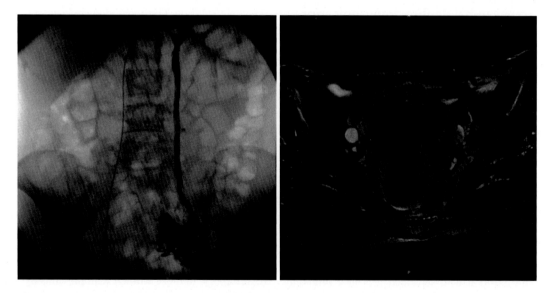

Fig. 11.5 Phlebography and MRI that show pelvic varicosities

degree of obesity and the ability and experience of the surgeons. If anyone starts a NOTES programme in their department, it would not be advisable to select obese patients with a BMI above 26 or 27. Although these patients can be offered a minimally invasive approach, the difficulties in retracting organs are worsened by a larger amount of fat. Furthermore, the peri-renal fat that in some cases is difficult to release might lead us to obtain a too large kidney to be removed harmless through the vagina. The more experience the surgeon gets in this technique, the more BMI he is able to accept, always keeping in mind that surgery will be more difficult.

Finally, another consideration to take into account is the history of previous abdominal surgery. As known by all surgeons, previous surgeries might turn an easy surgery into a very difficult one. Of special interest in this case is a previous hysterectomy, which would not contraindicate a transvaginal NOTES approach but would compel us to get some precautions during transvaginal trocar introduction (see later).

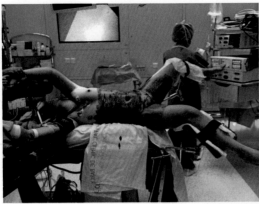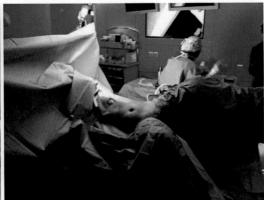

Fig. 11.6 Patient positioning and wrapping

Considerations for a Correct Transvaginal Nephrectomy Indication

- BMI
- Vaginal exam (distensibility)
- Anatomy of the specimen (size, vascular pedicle, etc.)
- Pelvic varicosities
- Previous surgeries

Patient Placement

Before starting any procedure, it is very important to make a correct patient placement, especially in any transvaginal approach.

The patient has to be placed in a semilumbotomy position with separated legs in a lithotomy position to allow vaginal access. Placing the patient at the edge of the table will permit the manipulation through the vagina (introduction of instruments, camera and bag). The contralateral leg of the surgery site must be placed lower than the other site (Fig. 11.6), and all pressure points have to be well protected to avoid any pressure injury.

Transvaginal Radical Nephrectomy

Trocar Placement and Surgery

Under general anaesthesia, the patient has to be placed in a semilumbotomy position as described previously. The vagina has to be prepped with povidone solution. Our technique consists in the placement of the first trocar (12 mm) under direct vision laterally 5 cm from the umbilicus. After the correct location is confirmed, we start the pneumoperitoneum insufflation and maintain it at 12 mmHg.

A zero-degree laparoscopic optic is used to place a 5-mm trocar in the flank. Finally, and under direct vision and retracting the uterus with a conventional grasper, an obesity port of 12 mm is placed through the vagina into the abdominal cavity, perforating the vaginal wall in the posterior cul-de-sac (Fig. 11.7). The continuous vision of the abdominal cavity permits a precise placement of the trocar that has to be in the midline, minimizing the risk of bowel and uterine vessel injury. In those women with previous hysterectomies, it is important to place the trocar far from the bladder to avoid possible injuries on it.

The trocar can be guided through the vagina using a conventional vaginal valve or the fingers of the contralateral hand.

Taking advantage of transabdominal camera, the deflectable optic (Deflectable-Tip EndoEYE, Olympus, Tokyo, Japan) with or without 3D (Olympus Exera 3D) can be easily introduced into the peritoneal cavity (Fig. 11.8).

After the initial setting, the nephrectomy can be done following the steps of a regular laparoscopic transabdominal nephrectomy, taking into account the peculiarities of the transvaginal vision (Fig. 11.9).

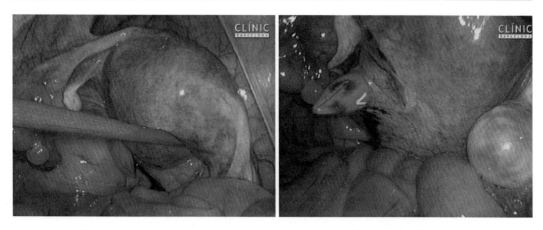

Fig. 11.7 Under direct vision, the uterus is retracted and the transvaginal trocar is inserted

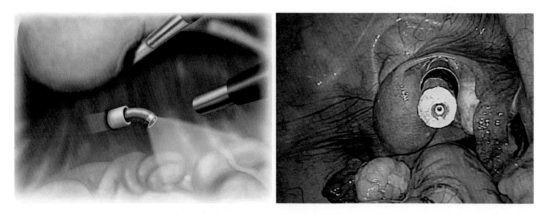

Fig. 11.8 Entrance of the camera into the abdominal cavity through the transvaginal trocar (From Alcaraz et al. [15]. Reprinted with permission from Elsevier Limited)

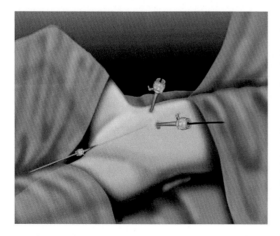

Fig. 11.9 Transvaginal mixed NOTES radical nephrectomy trocar setup (From Alcaraz et al. [15]. Reprinted with permission from Elsevier Limited)

We use the 5-mm abdominal trocar to enter a bipolar grasper and the 12-mm trocar to entrance monopolar scissors and LigaSure. Surgery starts by the incision of the Toldt's line, mobilizing the colon medially.

The ureter is localized, dissected and sectioned using the LigaSure device (Valleylab, Tyco Healthcare, Boulder, CO, USA). The renal hilum is reached by dissection of the lower pole of the kidney through cranial direction (Fig. 11.10). The renal artery is ligated with three Hem-o-lok clips (Weck Closure Systems, Research Triangle Park, NC, USA) and sectioned, keeping two clips in the patient side with enough distance between them. Ligation of the renal vein is done using the

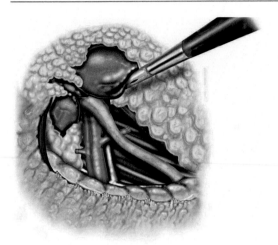

Fig. 11.10 Lower pole elevation that permits a better exposure of the renal hilum

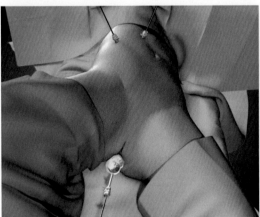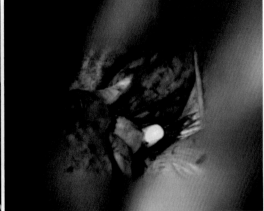

Fig. 11.11 Vaginal specimen removal inside the bag

same technique. The posterior wall and the upper pole of the kidney are then dissected, preserving the adrenal gland. After the whole specimen is detached, an organ bag is introduced through the trocar hole placed at the vagina under a direct vision using the 0° abdominal camera. The kidney is wrapped and removed under direct vision through an extended incision at the posterior wall of the vagina performed blindly with the fingers (Fig. 11.11). The vaginal wound is closed under direct vision using conventional open-surgery instruments. A running 2-0 absorbable suture or interrupted stitches can be done. It is really important to take all the vagina wall during clo-

sure. A gauze with epithelial cream is placed for 24 h into the vagina.

Transvaginal Living Donor Nephrectomy

Trocar Placement and Surgery

The transvaginal living donor nephrectomy has several modifications from the original radical nephrectomy. The woman's position is exactly the same (see previous description). The pneumoperitoneum is achieved by a 12-mm trocar placed in the umbilicus site under direct vision. A second

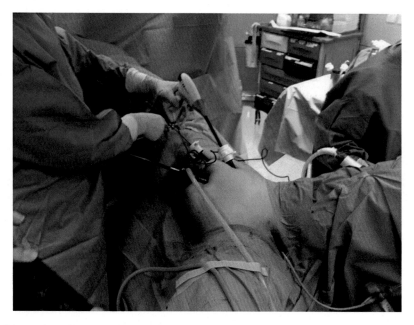

Fig. 11.12 Transvaginal mixed NOTES living donor nephrectomy trocar setup

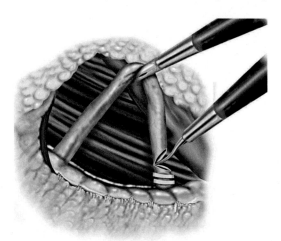

Fig. 11.13 Ureter section

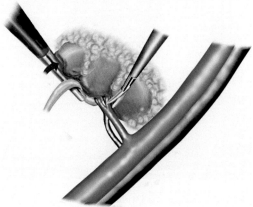

Fig. 11.14 Lower pole elevation (From Alcaraz et al. [15]. Reprinted with permission from Elsevier Limited)

10-mm trocar port is placed in the left iliac fossa and a 5-mm port next to the ribs. Finally, a 12-mm bariatric surgery trocar is placed through the vagina as described previously (Fig. 11.12). Retracting the uterus with a grasper through the 5-mm port facilitates this manoeuvre (Fig. 11.7). Kidney dissection is then performed following the steps of a regular laparoscopic transabdominal living donor nephrectomy using instruments through the vagina and the abdominal wall. After dissection of the colon, the ureter is located and carefully dissected distally until iliac vessels, where it is distally clipped and sectioned (Fig. 11.13). After the lower pole of the kidney is lifted with a forceps placed through the vaginal trocar, this manoeuvre is essential to facilitate vascular pedicle dissection (Fig. 11.14). Vascular dissection if very important in living donor nephrectomy. The vein has to be dissected totally taking the adrenal and gonadal vein with the LigaSure (Fig. 11.15). In the left site, almost always a lumbar vein surrounds the renal artery

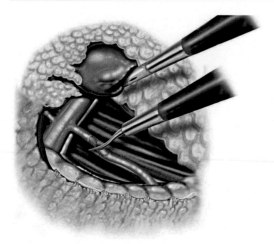

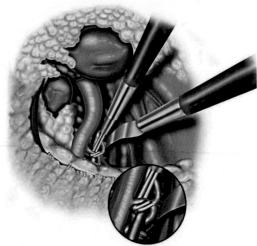

Fig. 11.15 Gonadal vein section

Fig. 11.16 Lumbar vein dissection. This manoeuvre permits to obtain a longer artery

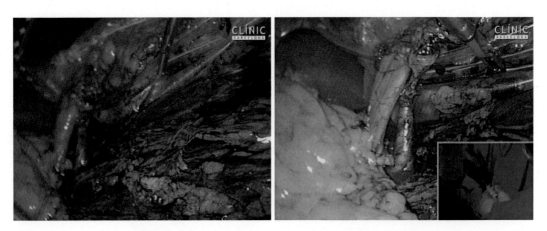

Fig. 11.17 Kidney wrap with the bag inserted through the vagina orifice. The metallic ring permits a gentle traction of the pedicle

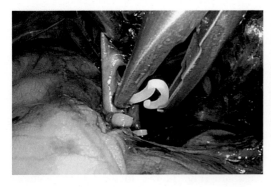

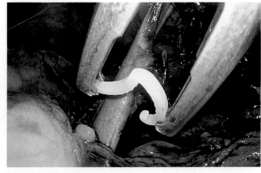

Fig. 11.18 Arterial clipping

Fig. 11.19 Vein clipping

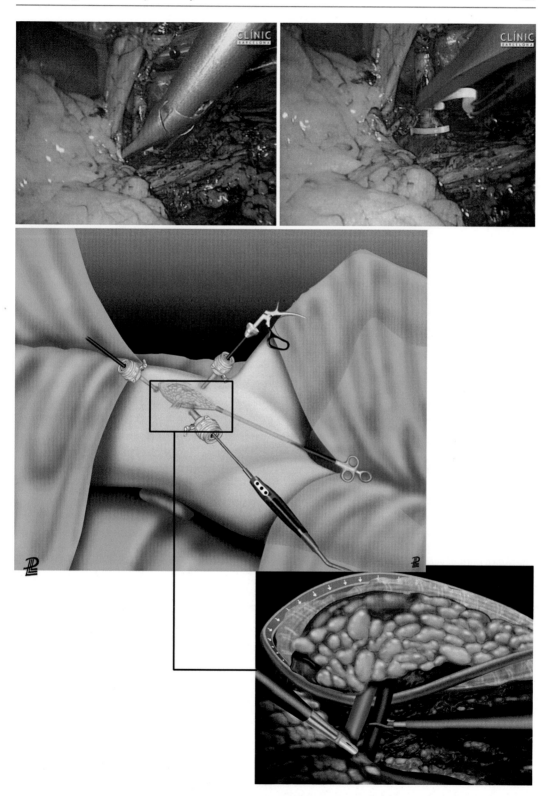

Fig. 11.20 Pedicle exposure and vessel clipping in a mixed NOTES transvaginal living donor nephrectomy (From Alcaraz et al. [20]. Reprinted with permission from Elsevier Limited)

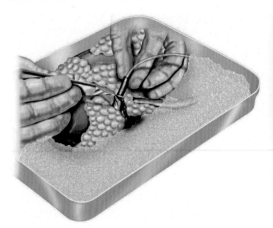

Fig. 11.21 Perfusion of the kidney after retrieval

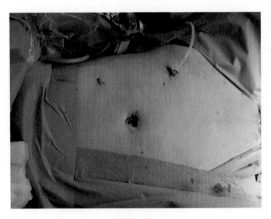

Fig. 11.22 Immediate results of a mixed NOTES transvaginal living donor nephrectomy

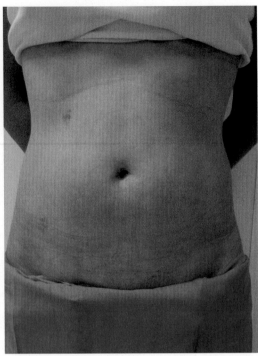

Fig. 11.23 4-month results after a mixed NOTES transvaginal living donor nephrectomy

external side to prevent contamination with vaginal bacteria. Finally, the kidney is transferred to a back table for perfusion and preparation for implantation (Fig. 11.21). The vagina wall is closed using the same technique previously described.

In Fig. 11.22 you can see the immediate final result and the result after 3 months in Fig. 11.23.

(Fig. 11.16). The section of this vein permits to get the artery until the aorta's ostium. Once the kidney and vascular pedicle are totally dissected, an EndoCatch (Covidien surgical) device is placed through the vaginal trocar incision (Fig. 11.17). The organ is wrapped inside the bag permitting us to apply a gentle traction with the metallic ring of the bag. This offers a good exposure of the pedicle for safe clipping and posterior section. Vessel clipation is done using Hem-o-lok clips (Teleflex Medical), metallic clips or staples in the proximal ends of the artery (Fig. 11.18) and vein (Fig. 11.19) before transection (Fig. 11.20). The kidney is removed inside the bag through the digitally extended incision in the posterior cul-de-sac. Then, the assistant has to remove the kidney from the bag carefully avoiding any contact with its

References

1. Clayman RV, Kavoussi LR, Soper NJ, et al. Laparoscopic nephrectomy: initial case report. J Urol. 1991;146(2):278–82.
2. Autorino R, Cadeddu JA, Desai MM, et al. Laparoendoscopic single-site and natural orifice transluminal endoscopic surgery in urology: a critical analysis of the literature. Eur Urol. 2011;59(1):26–45.
3. Lima E, Rolanda C, Autorino R, Correia-Pinto J. Experimental foundation for natural orifice transluminal endoscopic surgery and hybrid natural orifice transluminal endoscopic surgery. BJU Int. 2010;106(6 Pt B):913–8.
4. Gettman MT, Lotan Y, Napper CA, Cadeddu JA. Transvaginal laparoscopic nephrectomy: develop-

ment and feasibility in the porcine model. Urology. 2002;59(3):446–50.

5. Kalloo AN, Singh VK, Jagannath SB, et al. Flexible transgastric peritoneoscopy: a novel approach to diagnostic and therapeutic interventions in the peritoneal cavity. Gastrointest Endosc. 2004;60(1):114–7.

6. Pai RD, Fong DG, Bundga ME, Odze RD, Rattner DW, Thompson CC. Transcolonic endoscopic cholecystectomy: a NOTES survival study in a porcine model (with video). Gastrointest Endosc. 2006;64(3):428–34.

7. Lima E, Branco F, Parente J, Autorino R, Correia-Pinto J. Transvesical natural orifice transluminal endoscopic surgery (NOTES) nephrectomy with kidney morcellation: a proof of concept study. BJU Int. 2012;109(10):1533–7.

8. Bazzi WM, Stroup SP, Cohen SA, et al. Feasibility of transrectal hybrid natural orifice transluminal endoscopic surgery (NOTES) nephrectomy in the cadaveric model. Urology. 2012;80(3):590–5.

9. Bazzi WM, Wagner O, Stroup SP, et al. Transrectal hybrid natural orifice transluminal endoscopic surgery (NOTES) nephrectomy in a porcine model. Urology. 2011;77(3):518–23.

10. Box G, Averch T, Cadeddu J, et al. Nomenclature of natural orifice translumenal endoscopic surgery (NOTES) and laparoendoscopic single-site surgery (LESS) procedures in urology. J Endourol Endourol Soc. 2008;22(11):2575–81.

11. Breda G, Silvestre P, Giunta A, Xausa D, Tamai A, Gherardi L. Laparoscopic nephrectomy with vaginal delivery of the intact kidney. Eur Urol. 1993;24(1):116–7.

12. Gill IS, Cherullo EE, Meraney AM, Borsuk F, Murphy DP, Falcone T. Vaginal extraction of the intact specimen following laparoscopic radical nephrectomy. J Urol. 2002;167(1):238–41.

13. Branco AW, Branco Filho AJ, Kondo W, et al. Hybrid transvaginal nephrectomy. Eur Urol. 2008;53(6): 1290–4.

14. Ribal Caparros MJ, Peri Cusi L, Molina Cabeza A, Garcia Larrosa A, Carmona F, Alcaraz Asensio A. First report on hybrid transvaginal nephrectomy for renal cancer. Actas Urol Esp. 2009;33(3):280–3.

15. Alcaraz A, Peri L, Molina A, et al. Feasibility of transvaginal NOTES-assisted laparoscopic nephrectomy. Eur Urol. 2010;57(2):233–7.

16. Sotelo R, de Andrade R, Fernandez G, et al. NOTES hybrid transvaginal radical nephrectomy for tumor: stepwise progression toward a first successful clinical case. Eur Urol. 2010;57(1):138–44.

17. Kaouk JH, Haber GP, Goel RK, et al. Pure natural orifice translumenal endoscopic surgery (NOTES) transvaginal nephrectomy. Eur Urol. 2010;57(4):723–6.

18. Porpiglia F, Fiori C, Morra I, Scarpa RM. Transvaginal natural orifice transluminal endoscopic surgery-assisted minilaparoscopic nephrectomy: a step towards scarless surgery. Eur Urol. 2011;60(4):862–6.

19. Allaf ME, Singer A, Shen W, et al. Laparoscopic live donor nephrectomy with vaginal extraction: initial report. Am J Transplant. 2010;10(6):1473–7.

20. Alcaraz A, Musquera M, Peri L, et al. Feasibility of transvaginal natural orifice transluminal endoscopic surgery-assisted living donor nephrectomy: is kidney vaginal delivery the approach of the future? Eur Urol. 2011;59(6):1019–25.

21. Blondin D, Andersen K, Kroepil P, et al. Analysis of 64-row multidetector CT images for preoperative angiographic evaluation of potential living kidney donors. Radiologe. 2008;48(7):673–80.

22. Sebastia C, Peri L, Salvador R, et al. Multidetector CT of living renal donors: lessons learned from surgeons. Radiographics. 2010;30(7):1875–90.

LESS Pyeloplasty

12

Robert D. Brown, Humberto Laydner, Georges-Pascal Haber, and Robert J. Stein

Introduction

The creation of even smaller incisions for urologic surgery has been a goal since the introduction of laparoscopy for nephrectomy as described by Clayman et al. [1]. Never has this quest for decreasing incision size been so appropriate than for reconstructive procedures. No specimen extraction is necessary in making minimization of incisions in these cases a reasonable goal. In addition, many of these patients are younger and may be interested in a more cosmetic result.

R.D. Brown, MD
Department of Urology, Cleveland Clinic,
9500 Euclid Ave. Q10, Cleveland, OH 44195, USA
e-mail: rob.brown737@gmail.com

H. Laydner, MD
Department of Urology, University Hospitals Urology
Institute, Richmond Heights, Cleveland, OH, USA
e-mail: Laydner@icloud.com

G.-P. Haber, MD, PhD
Associate Staff, Department of Urology,
Center for Robotic and Image Guided Surgery,
Glickman Urological Institute, Cleveland Clinic,
Cleveland, OH, USA
e-mail: haberg2@ccf.org

R.J. Stein, MD (✉)
Associate Professor of Surgery, Department of
Urology, Center for Robotic and Image Guided
Surgery, Glickman Urological and Kidney Institute,
Cleveland Clinic, Cleveland, OH, USA
e-mail: steinr@ccf.org

Endoscopic options exist for treatment of primary ureteropelvic junction obstruction (UPJO), but pyeloplasty is associated with significantly higher success rates and is our preferred approach in these cases [2]. Multiple options are available for the reconstruction depending upon the etiology of the obstruction. For a UPJO due to an aperistaltic segment, a Fengerplasty with a Heineke-Mikulicz repair can be considered. For a high ureteral insertion, a Y-V plasty may be used. For any etiology of UPJO, an Anderson-Hynes dismembered pyeloplasty may be considered and is in fact our preferred approach for all primary UPJO. In this chapter we describe our technique for performing laparoendoscopic single-site surgery pyeloplasty (LESS-P).

Preoperative Evaluation

Hydronephrosis with a normal caliber ureter on axial imaging is the typical radiographic finding for UPJO. From the CT scan, note should also be taken of any nephrolithiasis present ipsilaterally. A diuretic radionuclide scan should be performed to assess the severity of obstruction and document the differential function of both renal units. Indications for repair include symptoms such as chronic discomfort or flank pain with caffeine or high-volume fluid intake (Dietl's crisis), pyelonephritis, loss of ipsilateral renal function, or stones. Patients are typically observed if they are

© Springer Science+Business Media New York 2017
J.H. Kaouk et al. (eds.), *Atlas of Laparoscopic and Robotic Single Site Surgery*,
Current Clinical Urology, DOI 10.1007/978-1-4939-3575-8_12

incidentally discovered to have hydronephrosis with none of the indications listed above by obtaining serial diuretic radionuclide scans.

Due to the higher failure rate and increased hemorrhagic risk, recognition of a crossing vessel prior to endopyelotomy is imperative [3]. As we typically perform dismembered pyeloplasty for primary UPJO, we do not routinely obtain angiographic imaging (MR or CT) to identify crossing vessels. Instead we assume a reasonable likelihood of the presence of crossing vessels (approximately 50 % of cases), and if encountered we carefully dissect and preserve them after which the UPJ repair is transposed anterior to them. It is important to note that crossing lower pole renal vessels usually consist of an artery and a vein, and therefore two vessels and not just one should be recognized.

Patient Selection

LESS-P can be considered for most patients with primary UPJO. Pyeloplasty for secondary UPJO can be especially challenging, and therefore we do not routinely suggest that a LESS approach should be considered for these cases. Relative contraindications for LESS-P include patients who are obese (BMI>35 kg/m^2) and patients who have undergone extensive prior upper abdominal surgery. Absolute contraindications are no different than that for conventional laparoscopic surgery and include bleeding diathesis.

Cystoscopy and Positioning

If LESS-P is elected, the patient is placed in dorsal lithotomy position after induction of general anesthesia. An ipsilateral retrograde pyelogram is performed to ensure no other ureteral pathology, and once the diagnosis is confirmed, a 4.7 Fr×28-cm double-J ureteral stent is placed over wire. A small caliber stent is used so that eventual sutured repair is not made more technically difficult by a bulky stent.

The patient is then placed in 60° modified flank position with the ipsilateral side up. The arms are placed on a double arm board, and the patient is taped after all pressure points are padded and an axillary roll is placed.

Access and Instrumentation

Our most common strategy for access involves the use of a single-port device, GelPoint (Applied Medical, Rancho Santa Margarita, CA, USA). We place this through an approximately 4-cm vertical incision directly through the umbilicus. All or nearly all of the incision should be contained within the umbilicus. The fascia is then incised with a scissor and the peritoneum is entered. The port is then placed as described elsewhere in this book. Alternatively, through the 4-cm skin incision, a 12-mm and two separate 5-mm ports may be placed for a single-incision approach with separate fascial stabs for port placement.

We most commonly use a flexible tip EndoEye laparoscope (Olympus, Center Valley, PA, USA) through one of the 5-mm ports. We use conventional laparoscopic instruments for dissection including a small bowel grasper in the left hand and a scissor or hook cautery dissector in the right hand. Prior to transecting the UPJ, we make a small puncture in the skin and place a 2-mm grasping instrument without using a port. The 2-mm grasper is held with the surgeon's left hand, so it is placed in the right lower quadrant for a right pyeloplasty and in the left upper quadrant for a left pyeloplasty. The grasper allows for triangulation while performing the more precise steps of UPJ transection, spatulation, and laparoscopic suturing. To this point we have found it unnecessary to use a liver retractor as we have found that the UPJ is always caudal to the edge of the liver especially from the vantage point of the umbilically placed laparoscope.

Dissection and Identification of the Ureter

The initial step is colon mobilization and on the right side the duodenum is kocherized. We tend to use a laparoscopic bowel grasper in the left hand and scissors in the right. In terms of

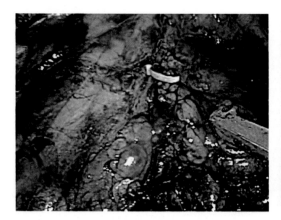

Fig. 12.1 Retraction of Gerota's fascia using a Hem-o-lok clip

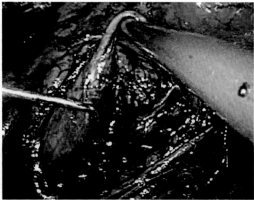

Fig. 12.2 Proximal ureter, UPJ, and renal pelvis dissected

clashing, the most advantageous configuration is usually working with the instruments in a vertical plane instead of horizontal. Therefore, within the patient's abdomen, the tip of the left-handed instrument usually is lateral or medial to the tip of the right-handed instrument.

We then dissect through Gerota's fascia just lateral to the inferior vena cava (IVC) on the right side and the aorta on the left side to identify the psoas muscle. The edge of Gerota's fascia is then grasped and held laterally. Using a suction device, the gonadal vein and ureter are swept medially, and the edge of Gerota's fascia is fixed to the lateral side wall using a Hem-o-lok clip (Weck Surgical Instruments, Teleflex Medical, Durham, NC) for retraction (Fig. 12.1).

A plane medial to the ureter and lateral to the gonadal vein is identified. This plane is developed superiorly using an electrocautery hook in the right hand until we approach the UPJ. At this point great care must be taken and the assumption must be that there may be crossing vessels. If crossing vessels are identified, they must be carefully dissected and preserved. The renal pelvis is also carefully dissected at this point and the rind is removed from the UPJ (Fig. 12.2). We find it useful to use a Maryland grasper in the left hand and scissors in the right hand for this more precise part of the dissection. The use of additional Hem-o-lok clips is often necessary for retraction of the Gerota's fascia overlying the lower pole of the kidney to the lateral side wall.

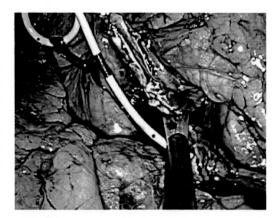

Fig. 12.3 UPJ dismembered

Dismembering of the UPJ

At this point the 2-mm grasper is introduced and is used to help manipulate tissue for transection of the UPJ. Special care is taken not to damage the indwelling ureteral stent (Fig. 12.3). The proximal curl of the stent is removed from the renal pelvis, and the ureter is spatulated laterally as the blood supply to the proximal ureter enters medially (Fig. 12.4). If the renal pelvis requires additional spatulation, it is done medially.

Anastomosis

A running anastomosis is created by using a dyed and an undyed 4-0 Vicryl suture, each placed in a half-moon configuration. The dyed suture is used

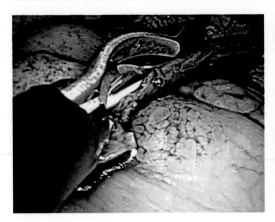

Fig. 12.4 Spatulation of the ureter laterally

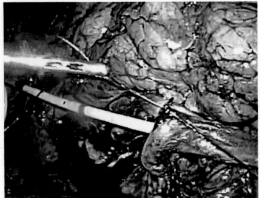

Fig. 12.5 Initial suture of the anastomosis

for the anterior and the undyed suture for the posterior portion of the anastomosis. The needle is manipulated using a laparoscopic needle driver in the right hand and a 2-mm grasper in the left hand. Initially a forehand orientation is used with the dyed suture, and the needle is passed through the lateral pelvis followed by a backhand pass of the needle at the apex of the ureteral spatulation. A knot is tied and the suture is passed for three to four throws on the anterior side of the anastomosis (Figs. 12.5 and 12.6). The needle can be grasped using a forehand grip during this part of the repair. The proximal curl of the stent is then replaced in the renal pelvis.

The undyed suture is then grasped with a backhand grip, and the dyed suture is retracted laterally with the 2-mm grasper to expose the posterior defect. The undyed suture is then passed through the lateral pelvis and apex of the ureteral spatulation, and a knot is tied next to the knot of the dyed suture. Using a backhand grip, the posterior anastomosis is completed using the undyed suture. Repair of the remaining anterior anastomotic defect is then accomplished with the dyed suture, and the two sutures are tied together. The initial two to three throws with each suture must be very precise to not include too much ureteral mucosa as this will narrow the anastomosis. After hemostasis is ensured, a closed-suction drain is brought through the single port and left transumbilically so that an additional incision need not be created.

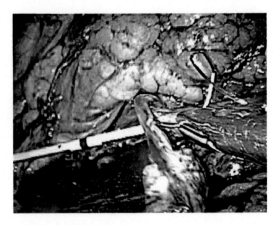

Fig. 12.6 Suturing of the anterior anastomosis

Renal Pelvis Tailoring

Renal pelvic tailoring is likely unnecessary in the majority of cases. In cases with a large redundant pelvis in which reduction is elected, we begin at the medial cut edge of the dismembered pelvis and continue cranially until further dissection is difficult due to nearby hilar anatomy. Great care is taken to recognize and not damage renal infundibula. The anastomosis of the UPJ is then completed as previously described. If the renal pelvis tissue to be discarded is completely excised, the upper edge of the pelvotomy may retract posterior to the renal vessels, and placement of the initial sutures may be difficult. Therefore we keep the dissected renal pelvis tissue attached by a small stalk cranially and use this as a handle to help place our first sutures for repair of the

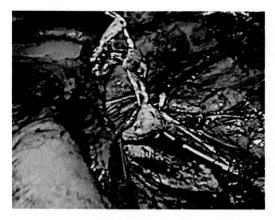

Fig. 12.7 Resected redundant renal pelvis still attached by a stalk of tissue superiorly

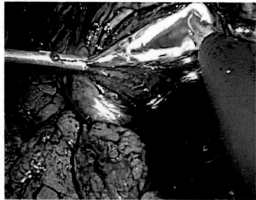

Fig. 12.9 Small pelvotomy for introduction of the flexible cystoscope

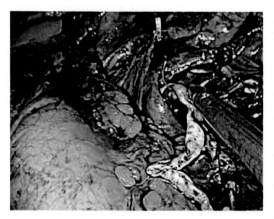

Fig. 12.8 Repair of the pelvotomy

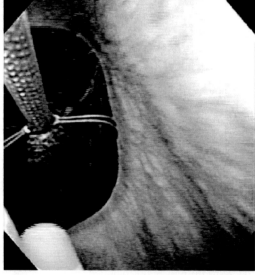

Fig. 12.10 Manipulation of renal calculus using a flexible cystoscope and stone basket

pelvotomy (Fig. 12.7). The dissected tissue may then be transected and we use a running barbed suture to repair the remaining defect (Fig. 12.8). This repair is completed when we reach the medial edge of the completed UPJ anastomosis.

Pyelolithotomy

Stones may be present in the renal collecting system and can be managed using pyeloscopy. After creating a small pelvotomy at the UPJ, a flexible cystoscope is introduced through one of the trocars of the single port and guided into the renal pelvis (Fig. 12.9). A separate camera and viewing tower are used to display the cystoscopic view. A stone basket is then used for stone

manipulation, and the anastomosis of the UPJ is then completed as previously described (Fig. 12.10).

Postoperative Care

Standardly, the Foley catheter is removed on the morning of the first postoperative day, and the drain fluid creatinine level is evaluated that evening. If no urine extravasation is confirmed, the drain is removed the next morning and the patient is discharged home. We typically remove the stent in 4 weeks and a diuretic radionuclide scan is obtained 1–2 months thereafter.

Analysis of Evidence for LESS-P

The first publication on LESS-P was reported in 2008 by Desai et al. and included 17 patients undergoing pyeloplasty [2]. The initial retrospective studies comparing LESS-P to conventional laparoscopic pyeloplasty (CL-P) demonstrated comparable functional outcomes and complication rates [3–5]; however, significant selection bias may have been present as LESS-P patients may have had fewer previous endoscopic treatments for ureteropelvic junction obstruction (UPJO) [3] and a lower BMI than CL-P patients [4]. In the only prospective randomized trial, Tugcu et al. demonstrated that LESS-P may decrease postoperative analgesic requirements and decrease the time to convalescence [6].

Loss of triangulation makes suturing in LESS-P a difficult task especially when using conventional laparoscopic instruments. To overcome this disadvantage, Ju et al., as in our technique, used a 2-mm subcostal port to facilitate triangulation similar to conventional laparoscopy with promising results [7]. Indeed, the idea of using a small assistant port has been used also in other institutions [8], with outcomes that are comparable to other LESS-P studies. Even when the assistant port is not planned, placement of a vconsidered without converting completely to CL-P [9]. Tsai et al. showed, with their ergonomic design, LESS-P could be performed with standard laparoscopic instruments without the use of an assistant port [10]. Other cost-saving techniques include the development of a reusable LESS port [11].

Given the technical difficulties associated with LESS-P, one might expect a steep learning curve for the procedure. In a case series of 28 patients, Best et al. found that 70 % of the complications they had occurred in the first ten patients [12]. This was confirmed by Ou et al. that found it took about 12 cases to complete the initial learning phase of the procedure [13].

The majority of LESS-P procedures are performed in a transperitoneal fashion with port placement in the umbilicus. However, Chen et al. first reported on a technique of retroperitoneal LESS-P with the port placement just below the 12th rib in the lumbar region [14]. Further studies have confirmed the utility of retroperitoneal LESS-P with outcomes comparable to the transperitoneal approach [13]. The retroperitoneal approach offers the advantages of providing more direct access to the UPJ and eliminating the need for bowel dissection. The downside to the retroperitoneal approach is that it does not have the cosmetic benefit seen with transumbilical port placement and provides a smaller working area.

Given that LESS-P is a novel procedure for which careful patient selection is necessary, most of the case series detailing it are small in size, and there is limited data on long-term follow-up. At a median of 24 months follow-up, Khanna et al. reported that 24 out of 25 LESS-P patients were asymptomatic or had improved symptoms after the procedure [15]. The number of LESS-P cases reported in the literature continues to grow (Tables 12.1 and 12.2). The largest LESS-P study to date is a multi-institutional study with a total of 140 patients; 109 patients had undergone pure LESS-P (the other 31 were robotic assisted) [16]. The outcomes of patients in the study were comparable to the historically reported outcomes in CL-P. Renal function following the procedure has been excellent with eGFR estimated around 80 (ml/min/1.73 m^2) [16, 17]. As skills and familiarity increase, LESS-P can be used in more complex cases such as with a horseshoe kidney [18] combined with pyelolithotomy [16].

LESS-P has been noted to be feasible in the pediatric population (Table 12.3). A case series by Tugcu et al. first examined the use of LESS-P in 11 children, and the outcomes were comparable to that of CL-P [19]. Further studies have confirmed that LESS-P can be a reasonable option for children and has even been performed in patients as young as 2 months [20–22]. Much like the adult population, conventional laparoscopic tools can be used for the surgery, decreasing costs [22]. However, long-term outcomes in the pediatric population are still unknown.

Table 12.1 Adult LESS-P patient demographics

Study	N	M	F	Age	BMI	L	R
Tracy et al. [3]	14	4	10	32	24	6	8
Best et al. [12]	28	11	14	33	24.6		
Tugcu et al. [6]	14	6	8	39		9	5
Kawauchi et al. [23]	1	0	1	30		1	0
Choi et al. [5]	4						
Ju et al. [7]	9	6	3	39	23.1	5	4
Ganpule et al. [9]	9	7	2	17.6	16.2	6	3
Chen et al. [14]	10	6	4	23.8	26.1	9	1
Tsai et al. [10]	2	1	1	39.5	24.8		
Faddegon et al. [18]	2	0	2	34	20.8	1	1
Schwentner et al. [11]	4	2	2	42.5		1	3
Nagabhushana et al. [24]	2			27			
Zou et al. [8]	9			28	24.9	5	4
Tugcu et al. [25]	19	10	9	35.9	25.1	11	8
Ou et al. [13]	27	16	11	36.8	24.1	17	10
Rais-Bahrami et al. [16]	109	57	83	39.9	24.8	68	72

Table 12.2 Outcomes of LESS-P in adults

Study	Mean operative time	EBL	Mean hospital stay (D)	Complications	Clavien score			Symptom resolution	Radiographic resolution obstruction
					1	2	3		
Tracy et al. [3]	202	35	3.2	5	2		3		10 of 10
Best et al. [12]	197		2.6	8	2	1	4		20 of 21
Tugcu et al. [6]	204.5	102	2	1	1				14
Kawauchi et al. [23]	240	low	6	0				1	
Choi et al. [5]	196	80	4.5	1					
Ju et al. [7]	252.2	150	6	4	2		0	9	9
Ganpule et al. [9]	204.6	70.6	3	0					6 of 6
Chen et al. [14]	148.4	31	5.7	2				9 of 9	9 of 9
Tsai et al. [10]	213			0					2 of 2
Faddegon et al. [18]	187.5	50	3.5	0				1 of 1	1 of 1
Schwentner et al. [11]	89.75	17.5	3.5	0					
Nagabhushana et al. [24]	135		3	0					
Zou et al. [8]	140	75	7	1			1		
Tugcu et al. [25]	195.2	55.7	2.1	1					18 of 19
Ou et al. [13]	175.9	83.3	3.7	3	3	0	0		25
Rais-Bahrami et al. [16]	202.1	61.2	2.4	26	7	8	11	128	119

EBL stands for estimated blood loss

Conclusion

LESS-P can be performed effectively and reproducibly using techniques such as those described in this chapter. Clashing due to lack of triangulation and ergonomic challenges can make these procedures demanding, and therefore significant experience in conventional laparoscopy is recommended prior to embarking on these cases.

Table 12.3 Pediatric LESS pyeloplasty

	N	Sex		Age (years)	Side		Mean operative time	EBL	Mean hospital stay (D)	Complications	Symptom resolution	Radiographic resolution obstruction
		M	F		L	R						
Tugcu et al. [6]	11	7	4	10	6	5	182.5	97.3	2	2	11	11
Bi et al. [20]	22	18	4	4.7	20	2	198		6.4	3	21	
Zhou et al. [21]	24	16	8	1.2	18	6	145	10	7	2	24	23
Uygun et al. [22]	3	2	1	1.7			63		4			

References

1. Clayman RV, Kavoussi LR, Soper NJ, Dierks SM, Meretyk S, Darcy MD, et al. Laparoscopic nephrectomy: initial case report. J Urol. 1991;146:278–82.
2. Desai MM, Berger AK, Brandina R, Aron M, Irwin BH, Canes D, Desai MR, Rao PP, Sotelo R, Stein R, Gill IS. Laparoendoscopic single-site surgery: initial hundred patients. Urology. 2009;74(4):805–12.
3. Tracy CR, Raman JD, Bagrodia A, Cadeddu JA. Perioperative outcomes in patients undergoing conventional laparoscopic versus laparoendoscopic single-site pyeloplasty. Urology. 2009;74(5):1029–34.
4. Stein RJ, Berger AK, Brandina R, Patel NS, Canes D, Irwin BH, Aron M, Autorino R, Shah G, Desai MM. Laparoendoscopic single-site pyeloplasty: a comparison with the standard laparoscopic technique. BJU Int. 2011;107(5):811–5.
5. Choi KH, Ham WS, Rha KH, Lee JW, Jeon HG, Arkoncel FR, Yang SC, Han WK. Laparoendoscopic single-site surgeries: a single-center experience of 171 consecutive cases. Korean J Urol. 2011;52(1):31–8.
6. Tugcu V, Sönmezay E, Ilbey YO, Polat H, Tasci AI. Transperitoneal laparoendoscopic single-site pyeloplasty: initial experiences. J Endourol. 2010;24(12):2023–7.
7. Ju SH, Lee DG, Lee JH, Baek MK, Jeong BC, Jeon SS, Lee KS, Han DH. Laparoendoscopic single-site pyeloplasty using additional 2 mm instruments: a comparison with conventional laparoscopic pyeloplasty. Korean J Urol. 2011;52(9):616–21.
8. Zou X, Zhang G, Xue Y, Yuan Y, Xiao R, Wu G, Wang X, Wu Y, Long D, Yang J, Xu H, Liu F, Zhang X. Suprapubic-assisted laparoendoscopic single-site surgery (LESS) in urology: our experience. BJU Int. 2013;112(2):E92–8.
9. Ganpule AP, Sharma R, Kurien A, Mishra S, Muthu V, Sabnis R, Desai MR. Laparoendoscopic single site surgery in urology: a single centre experience. J Minim Access Surg. 2012;8(3):79–84.
10. Tsai YC, Lin VC, Chung SD, Ho CH, Jaw FS, Tai HC. Ergonomic and geometric tricks of laparoendoscopic single-site surgery (LESS) by using conventional laparoscopic instruments. Surg Endosc. 2012;26(9):2671–7.
11. Schwentner C, Todenhöfer T, Seibold J, Alloussi S, Aufderklamm S, Mischinger J, Stenzl A, Gakis G. Cost effective laparoendoscopic single-site surgery with a reusable platform. JSLS. 2013;17(2):285–91.
12. Best SL, Donnally C, Mir SA, Tracy CR, Raman JD, Cadeddu JA. Complications during the initial experience with laparoendoscopic single-site pyeloplasty. BJU Int. 2011;108(8):1326–9.
13. Ou Z, Qi L, Yang J, Chen X, Cao Z, Zu X, Liu L, Wang L. Preliminary experience and learning curve for laparoendoscopic single-site retroperitoneal pyeloplasty. J Laparoendosc Adv Surg Tech A. 2013;23(9):765–70.
14. Chen Z, Chen X, Wu ZH, Luo YC, He Y, Li NN, Xie CQ, Lai C. Feasibility and safety of retroperitoneal laparoendoscopic single-site dismembered pyeloplasty: a clinical report of 10 cases. J Laparoendosc Adv Surg Tech A. 2012;22(7):685–90.
15. Khanna R, Isac W, Laydner H, Autorino R, White MA, Hillyer S, Spana G, Shah G, Desai MM, Haber GP, Kaouk JH, Stein RJ. Laparoendoscopic single site reconstructive procedures in urology: medium term results. J Urol. 2012;187(5):1702–6.
16. Rais-Bahrami S, Rizkala ER, Cadeddu JA, Tugcu V, Derweesh IH, Abdel-Karim AM, Kawauchi A, George AK, Autorino R, Bagrodia A, Sonmezay E, Elsalmy S, Liss MA, Harrow BM, Kaouk JH, Richstone L, Stein RJ. Laparoendoscopic single-site pyeloplasty: outcomes of an international multi-institutional study of 140 patients. Urology. 2013;82(2):366–72.
17. Harrow BR, Bagrodia A, Olweny EO, Faddegon S, Cadeddu JA, Gahan JC. Renal function after laparoendoscopic single site pyeloplasty. J Urol. 2013;190(2):565–9.

18. Faddegon S, Tan YK, Olweny EO, Park SK, Best SL, Cadeddu JA. Laparoendoscopic single-site (LESS) pyeloplasty for horseshoe ureteropelvic junction obstruction. JSLS. 2012;16(1):151–4.

19. Tugcu V, Ilbey YO, Polat H, Tasci AI. Early experience with laparoendoscopic single-site pyeloplasty in children. J Pediatr Urol. 2011;7(2):187–91.

20. Bi Y, Lu L, Ruan S. Using conventional 3- and 5-mm straight instruments in laparoendoscopic single-site pyeloplasty in children. J Laparoendosc Adv Surg Tech A. 2011;21(10):969–72.

21. Zhou H, Sun N, Zhang X, Xie H, Ma L, Shen Z, Zhou X, Tao T. Transumbilical laparoendoscopic single-site pyeloplasty in infants and children: initial experience and short-term outcome. Pediatr Surg Int. 2012;28(3):321–5.

22. Uygun I, Okur MH, Aydogdu B, Arslan MS, Cimen H, Otcu S. Transumbilical scarless surgery with thoracic trocar: easy and low-cost. J Korean Surg Soc. 2013;84(6):360–6.

23. Kawauchi A, Kamoi K, Soh J, Naitoh Y, Okihara K, Miki T. Laparoendoscopic single-site urological surgery: initial experience in Japan. Int J Urol. 2010;17(3):289–92.

24. Nagabhushana M, Kamath AJ, Manohar CS. Laparoendoscopic single-site surgery in urology using conventional instruments: our initial experience. J Endourol. 2013;27(11):1354–60.

25. Tugcu V, Ilbey YO, Sonmezay E, Aras B, Tasci AI. Single-site versus conventional transperitoneal laparoscopic pyeloplasty: a prospective randomized study. Int J Urol. 2013;20(11):1112–7.

LESS Ileal Interposition

13

Robert D. Brown, Oktay Akca, Homayoun Zargar, and Robert J. Stein

Introduction

For complex cases involving long or multiple ureteral strictures or extensive ureteral neoplasm associated with a solitary kidney, few options exist clinically. Depending on the ipsilateral renal function and solitary kidney status, simple nephrectomy, transureteroureterostomy, ileal interposition, or renal autotransplantation can be considered. Historically ileal interposition has been done as an open procedure; however, cases have been reported of laparoscopic techniques being used as early as the year 2000 [1–3]. In a retrospective comparison of seven laparoscopic to seven open procedures, narcotic requirements (median 38.9 vs 322.2 mg, $p = 0.035$) and time to convalescence (median 4 vs 5.5 weeks, $p = 0.03$) were less for the laparoscopic group.

The evidence for using laparoendoscopic single-site surgery (LESS) for ileal interposition is even more limited. The initial case and technique were reported by Desai et al. [4]. Khanna et al. published a series of three patients that underwent ileal interposition, two for strictures secondary to recurrent calculi and one with a ureteral injury [5]. Mean operative time was 400 min and the average hospital stay was 3.7 days. The ureterovesical anastomosis took place extracorporeally. At 35 months follow-up, the two patients with calculi continued to pass stones but no longer had symptoms. The other patient died 6 months later due to a thromboembolic event. One complication of an anastomotic leak requiring prolonged drainage with a nephrostomy tube was noted.

R.D. Brown, MD
Department of Urology, Cleveland Clinic,
9500 Euclid Ave. Q10, Cleveland, OH 44195, USA
e-mail: rob.brown737@gmail.com

O. Akca, MD
Department of Urology, Glickman Urological
and Kidney Institute, Cleveland Clinic,
Cleveland, OH, USA
e-mail: akcao@ccf.org

H. Zargar, MBChB, FRACS
Department of Urology, Glickman Urology and Kidney
Institute, Cleveland Clinic, Cleveland, OH, USA
e-mail: homi.zargar@gmail.com

R.J. Stein, MD (✉)
Associate Professor of Surgery, Department of
Urology, Center for Robotic and Image Guided
Surgery, Glickman Urological and Kidney Institute,
Cleveland Clinic, Cleveland, OH, USA
e-mail: steinr@ccf.org

Patient Evaluation

Initial evaluation should be performed with CT in order to help determine the etiology of obstruction and evaluate for neoplasm or stones. Radionuclide scanning is useful to evaluate differential renal function and assess for obstruction. If a stricture is noted, further evaluation with retrograde pyelogram and possibly ureteroscopy

© Springer Science+Business Media New York 2017
J.H. Kaouk et al. (eds.), *Atlas of Laparoscopic and Robotic Single Site Surgery*,
Current Clinical Urology, DOI 10.1007/978-1-4939-3575-8_13

are useful to assess the length of stricture and location of ureteral involvement. Ureteroscopy can also be used to obtain biopsies of any suspicious areas.

Operative correction is indicated if the patient is symptomatic and has history of pyelonephritis or there is ipsilateral loss of kidney function. Endoscopic treatment, ureteroneocystostomy, or ureteroureterostomy should be considered before discussing ileal interposition. If the diseased ureteral segment is long or especially proximal and renal function is adequate, then ileal interposition, autotransplantation, or transureteroureterostomy may be considered. Relative contraindications to ileal interposition include inflammatory bowel disease and renal insufficiency due to concerns of metabolic derangements.

Patient Positioning

The patient is placed in 45° modified flank position with no flex in the table and with the affected side up. After padding all pressure points and placing an axillary roll, the patient is taped securely so that the bed can be tilted to full flank position for the upper tract portions of the case and to supine position for the pelvic portion of the procedure.

Port Positioning and Instrumentation

A 4–5 cm vertical incision directly through the umbilicus is created and the fascia is incised with scissors. A GelPOINT single-port device (Applied Medical, Rancho Santa Margarita, CA, USA) is introduced after access to the peritoneum is obtained. Standard laparoscopic instruments including small bowel graspers, scissors, and electrocautery hook are used for dissection. A laparoscopic needle holder and 2 mm grasper, which are introduced through a separate pinpoint incision, are used for suturing of the proximal and distal anastomoses.

Dissection

The table is initially tilted to flank position and the colon mobilized medially. The ureter is identified and the area of proximal narrowing is dissected. In our experience, there is a significant amount of extrinsic scar in this area, and it has not been necessary to use stents or ureteroscopy in order to reliably identify the area of concern. The ureter is then transected just cranial to the diseased area which results in a widely dilated ureter proximally.

At this point, the table is tilted so that the patient is in supine position and the bladder is mobilized using the electrocautery hook. Dissection is carried to the superior vesical pedicles bilaterally. The dome of the bladder is then cleared of overlying fat and an area ipsilateral to the pathology is prepared for the eventual distal anastomosis by clearing the detrusor muscle.

Isolation of the Ileal Segment

The ileum is marked with a suture 20 cm proximal to the ileocecal valve. The GelCap is then removed from the single-port device, and the ileum is exteriorized by grasping the suture with a grasper. We ensure knowledge of the orientation of the ileum at all times.

All bowel isolation is performed extracorporeally. First the mesentery is divided and a 15–20 cm ileal segment is isolated using GIA staplers (Fig. 13.1). Bowel continuity is restored by performing a two-layer handsewn anastomosis with permanent suture. A 7Fr ×24 cm double pigtail ureteral stent is placed through the isolated ileal segment and secured at both ends with a 3-0 chromic suture after portions of the staple line are removed. A Penrose drain is sutured near the proximal edge of the bowel to use as a handle and to mark proper orientation of the isolated segment. All bowel components are then returned to the peritoneum through the Alexis wound protector component of the GelPOINT device (Fig. 13.2). The GelCap is replaced and pneumoperitoneum restored.

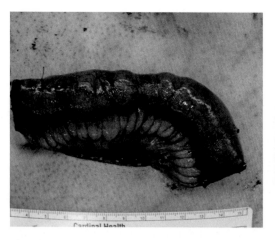

Fig. 13.1 Extracorporeal isolation of the ileal segment

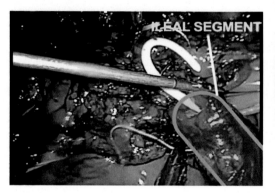

Fig. 13.2 Isolated ileal segment with preplaced stent within the peritoneum

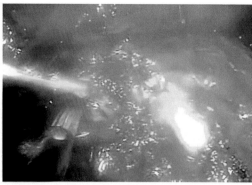

Fig. 13.3 Creation of cystotomy in the bladder dome

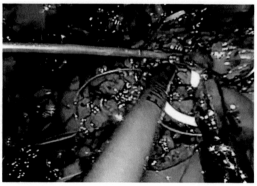

Fig. 13.4 Placement of distal curl of ureteral stent into the bladder after initial anastomotic sutures placed

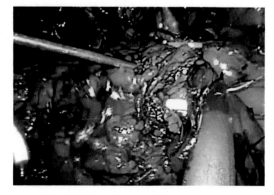

Fig. 13.5 Completion of ileovesical anastomosis

Anastomoses

The ileal segment must be oriented properly so the passage of urine occurs in an isoperistaltic direction. With the patient still in supine position, a cystotomy is created in the bladder dome (Fig. 13.3). The 2 mm grasper is positioned in the left lower quadrant and is used to improve triangulation. The posterior ileovesical anastomosis is completed with a running 3-0 barbed suture. The distal curl of the ureteral stent is placed in the bladder (Fig. 13.4) and the anterior anastomosis is completed with a separate running suture (Fig. 13.5).

The table is then tilted so that the patient is once again in flank position. The Penrose drain is then fixed to lateral side wall so that the proximal end of the ileal segment is in close apposition to the transected proximal ureter. The 2 mm grasper is also used to assist with completion of the

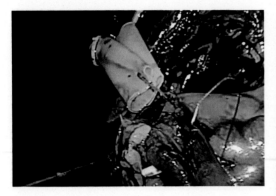

Fig. 13.6 Completion of ureteroileal anastomosis

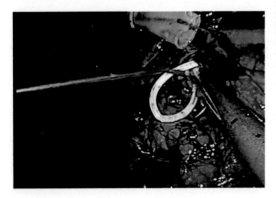

Fig. 13.7 Placement of proximal curl of ureteral stent into the ureter after initial ureteroileal anastomotic sutures placed

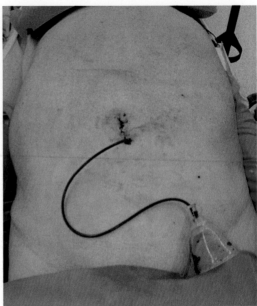

Fig. 13.8 Postoperative image with closed suction drain positioned in the umbilical incision

Postoperative Management

The diet is advanced upon return of bowel function. Prior to discharge from the hospital, the drain fluid is evaluated for creatinine level and removed if there is no urine extravasation. The Foley catheter is removed 10 days postoperatively and the ureteral stent is removed 1 month postoperatively. A cystogram at the time of Foley catheter removal is optional.

ileoureteral anastomosis. For a left-sided case, the 2 mm grasper is placed in the left upper quadrant. For a right-sided case, the grasper is placed in the right lower quadrant. Two separate 4-0 Vicryl running sutures are then used to complete the anastomosis (Fig. 13.6). The proximal curl of the ureteral stent is placed in the ureter and renal pelvis when half of the anastomosis is finished (Fig. 13.7).

After hemostasis is ensured, the Foley catheter is irrigated in order to test both anastomoses. If a nephrostomy tube is still in place, this can also be irrigated to evaluate the proximal anastomosis. A closed suction drain is passed through the umbilical incision and curled so that it is near both anastomoses. The umbilical incision is then closed (Fig. 13.8).

Conclusions

Ileal interposition is a rarely performed reconstructive procedure which can be demanding due to the multiple surgical steps required as well as extensive suturing involved. Likely for these reasons, the procedures are usually performed using an open technique. Nevertheless, significant advantages for recovery and postoperative pain have been noted if these surgeries are completed laparoscopically. Minimizing incisions even further to only include the incision to exteriorize the bowel is the goal of

LESS. Further evaluation is required to determine if there are advantages to this approach over conventional laparoscopy.

References

1. Gill IS, Savage SJ, Senagore AJ, et al. Laparoscopic ileal ureter. J Urol. 2000;163:1199.
2. Kamat N, Khandelwal P. Laparoscopy-assisted ileal ureter creation for multiple tuberculous strictures: report of two cases. J Endourol. 2006;20:388.
3. Castillo OA, Sanchez-Salas R, Vitagliano G, Diaz MA, Foneron A. Laparoscopy-assisted ureter interposition by ileum. Endourology. 2008;22(4): 687–92.
4. Desai MM, Stein R, Rao P, Canes D, Aron M, Rao PP, Haber GP, Fergany A, Kaouk J, Gill IS. Embryonic natural orifice transumbilical endoscopic surgery (E-NOTES) for advanced reconstruction: initial experience. Urology. 2009;73(1):182–7.
5. Khanna R, Isac W, Laydner H, Autorino R, White MA, Hillyer S, Spana G, Shah G, Desai MM, Haber GP, Kaouk JH, Stein RJ. Laparoendoscopic single site reconstructive procedures in urology: medium term results. J Urol. 2012;187(5):1702–6.

Robotic-LESS Radical Prostatectomy

Ernesto R. Cordeiro Feijoo, Rafael Sanchez-Salas, and Eric Barret

Introduction

Since the first published outcomes on laparoscopic RP by Gillonneau et al., this technique has been continuously evolving worldwide [1–4]. The main goal of RP is to treat the cancer while preserving patients' quality of life (QoL), by reducing the risks of incontinence and erectile dysfunction. The introduction of *laparoendoscopic single-site surgery* (LESS) to this minimally invasive field represented a significant challenge compared to standard laparoscopy. However, despite the technical difficulties inherent to the procedure, different authors have demonstrated the feasibility of this surgery by a single access [5–7]. Since the first published successful cases of robotic-LESS (R-LESS) RP [1, 8], the number of clinical series has been considerably growing [7–12].

Along this section, we will present the laparoendoscopic single-site surgery robotic-assisted radical prostatectomy (LESS-RARP) technique in a comprehensive approach, based on the existing evidence in terms of technical features, indications and procedural highlights.

E.R.C. Feijoo, MD, FEBU • R. Sanchez-Salas, MD
E. Barret, MD (✉)
Department of Urology, Institut Montsouris
Université Paris-Descartes, Paris, France
e-mail: uro@imm.fr; ercordeiro@hotmail.com; eric.barret@imm.fr

Technical Features

Since its inception, LESS has been challenging due to reduced working space, loss of triangulation and instrument clashing. Therefore, specialized access devices and instruments have been continuously developed. R-LESS seem to have overcome some of these limitations with technological advantages such as articulated wristed motion instruments, tremor filtration, stereoscopic three-dimensional view and overall ergonomic benefits that could improve surgeon comfort significantly.

We will briefly describe the most used access platforms and technological innovations on R-LESS developed during the last years.

Access Techniques

For pelvic R-LESS procedures, the patient is placed in the Trendelenburg dorsal lithotomy position, and an omega-like or midline umbilical incision is created [13]. As for RP, either conventional or robotically assisted, two types of accesses have been described: the transperitoneal and the extraperitoneal approaches [14].

Across the literature, surgeons reported pneumoperitoneum leakage commonly experienced with robotic trocars placed through a single-port device, which may represent an important issue especially in cases of extraperitoneal approaches. Therefore, placement of the robotic instrument trocars via separate fascial stabs alongside the device or through a single incision without a commercially available device has been described [15].

Access Platforms

A wide variety of access platforms from homemade to commercially available have been used in R-LESS. The most common are (a) QuadPort® (Advanced Surgical Concepts, Wicklow, Ireland) which contains 5(1)-, 10(2)- and 15(1)-mm ports and is placed through a 2–7 cm incision [6]; (b) SILS® port (Covidien, Mansfield, MA, USA) which contains four sites for port placement and is introduced through a 3–4 cm incision; (c) TriPort® (Olympus Medical Systems Europa GmbH); and (d) GelPort/GelPoint® (Applied Medical, Rancho Santa Margarita, California, USA) which includes a gel cap through which various ports in any arrangement may be introduced [16].

The use of homemade access platforms composed of a wound retractor as an inner ring covered by an intact surgical glove with trocars introduced through the fingers of the glove has been also described [17].

Recently, a novel platform for R-LESS has been developed by the da Vinci Single-Site Surgery group and is composed by a multichannel access port with a room for four cannulas and an insufflation valve. Two curved cannulas are for robotically controlled instruments, and the other two cannulas are straight; one cannula is 8.5 mm and accommodates the robotic endoscope, and the other cannula is a 5-mm bedside-assistant port. The curved cannulas are integral to the system, since their configuration allows the instruments to be positioned to achieve triangulation of the target anatomy, as they cross the midway through the access port. Special software enables same-sided hand–eye control of the instruments despite the crossed cannulas. The second part of the platform is a set of semirigid, non-wristed instruments with standard da Vinci instrument tips [18].

In our experience, we usually use the GelPoint® device due to its easy placement and the possibility of changing the port placement while limiting leaks [10].

Indications

The indications for LESS-RARP are similar to those accepted for radical retropubic prostatectomy (RRP), laparoscopic radical prostatectomy (LRP) and RARP which are: patients with low- and intermediate-risk localized PCa, with life expectancy over 10 years who accept the potential risks and complications related to RP, and highly selected patients with high-risk localized PCa in the context of multimodal treatment [19].

No specific guidelines for LESS-RARP are yet available, but in the context of intermediate- and high-risk patients, in whom pelvic lymph node dissection (PLND) is indicated, special consideration needs to be taken on the decision-making process due to the added technical difficulty that this procedure may present, thus reserving this technique for more suitable low-risk PCa patients.

Across the available literature, case series on LESS-RARP involved patients with a body mass index (BMI) in the range of 23–30 kg/m² [20]. Thus, one could assume that obese patients are not, to date, suitable candidates for LESS-RARP.

Procedural Highlights

Main differences from the standard RARP technique are related to the port entry and the access platforms used, which varies among the different centres. Another minor drawback is related to the inability to use the fourth robotic arm, thus decreasing some aspects of the surgeon's dexterity and autonomy.

Patient Positioning

Patients are positioned in supine with or without steep Trendelenburg. An 18 F Foley-like bladder catheter is placed. Legs are extended and abduced. The robot (da Vinci S or Si) is approached to the

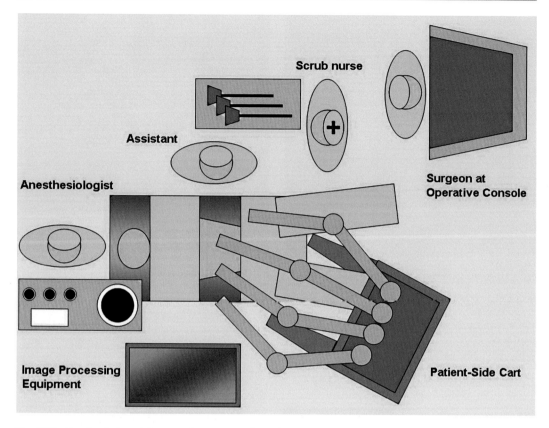

Fig. 14.1 Overhead view of the operating room configuration

operating table between the legs of the patient or in an acute angle from the right leg's longitudinal axis (side docking).

According to our experience, we choose the robot's right side docking in order to allow better deployment of the robotic arms, while the assistant is standing at the left patient's bedside, thus providing him a more comfortable position. The scrub nurse is standing next to him, at the level of the patient's legs (Fig. 14.1).

Port Placement

Based on our experience, we usually recommend performing an extraperitoneal access, avoiding the bladder mobilization needed during transperitoneal approaches.

A single 3–5 cm infraumbilical 'Y'-shaped incision is performed (Fig. 14.2). The anterior rectus fascia is exposed and incised; a balloon dilator is used to develop the extraperitoneal space. At this point, trocar placement can be achieved alternatively in different fashions:

(a) A 12-mm camera port, two 8-mm robotic trocars and a 5-mm port are placed in a rhomboid shape, through the same skin incision but through different fascial stabs, as described by Barret et al. [10, 11].

(b) A R-port is used, placed between two robotic trocars (8 and 5 or 8 mm), thus allowing suction and suture insertion through the same port [9].

(c) A SILS port is placed through a 3–5 cm incision, between two robotic trocars of 5 mm aside the device and inserted through the same fascial stab used for the port [21].

(d) Use of GelPort/GelPoint device, through which one 12-mm port for the robotic endoscope (opposite side of the umbilicus), two robotic 8-mm trocars and one 10-mm trocar (next to the umbilicus) for the bedside assistant are placed.

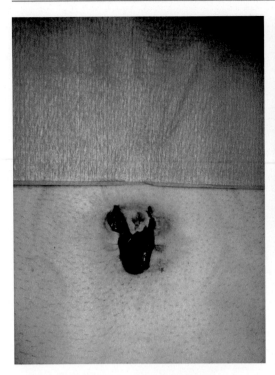

Fig. 14.2 Y-shaped skin incision for LESS-RARP

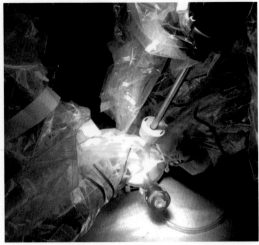

Fig. 14.4 Da Vinci Si docked

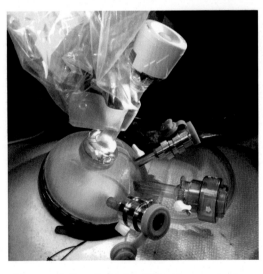

Fig. 14.3 GelPort device installed with trocars in place

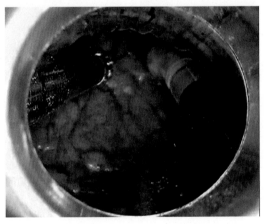

Fig. 14.5 Endoscopic view from the camera trocar. Maryland grasper on the left and monopolar scissors on the right

insufflation up to a pressure of 12–15 mmHg; then, the robot is docked and the instruments inserted into the abdominal cavity under direct vision (Fig. 14.4).

As described by Barret et al. [22], according to our experience, we prefer to use the GelPort® device given its ergonomic features and its facility for trocar introduction through the gel platform (Fig. 14.3).

Once the access platform is in place, pneumoperitoneum is created by high-flow CO2

Instrument Introduction

A robotic bipolar Maryland grasper is introduced through the left robotic trocar and robotic monopolar scissors through the right robotic trocar for the left and right surgeon's hands, respectively (Fig. 14.5). Then, according to our

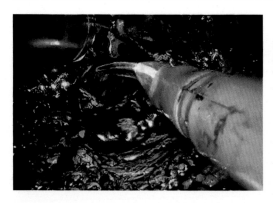

Fig. 14.6 Bladder neck preservation and section of the posterior detrusor fibres

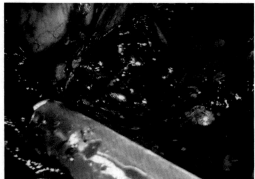

Fig. 14.8 Exposure of the posterior prostatic contour

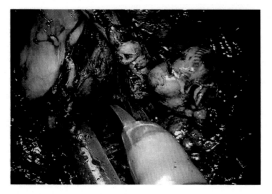

Fig. 14.7 Seminal vesicle mobilization and exposure of the Denonvillier's fascia

institution, an antegrade approach to RARP is performed. A Beniquet sound will also be deployed to mobilize the gland during the procedure, in order to facilitate its dissection.

Bladder Neck and Seminal Vesicle Dissection

The anterior aspects of the bladder and the prostate are dissected in order to identify the anatomical landmarks. The balloon of the bladder catheter is deflated. Dissection is performed following the natural plane between the prostate and the bladder in order to preserve the bladder neck, which constitutes a crucial step to improve the urethrovesical coupling during anastomosis. After anatomic bladder neck preservation, a Beniquet is introduced into the ure-

thra, thus allowing prostate's mobilization. Then, division of the posterior longitudinal detrusor fibres is performed (Fig. 14.6) until the vas deferens, which are sharply divided bilaterally.

The artery of the vas typically courses between the vas and the medial aspect of the seminal vesicles, and it is controlled by either inclusion with a clip or with bipolar cautery. The absence of a fourth arm makes anterior traction of the SV difficult. Then, blunt dissection is used to define the medial SV contour, which is typically avascular. The SV dissection then proceeds laterally. SV arterial blood supply originates inferolaterally, and bipolar cautery is used sparingly to control arterioles located on the SV surface proximal to the SV tip. After sharp division, the arterioles are gently peeled downward and away from the SV tip, which allows full mobilization of the SVs. After bilateral SV dissection, upwards traction of both SVs allows exposure of the Denonvillier's fascia (Fig. 14.7).

Posterior Dissection and Development of the Posterior Prostatic Contour

The Denonvillier's fascia is sharply incised in the midline; the anatomic plane between the prostatic fascia (PF) and the Denonvillier's fascia is separated to define the posterior prostatic contour (Fig. 14.8). Dissection is performed laterally, especially in the case of a nerve-sparing surgery

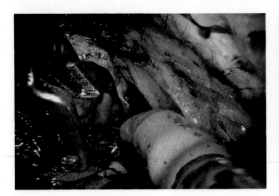

Fig. 14.9 Lateralization of levator fascia and fibres allows exposure of the anterolateral prostate contour (*right side*)

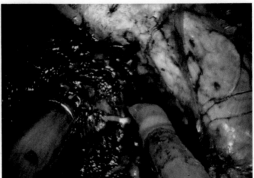

Fig. 14.10 Division of the lateral vascular pedicles (*right side*)

technique. The posterior contour is then developed laterally and towards the apex.

Periprostatic Fascia Dissection and Development of the Anterolateral Prostatic Contour

At this point, the pelvic fascia is incised at the mid-part of the prostate contour. The attachments of the periprostatic fascia are freed by lateralizing the levator fascia (LF) and levator ani fibres, thus defining the anterolateral prostate contour. Nerves running along the medial border of the LF are pushed posterolaterally using blunt dissection, which permits identification of the neurovascular bundles (NVB) (Fig. 14.9). Rubbing towards the prostate base defines the distal fold of the lateral pedicle.

Division of the Lateral Vascular Pedicles

The aforementioned manoeuvres create a window defined by the confluence of the anterior and posterior prostate contours and the distal fold of the lateral pedicle. At this point, the latter is clamped with Hem-o-lok® clips and sharply divided with cold scissors (Fig. 14.10). Clips are placed up to the distal lateral pedicle fold, beyond which intrafascial versus interfascial nerve sparing is executed.

Antegrade Neurovascular Bundle Dissection

At this point, an intrafascial, interfascial or extrafascial technique can be used according to the patient's risk group, surgeon's preference and ultimately to technical feasibility. This surgical step varies among the authors in terms of nerve-sparing approaches and the use of different types of energy for dissection and haemostasis.

Barret et al. described the use of bipolar cautery and metallic clips to perform an antegrade full nerve-sparing dissection of the prostate [11].

An antegrade non-nerve-sparing dissection was reported by Kaouk et al., using a Harmonic scalpel [9].

White et al. described both the use of robotically placed Hem-o-lok® clips and sharp interfascial dissection and a non-nerve-sparing approach using a 5-mm harmonic scalpel [21].

Dorsal Vascular Complex Control and Apex Dissection

After achieving bilateral NVB release up to or beyond the mid prostate, apical dissection is achieved, while mobilizing the gland with the Beniquet sound.

The puboprostatic ligaments are divided and the dorsal vascular complex (DVC) is sharply divided and mobilized anteriorly to expose the prostatic apex. The urethra is then sharply divided

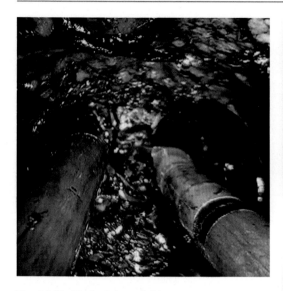

Fig. 14.11 Urethral sharp division

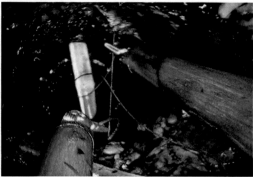

Fig. 14.12 Dorsal vascular complex control by using Vicryl® running sutures

(Fig. 14.11). Immediately, the DVC is selectively sutured by using 2/0 polyglactin (Vicryl®) stitches (Fig. 14.12). Gentle rotation of the prostate medially allows completion of antegrade apical nerve sparing.

Urethrovesical Anastomosis

Robotic needle drivers in the left and right hands are used to complete the urethrovesical anastomosis. Also at this point, the anastomosis between the bladder neck and the urethra can be achieved in different fashions. As initially described by Barret et al., the anastomosis can be performed by using separate single stitches [11]. Other authors describe the use of 3/0 poliglecaprone (Monocryl®), to place two running sutures from hours 6 to 12 bilaterally and tie the knot between them.

Based on our experience, we prefer to perform two running 3/0 barbed sutures (V-Loc®) to secure the anastomosis (Fig. 14.13). Primarily, the posterior running suture between hours 3 and 9 is performed, which constitutes probably the most important step during the anastomosis, which secures the posterior plate. Consecutively, the anterior running suture between hours 3 and 9 is performed for final closure and coupling of the vesico-urethral anastomosis.

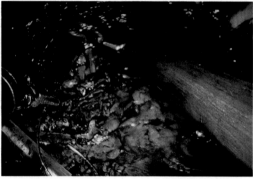

Fig. 14.13 Vesicourethral anastomosis by using running barbed sutures

An 18/20 F Foley catheter is inserted under vision into the bladder before completion of the anastomosis. After completion of the suture, the anastomosis is verified to be watertight.

End of the Procedure

The specimen is placed into an endoscopic bag and grasped firmly. A silicon drainage tube is inserted and placed percutaneously in the pelvis. Trocars are extracted under direct vision. The single-port device is removed. The endoscopic bag containing the surgical specimen is extracted through the same incision. The pneumoperitoneum is evacuated, fascial closing is performed and the Y-shaped skin incision is finally sutured (Fig. 14.14).

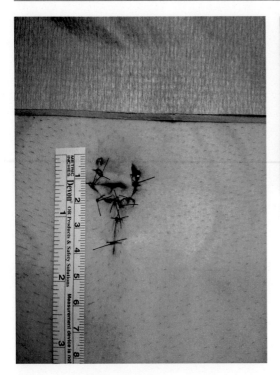

Fig. 14.14 Final skin closure

Transperitoneal LESS-RARP

During this approach, both the platform access and ports are placed using the same fashion as described for the extraperitoneal technique. In addition, the main surgical steps remain the same. The essential difference lies on the bladder mobilization at the beginning of the procedure. In this context, lateral incision of the anterior parietal peritoneum at level of the umbilical arteries and the urachus is performed in order to free the bladder and to gain access to the Retzius avascular space (Fig. 14.15). The anterior aspect of the bladder, along with the anterior aspect of the prostate and the bladder neck, is consequently exposed.

Tips and Pitfalls of R-LESS

Recent technological advances have led to an increase in LESS and therefore an additional option for patients willing to undergo minimally invasive surgery. Although not enough

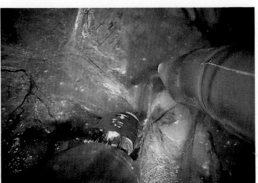

Fig. 14.15 Bladder mobilization by Retzius space dissection

randomized data are available in the literature, this technique appears to be promising in terms of per operative outcomes [23].

However, it is important to remember the pitfalls of this technique and its inherent difficulties. Although the da Vinci R-LESS platform provides benefits in terms of instrument crossing, ergonomics and instrument tip articulation, considerable instrument clashing limits precise tissue handling and retraction. Instruments are placed in-line, turning triangulation difficult. In this context, it has been suggested to displace the robotic trocars in a slightly unparallel position to reduce clashing. In addition, maximization of the distance between robotic trocars in the skin incision can be obtained by clutching the whole robotic arms, dragging them laterally [21].

Another challenging step of the procedure is the division of the lateral vascular pedicles. The use of an 8-mm robotic Hem-o-lok® clip applier has been reported in order to allow the operating surgeon to place clips, thus overcoming the clashing encountered by the assistant [21].

The use of 30° optics may be useful as it can be rotated to provide endoscopic vision from an angle away from the other instruments avoiding clashing.

The absence of the fourth robotic arm hampers adequate tissue retraction. It has been suggested that straight needle sutures can be passed percutaneously either through the bladder neck or the prostatic base to allow external traction in a 'marionette' fashion, thus facilitating exposure [21].

Suction can be obtained both by a standard laparoscopic sucker or by using a drainage tube located in the pelvis. Continuous drainage by the tube reduces the instrument conflict between the assistant and the operating surgeon.

Finally, as it was stated before, LESS-RARP may be limited by the specific anatomical features of the male pelvis, constituting a burden for the technique in terms of exposition and suturing, which are ultimately the key points of the procedure [12].

Conclusions

Radical prostatectomy constitutes an essential surgical intervention in urological daily practice. The key points of the procedure are the dorsal vein control, apex exposure and cavernosal nerve sparing. They are particularly difficult to perform and may have significant implications on oncological and functional results. Thus, a robotic interface may represent the key factor in overcoming the critical restrictions related to LESS. Encouraging robotic innovations are imminent and will shed light to the current landscape of scarless surgery.

References

1. Guillonneau B, Cathelineau X, Barret E, Rozet F, Vallancien G. Laparoscopic radical prostatectomy. Preliminary evaluation after 28 interventions. Presse Med. 1998;27(31):1570–4.
2. Guillonneau B, Cathelineau X, Barret E, Rozet F, Vallancien G. Laparoscopic radical prostatectomy: technical and early oncological assessment of 40 operations. Eur Urol. 1999;36(1):14–20.
3. Guillonneau B, Vallancien G. Laparoscopic radical prostatectomy: initial experience and preliminary assessment after 65 operations. Prostate. 1999;39(1):71–5.
4. Guillonneau B, Vallancien G. Laparoscopic radical prostatectomy: the Montsouris technique. J Urol. 2000;163(6):1643–9.
5. Kommu SS, Rane A. Devices for laparoendoscopic single-site surgery in urology. Expert Rev Med Devices. 2009;6(1):95–103.
6. Granberg CF, Gettman MT. Instrumentation for natural orifice translumenal endoscopic surgery and laparoendoscopic single-site surgery. Indian J Urol. 2010;26(3):385–8.
7. Autorino R, Kaouk JH, Stolzenburg JU, Gill IS, Mottrie A, Tewari A, et al. Current status and future directions of robotic single-site surgery: a systematic review. Eur Urol. 2013;63(2):266–80.
8. Desai MM, Aron M, Berger A, Canes D, Stein R, Haber GP, et al. Transvesical robotic radical prostatectomy. BJU Int. 2008;102(11):1666–9.
9. Kaouk JH, Goel RK, Haber GP, Crouzet S, Stein RJ. Robotic single-port transumbilical surgery in humans: initial report. BJU Int. 2009;103(3):366–9.
10. Barret E, Sanchez-Salas R, Kasraeian A, Benoist N, Ganatra A, Cathelineau X, et al. A transition to laparo-endoscopic single-site surgery (LESS) radical prostatectomy: human cadaver experimental and initial clinical experience. J Endourol. 2009;23(1):135–40.
11. Barret E, Sanchez-Salas R, Cathelineau X, Rozet F, Galiano M, Vallancien G. Re: initial complete laparoendoscopic single-site surgery robotic assisted radical prostatectomy(LESS-RARP). Int Braz J Urol. 2009;35(1):92–3.
12. Sanchez-Salas R, Clavijo R, Barret E, Sotelo R. Laparoendoscopic single site in pelvic surgery. Indian J Urol. 2012;28(1):54–9.
13. White MA, Haber GP, Autorino R, Khanna R, Altunrende F, Yang B, et al. Robotic laparoendoscopic single-site surgery. BJU Int. 2010;106(6 Pt B):923–7.
14. Kumar P, Kommu SS, Challacombe BJ, Dasgup-Ta P. Laparoendoscopic single-site surgery (LESS) prostatectomy – robotic and conventional approach. Minerva Urol Nefrol. 2010;62(4):425–30.
15. Verit A, Rizkala E, Autorino R, Stein RJ. Robotic laparoendoscopic single-site surgery: from present to future. Indian J Urol. 2012;28(1):76–81.
16. Stein RJ, White WM, Goel RK, Irwin BH, Haber GP, Kaouk JH. Robotic laparoendoscopic single-site surgery using GelPort as the access platform. Eur Urol. 2010;57(1):132–6.
17. Jeon HG, Jeong W, Oh CK, Lorenzo EI, Ham WS, Rha KH, et al. Initial experience with 50 laparoendoscopic single site surgeries using a homemade, single port device at a single center. J Urol. 2010;183(5):1866–71.
18. Haber GP, White MA, Autorino R, Escobar PF, Kroh MD, Chalikonda S, et al. Novel robotic da Vinci instruments for laparoendoscopic single-site surgery. Urology. 2010;76(6):1279–82.
19. Merseburger AS, Herrmann TR, Shariat SF, Kyriazis I, Nagele U, Traxer O, et al. EAU guidelines on robotic and single-site surgery in urology. Eur Urol. 2013;64(2):277–91.
20. De SM, Quattrone C, Damiano R, Tanabalan C, Rane A. Patient selection for LESS urological surgery. Arch Esp Urol. 2012;65(3):280–4.
21. White MA, Haber GP, Autorino R, Khanna R, Forest S, Yang B, et al. Robotic laparoendoscopic single-site radical prostatectomy: technique and early outcomes. Eur Urol. 2010;58(4):544–50.

22. Barret E, Sanchez-Salas R, Ercolani MC, Rozet F, Galiano M, Cathelineau X. Natural orifice transendoluminal surgery and laparoendoscopic single-site surgery: the future of laparoscopic radical prostatectomy. Future Oncol. 2011;7(3):427–34.

23. Sanchez-Salas RE, Barret E, Watson J, Stakhovskyi O, Cathelineau X, Rozet F, et al. Current status of natural orifice trans-endoscopic surgery (NOTES) and laparoendoscopic single site surgery (LESS) in urologic surgery. Int Braz J Urol. 2010;36(4):385–400.

LESS Radical Cystectomy

15

Javier C. Angulo, Felipe Cáceres,
and Pedro M. Cabrera

Introduction

Urothelial bladder cancer is a very common malignancy in the elderly population of both the USA and Europe, and Spain is one of the territories of Western Europe with the highest incidence of bladder cancer among men and one of the lowest among women [1]. Complete removal of the bladder within the standard limits, and thorough extirpation of pelvic lymph nodes, remains the preferred therapeutic option for muscle-invasive disease in our environment, also in the elderly population [2].

Laparoscopic radical cystectomy (LRC) and robot-assisted LRC appear feasible alternatives and have been recently promoted over open surgery for they definitely allow earlier return to normal bowel function and shorten hospital stay, and an increasing number of series provide excellent long-term oncologic results equivalent to those of open surgery [3–7]. However, regardless of its minimally invasive character, robotic cystectomy especially with construction of intestinal neobladder is a time-consuming difficult procedure still with significant morbidity [8–10]. However, due to financial circumstances in our environment, the cost of robotic approach has become unbearable.

Laparoendoscopic single-site surgery (LESS) has become widely applicable in different urological settings and for many different procedures [11]. New technical developments that include the application of robots and precise manual systems are contributing to further development of this new field, also in urologic pelvic surgery where LESS surgery has not been so popular [12, 13]. However, it is evident that LESS application for bladder cancer surgery remains one of the least used indications, possibly for the drawback that constitutes performance of again such time-consuming and complex procedure like radical cystectomy and urinary diversion [14]. This challenge relates to the exigent steps of an accurate reconstructive surgery (ileal conduit and specially orthotopic neobladder) that must complete the extirpative procedure [15].

Since its original description in 2009 [16], laparoendoscopic radical cystectomy (LESS-RC) through different single-port systems has been reported worldwide in less than 30 cases, using either robotic, manual, or handmade platforms [11, 14, 16–21]. Since October 2011 we have

J.C. Angulo, MD, PhD (✉)
Jefe de Servicio de Urología, Department of Urology,
Hospital Universitario de Getafe, Profesor Titular de
Urología, Universidad Europea de Madrid,
Laureate Universities, Madrid, Spain
e-mail: javier.angulo@salud.madrid.org;
jangulo@futurnet.es

F. Cáceres, MD • P.M. Cabrera, MD
Department of Urology, Hospital Universitario
de Getafe, Madrid, Spain
e-mail: fcaceresj74@hotmail.com;
pmcabreracastillo@gmail.com

© Springer Science+Business Media New York 2017
J.H. Kaouk et al. (eds.), *Atlas of Laparoscopic and Robotic Single Site Surgery*,
Current Clinical Urology, DOI 10.1007/978-1-4939-3575-8_15

performed LESS-RC in 30 cases, 28 of them with reusable manual single-port system that incorporates bended instruments with double rotation, thus allowing precise movements, recovering triangulation, and avoiding clashing and two with straight laparoscopic instruments and a disposable single-port platform. Besides, partial cystectomy has been performed in three additional cases, one for tumor in a diverticulum and two cases for benign disease. Always the multichannel platform has been placed in the umbilicus and an additional 10-mm lateral port placed on right iliac fossa has been used to facilitate intracorporeal suture and extraction of drainage and ureteral catheters. Other authors prefer a homemade disposable multichannel port made from two stretchable rings or a cone and a surgical glove with trocars and valves attached to its fingers through which straight elements are used [20, 21] or even inserting several ports through a single aponeurotic incision (single-incision triangulated umbilical surgery) [22].

Pure LESS-RC without any accessory port has been performed, either using specific flexible steerable laparoscope and flexible monopolar scissors [17] or straight instruments through a multichannel homemade device [21] at a reasonable time, but always performing cutaneous ureterostomy or ileal conduit, thus revealing the actual technical limitations to perform LESS-RC and continent urinary diversion through a single port exclusively. We therefore prefer to use the two-port technique we describe.

Patient Preparation

Detailed informed consent and counseling is mandatory before a patient is considered for LESS-RC. We do not use specific preoperative bowel preparation with antibiotic, except for large bowel enema and perioperative antibiotic prophylactic cover with 2 g parenteral amoxicillin plus clavulanic 30 min before at the time of anesthesia induction and repeat 1 g dose every 8 h (three doses total) according to our hospital policy. Patients allergic to β-lactams use metronidazole and gentamicin also in the first 24 h. The abdomen is shaved, prepped, and draped in the regular fashion. Under general endotracheal anesthesia, the patient is catheterized and placed in forced 30° Trendelenburg position with the arms tucked at the sides. In females a modified lithotomy position where the legs are gently abducted and placed in stirrups, in a steep Trendelenburg position, is used. The operating room is positioned with the surgeon standing close to the patient's head on the left side and the assistant on the right. Video monitors are placed at the foot of the bed in direct line of sight with the surgeons and laparoscopic instruments (Fig. 15.1). The nurse assistant is placed at the right side of

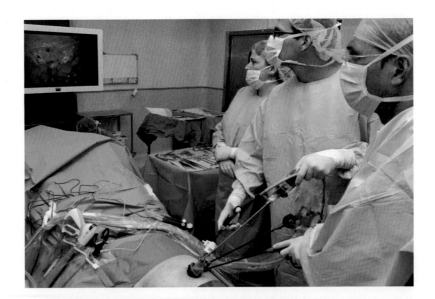

Fig. 15.1 Operating room placement, patient positioning, and distribution of surgeons

the patient close to the surgeons, and the anesthesiologist is placed behind the surgeons with open access to the head and the left size of the patient. The patient is secured to the table with padded shoulders. Compression stockings and intermittent pneumatic compression devices are applied to prevent thromboembolism.

Obtaining Access

The umbilicus is grasped with an Allis forceps, everted in a nipple fashion, to make a small 2.5-cm incision. When the skin is released, the wound will be limited to the inside of the umbilical scar (Fig. 15.2). The access to the abdominal cavity is gained by inserting a reusable rigid trocar, KeyPort© (Richard Wolf GmbH, Knittlingen, Germany), sized 2.5 cm at the tip and 3.5 cm at the base that fits the umbilical opening without need of external or internal fixation, in a screw-driven fashion (Fig. 15.3). Alternatively S-Port© (Karl Storz GmbH, Tuttlingen, Germany)

modular system can be used but needs a somewhat bigger umbilical incision and a disposable draping as wound protector. Inner element of KeyPort is removed (Figs. 15.4 and 15.5), and the soft multichannel cover with three openings (5, 10, and 15 mm, respectively) is closed to insert curved instruments composed of inner sheath, outer element, and handle. These elements incorporate a new DuoRotate© system (Richard Wolf) that allows precise movements of the tips after alignment of the arms (Fig. 15.6). A 5.5-mm wide, 50-cm long, 0° lens laparoscope and two operative curved instruments are used (atraumatic prehension forceps and Metzenbaum scissors) in turns with LigaSure© or ForceTriad© (Covidien, Dublin, Ireland) (5 or 10 mm if desired), Hem-o-lok© (Teleflex Inc., Research Triangle Park, NC, USA) clip applier, and Endopouch Retriever© (Johnson & Johnson, New Brunswick, NJ, USA).

The procedure is always performed through a transperitoneal approach. Right-handed surgeons use forceps grasper with the left hand, and it

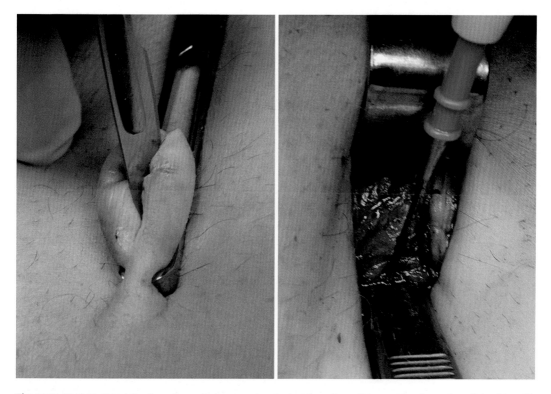

Fig. 15.2 Umbilical incision is performed after grasping the inside surface of the navel and eversion of the skin with an Allis clamp. The aponeurosis is opened with cautery

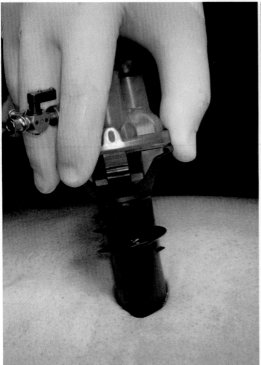 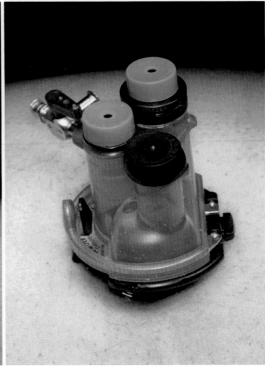

Fig. 15.3 Insertion in a screw fashion of reusable multichannel port KeyPort mounted in one piece fit into the umbilical incision without leakage and providing ample

mobility. The soft multichannel cover has three openings (5, 10, and 15 mm) and gas valve

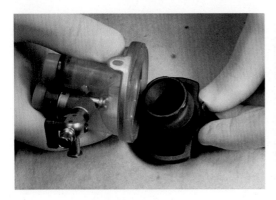 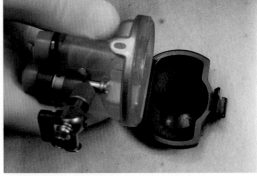

Fig. 15.4 The soft ceiling is opened to remove the inner rigid sheath

Fig. 15.5 The abdominal content is seen and the cap is closed ready to insert the working instruments

appears on the right side of the screen, and scissors with the right hand that appears on the left. Umbilical placement of the system hides the surgical scar in the navel, giving the final appearance of a scar-free surgery. The second surgeon uses a 10–12-mm additional port placed in the right iliac fossa and holds the lens. This access is ideal to insert the suction irrigation system and

5–10-mm material including straight grasping forceps, needle holder, ForceTriad© (5 or 10 mm if desired), and Hem-o-lok® clip applier. This accessory port is very useful to perform the anastomosis with a straight needle holder and to extract the drainage and ureteral stents distant from the umbilicus preventing hematoma formation or infection. This port also facilitates proper

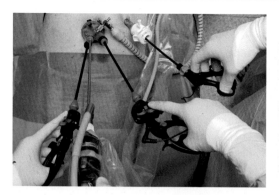

Fig. 15.6 Two curved working instruments and long 5-mm lens are inserted. The handle of the elements incorporates a system that allows precise rotation of the tip of the instruments (DuoRotate)

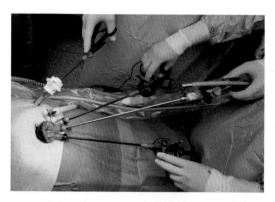

Fig. 15.7 The incorporation of the accessory port allows excellent triangulation and permits the distribution of the working space with no clashing. During the resection the surgeon stays on the left and manages the curved instruments, while the assistant takes the camera and manages the additional port. During the reconstruction the surgeon moves to the right side and uses the accessory port for suturing

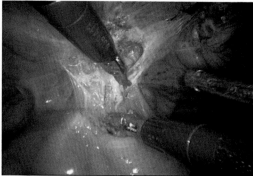

Fig. 15.8 Intestinal adherence if present must be freed before the procedure starts

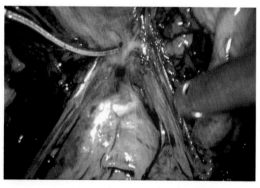

Fig. 15.9 Opening of retrovesical peritoneum to expose Denonvilliers' fascia and develop the space between the rectum and bladder

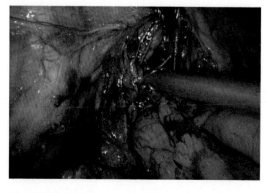

Fig. 15.10 Identification and dissection of the ureter toward its insertion in the bladder

working angle and avoids clashing of the laparoscope with the instruments and provides additional very effective double triangulation that is useful both in the excisional time and especially the reconstructive step of the operation (Fig. 15.7).

Cystectomy

Often intestinal adherences must be freed before initiating the procedure (Fig. 15.8). Surgery begins with the opening of the parietal pelvic peritoneum, ureteral identification as they cross over the common iliac artery, opening of the pouch of Douglas, and dissection of the seminal case (Fig. 15.9). The ureters are mobilized inferiorly to the level of the ureterovesical junction (Fig. 15.10). Careful dissection of the distal portion of each ureter is completed before double ligation with Hem-o-lok© and section (Fig. 15.11). Biopsies are sent for intraoperative evaluation of ureteral margin status to rule out residual tumor (Fig. 15.12).

The superior vesical pedicles are identified on each side by tracing the median umbilical ligament that continues as superior vesical artery and terminate to internal iliac vessel. Ligation of the vas deferens and superior vesical pedicles (Fig. 15.13) is performed with Hem-o-lok© and ForceTriad®. The ejaculatory organs are left en bloc and held anteriorly to separate the rectum from the specimen.

The dissection proceeds more distally by entering the plane between the bladder base and the prostate. The seminal vesicles and their attachment with Denonvilliers' fascia and adjacent tissues are freed. Incision of the plane of Denonvilliers' is essential to ensure visualization of posterior and inferior vesical pedicles. Hemostasis of these pedicles is completed with a 10-mm ForceTriad© (Fig. 15.14). The bladder is liberated and mobilized from the attachment of the urachus (Fig. 15.15), and the space of Retzius to the prostatic apex is developed by depressing the bladder, exposing white endopelvic fascia on either side of the prostate (Fig. 15.16). The endopelvic fascia is then incised bilaterally to expose the puboprostatic ligaments and the dorsal venous complex. This plexus of Santorini is gently dissected with right-angle forceps and suture ligated or controlled with ForceTriad© (Fig. 15.17).

In case a nerve-sparing LESS-RC is intended, the lateral aspect of the prostate is dissected and exposed precisely by placing countertraction on the prostatovesical junction. The nerve branches

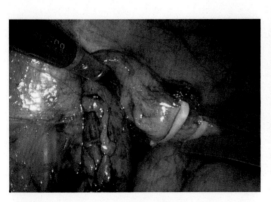

Fig. 15.11 Double ligation with Hem-o-lok and division of the distal portion of the ureter

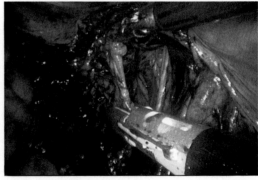

Fig. 15.13 Superior vesical pedicle is divided with ForceTriad, and the superior vesical artery is prepared for ligation with Hem-o-lok

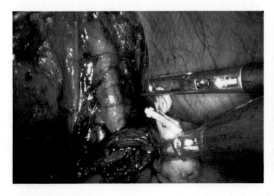

Fig. 15.12 Biopsy sent for intraoperative frozen section to evaluate ureteral margin status

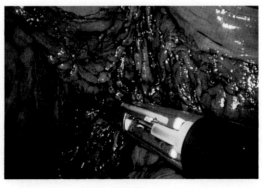

Fig. 15.14 Hemostasis of inferior vesical pedicle is performed with the application of ForceTriad

from the hypogastric plexus are located below the vesicoprostatic pedicles. The visceral pelvic fascia is exposed on the lateral aspects of the prostate and the neurovascular bundle, and

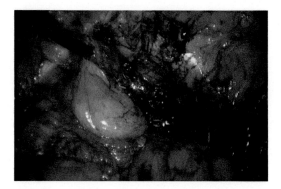

Fig. 15.15 The bladder is freed and mobilized from the urachus to develop the space of Retzius

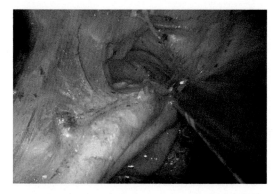

Fig. 15.16 The space of Retzius is opened with visualization of endopelvic fascia

periprostatic fascia is dissected up to the apex on either side with minimum hemostasis with harmonic scalpel, Enseal® G2 Tissue Sealer (Johnson & Johnson), to cause less lateral thermal damage.

At this point the urethra dissected just distal to the apex of the prostate and cut-sectioned (Fig. 15.18). When an orthotopic bladder reservoir is planned, only a Hem-o-lok is placed proximally, and when heterotopic urine derivation is planned in the form of ileal conduit, ureterosigmoidostomy, or cutaneous ureterostomy, two Hem-o-loks are placed, and the urethra is sectioned between them. The specimen is placed into a bag and left in the abdominal cavity. Precise hemostasis of any bleeding area is performed and testing of rectum integrity with both digital exam and visual inspection after methylene blue instillation through a Pezzer rectal catheter.

LESS anterior pelvic exenteration in females has several distinctive features from male LESS-RC. The differences stand in the fact that the specimen includes the bladder, ovaries, fallopian tubes, uterine cervix, and vaginal dome and also that it is extracted through the vagina. The procedure starts with coagulation and section of the round ligament and ovarian vessels (Fig. 15.19). Then the ureter is dissected from the iliac vessels down to the bladder wall, distally clipped and cut. Distal ureteral margin is intraoperatively sent for frozen section to ensure that the ureteral margin is free of neoplasm. An external

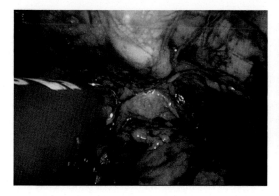

Fig. 15.17 The endopelvic fascia is incised to expose the prostatic apex and control the plexus of Santorini using ForceTriad or alternatively suture ligation

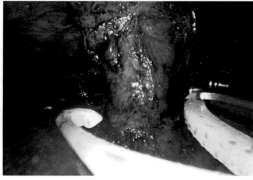

Fig. 15.18 The urethra is dissected close to the prostatic apex and after catheter removal clipped with Hem-o-lok. The urethral stump is left opened when orthotopic neobladder is planned

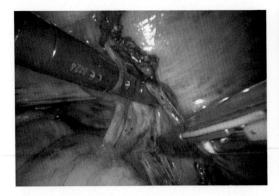

Fig. 15.19 Coagulation and section of the round ligament and ovarian vessels as the first step of pelvic exenteration in female

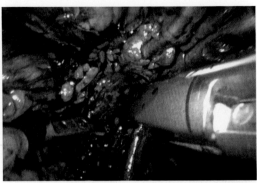

Fig. 15.21 Uterine artery is sealed and cut with ForceTriad application

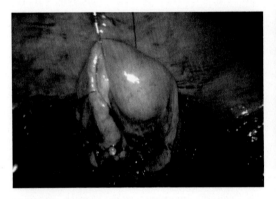

Fig. 15.20 "Marionette" suture to fix the uterus to the abdominal wall facilitates dissection of the bladder

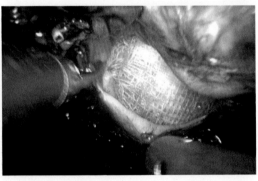

Fig. 15.22 The posterior vaginal wall is cut and a sponge placed in the vaginal cavity is exposed. This sponge facilitates dissection of the bladder

suture in a "marionette" fashion is used to fix the uterus to the abdominal wall (Fig. 15.20). Douglas pouch is opened, and cold-cutting dissection of the plane between uterus and rectum is performed. The uterine pedicle is sealed and cut, and the same procedure is worked out with the superior vesical arteries (Fig. 15.21). Later the posterior vaginal wall is cut (Fig. 15.22), and the anterior side of the bladder is dissected. A sponge in the vagina facilitates this dissection. The dorsal vein complex is sealed and cut with 10-mm ForceTriad©. Anterior vaginal plane is completed and the urethra isolated before occlusion with two Hem-o-loks© to be sectioned between them (Fig. 15.23). The specimen is

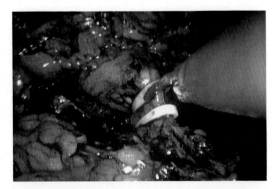

Fig. 15.23 A portion of the anterior vaginal wall is included in the specimen, and the bladder is totally dissected. Dorsal vein complex is coagulated, and the urethra is exposed and clipped with two Hem-o-loks before sectioning in the middle

pouched. The closing thread of the retrieval system is laparoendoscopically transferred out through the introitus, and gently external traction is applied to complete atraumatic specimen extraction through the vagina, thus combining the concepts of LESS and NOTES (Fig. 15.24). Strictly speaking, LESS anterior exenteration in females should be termed "transvaginal NOTES-assisted LESS radical cystectomy." Careful hemostasis is carried out, and the vaginal wound is closed laparoendoscopically with a running 90 2/0 30-cm V-Loc™ suture (Covidien, Dublin, Ireland) (Fig. 15.25).

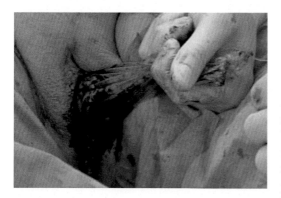

Fig. 15.24 The anterior exenteration specimen is bagged, and the purse is transferred out of the vaginal hiatus to be extracted from outside the vagina

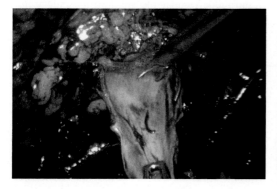

Fig. 15.25 The posterior side of the vagina is plicated to close the vaginal defect. The suture is performed laparoendoscopically with absorbable wound closure device V-Loc

Pelvic Lymph Node Dissection

Nodal dissection is performed after the cystectomy because the situation of finding surprising bulky nodal disease precluding surgery is now very exceptional in the era of imaging techniques. The pelvic lymph node (obturator, internal iliac, external iliac, common iliac, and presacral, bilaterally; and also preaortic and precaval) dissection is from an oncological perspective as important and time-consuming as the cystectomy itself and must be performed systematically. The procedure can begin caudally and extend cephalad. Obturator nodal dissection distally starts with the node of Cloquet (Fig. 15.26). Careful attention must be paid to the circumflex vessels because they can be easily injured by excessive traction or cautery. Obturator nerve and artery are skeletonized (Fig. 15.27). Obturator vein may be sacrificed to allow complete dissection below the obturator nerve. At this point obturator nodes mix with paravesical nodes, both in the lateral rectal sulci and those already extracted with the bladder. Certainly the amount of nodes obtained in this area depends on the lateral extent of the resection at the time of cystectomy. The nodal packet with its caudal portion detached is mobilized upward to the origin of the bifurcation of the common iliac nodes. Careful medial retraction of the external iliac vessels gives access to

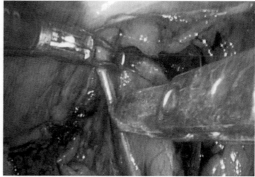

Fig. 15.26 Pelvic lymph node dissection in a caudocranial fashion starts with the dissection of the node of Cloquet closed to the circumflex vessels

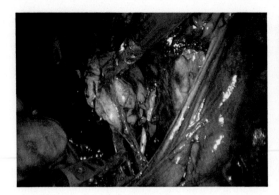

Fig. 15.27 Lymph node dissection continues cleaning the obturator fossa where obturator nerve and artery are skeletonized

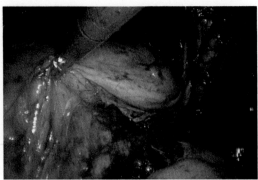

Fig. 15.29 Medial retraction of descending colon exposes common and internal iliac vessels

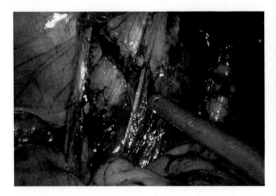

Fig. 15.28 Lymph node dissection continues at the level of the external iliac vessel

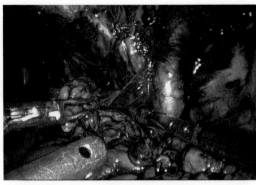

Fig. 15.30 The internal iliac territory is dissected. Nodal tissue medial to the artery is separated from the vessel with a "split and roll" technique

the triangle of Marcille (Fig. 15.28), crossed by the obturator nerve and limited laterally by the medial border of the psoas muscle and the genito-femoral nerve and below by the lateral margin of the vertebral column and the iliolumbar ligament. Large lumbar veins are often present in this area, and their bleeding can be very troublesome.

At this time internal iliac nodal chain dissection follows, initiating at the bifurcation of the common iliac artery where the origin of the hypogastric artery is identified. Descending colon must be retracted medially to facilitate exposure (Fig. 15.29), and precise dissection is performed with scissors on the right hand and bipolar cautery on the left. Dissection is carried out distally, and the nodal tissue lateral to the external iliac vessels is removed. Inspection of the contralateral presacral region gives additional

tissue hidden under the sigmoid mesentery that must be rotated to allow presacral dissection.

To complete the external iliac node dissection, posterior peritoneal tissue is divided, and the genitofemoral nerve is again identified lateral to the external iliac artery. The nodal tissue medial in the territory of the hypogastric artery is also lifted off the vessel with "split and roll" technique (Fig. 15.30). Later common iliac nodes are dissected removing the tissue anterior, medial, and lateral to the common iliac artery (Fig. 15.31). The posterior peritoneum over the common iliac artery is divided, and dissection progresses cephalic to identify the aortic bifurcation. Again split and roll over both common iliac arteries allow resection of the nodal tissue at the level of the aortic bifurcation. Next, resection of the

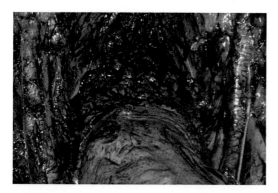

Fig. 15.31 Iliac lymph node dissection is completed on both sides

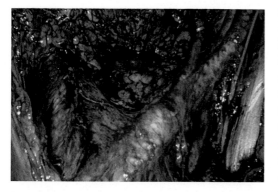

Fig. 15.32 The vena cava, aortic bifurcation, and presacral space are dissected together. Presacral nodes are included to complete extended pelvic lymph node dissection

nodes anterior to the inferior vena cava is undertaken (Fig. 15.32). The vena cava bifurcation is often more distal than the aortic bifurcation, and these nodes sometimes can be dissected en bloc with the presacral nodes. At this point one must be especially cautious to avoid bleeding from presacral veins. Change to 30° lens aids with the proximal part of the operation.

The cephalad boundary of the extended nodal dissection we perform is the aortic bifurcation, the caudal limit is the node of Cloquet and circumflex vessels coming from the external iliac arteries, the lateral borders are the genitofemoral nerves, and the medial boundaries are the paravesical and pararectal nodes left after the cystectomy. The median number of nodes we obtain with this procedure is 19 (IQR 16–32). To summarize, LESS-extended pelvic lymph node

dissection is possible and must be performed adequately and precisely because the number of nodes is a surrogate for the oncologic efficacy independently of the approach used [2, 10, 23] and also because morbidity at this time of the surgery is significant.

We bag the nodal tissue together with the cystectomy specimen, and this pouch will be extracted at a later stage out through the umbilicus in males after removal of the reusable port. In females where the cystectomy specimen has already been extracted, nodal retrieval can be performed directly at this point.

Reconstructive stage to perform urinary diversion follows pelvic lymph node dissection. Several options are possible, either using the intestine to construct a neobladder or an ileal loop to perform cutaneous ureteroileostomy or avoiding the intestine and perform a cutaneous ureteroureterostomy. This last option is very rarely recommended to avoid late estenotic complications. We have performed it only in a case of our series, due to elevated age and morbidity and the presence of very advanced disease. Ileal conduit, using 15 cm of bowel, or neobladder, with a longer segment of 45–50 cm, is preferred. The election depends on patient counseling, age, and condition. In tumors with negative urethral biopsy, an ortothopic reservoir is always recommended as first choice.

Orthotopic Neobladder

Before extraction of the umbilical platform and specimen, the intestine is marked with a reference suture and Hem-o-lok© 15 cm from the ileocecal valve, which will help to properly select and work out the intestinal segment (Fig. 15.33). Then the umbilical reusable platform is extracted, and after minimal enlargement of the aponeurotic and skin incisions (Fig. 15.34) the cystoprostatectomy and nodal specimen is retrieved (Fig. 15.35). The KeyPort is placed again in the umbilicus, sometimes needing a fixation stitch if the wound has been significantly enlarged. The stay suture is pulled out through the umbilical platform using the curved instrument and,

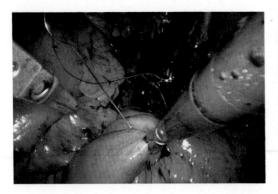

Fig. 15.33 The intestine is marked with a reference suture 15 cm from the ileocecal valve that will help properly extract and select the intestinal segment to perform the urinary diversion

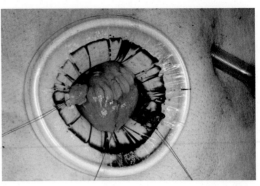

Fig. 15.36 Alexis wound retractor placed in the umbilicus allows small bowel and ureteral extracorporeal position to perform the urinary diversion, either neobladder or ileal conduit

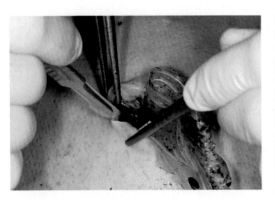

Fig. 15.34 Slight enlargement of the aponeurotic and skin incisions after extraction of umbilical reusable platform facilitates organ retrieval

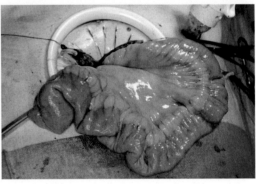

Fig. 15.37 A 45–50-cm intestinal segment chosen to perform Studer's reservoir after intestinal continuity has been restored

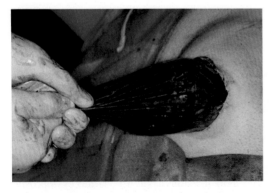

Fig. 15.35 The purse with the cystoprostatectomy specimen is extracted off the umbilicus by gentle traction

simultaneously, with the help of straight material through the 10-mm accessory trocar, and the endings of the ureters are carefully grasped out through the umbilical KeyPort. Once again the

umbilical platform is taken out, and two additional stay sutures are placed on the distal end of each ureter to avoid them being lost in the abdominal cavity.

An Alexis® wound retractor (Applied Medical, Rancho Santa Margarita, CA, USA) is placed into the umbilical incision to facilitate extracorporeal intestinal stage of the operation with construction of the reservoir and reestablishment of intestinal continuity. The marking intestinal suture and the tip end of both ureters come out from the umbilical incision (Fig. 15.36). The small bowel is extracted, and the 45–50-cm intestinal segment that will serve to do the neobladder is identified (Fig. 15.37). The intestine is cut and ileoileal anastomosis performed with mechanical sutures. The afferent limb of the intestinal segment is closed using a GIA stapler

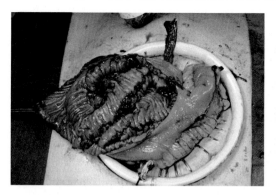

Fig. 15.38 Detubulization and reservoir configuration with preservation of an afferent segment to which the ureters are anastomosed

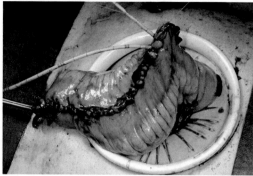

Fig. 15.40 The neobladder is completed and urinary diversion catheters come out of the reservoir. The distal end of the reservoir is left open to be later anastomosed to the urethral stump

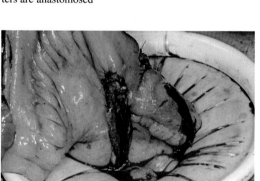

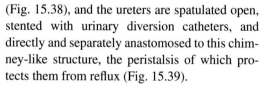

Fig. 15.39 Ureters are spatulated, stented, and individually anastomosed to the afferent limb of the reservoir

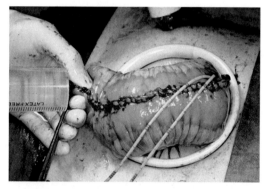

Fig. 15.41 Watertightness of the reservoir is tested before introduction in the abdominal cavity

(Fig. 15.38), and the ureters are spatulated open, stented with urinary diversion catheters, and directly and separately anastomosed to this chimney-like structure, the peristalsis of which protects them from reflux (Fig. 15.39).

The rest of the excluded segment is detubularized to construct extracorporeal Studer's reservoir with straight needle absorbable suture (Fig. 15.40). Watertightness of the reservoir is confirmed with instillation of 100–200 ml of saline into the neobladder (Fig. 15.41). A distal hole to face the urethral end and a pulling suture are left before the neobladder is introduced into the pelvic cavity. The sutures that will be used to perform the urethro-neovesical anastomosis are also left in place before the neobladder is introduced in the pelvis (Fig. 15.42). These tricks will later facilitate very much traction of the neobladder and the initiation of the anastomosis. Also it

is important to take into account that the intestinal time must be performed fast to avoid mesenteric edema causing difficultness to insert the reservoir into the pelvis.

After neobladder insertion the KeyPort is for the last time reintroduced in the umbilicus to perform the urethral anastomosis with the two barbed Glycomer V-Loc™ 90 2–0 hemi-sutures already mentioned crossed at 6 o'clock position, until they meet at 12 o'clock over a silicone urethral catheter (Fig. 15.43). Urethropexy with suture fixation to the pubic bone is developed by traction with Hem-o-lok placement at the end of the anastomosis, as an attempt to facilitate continence recovery [24] (Fig. 15.44). Finally, integrity of the catheter and correct filling and emptying of the reservoir are confirmed once more with instillation of saline into the neobladder from the urethral meatus (Fig. 15.45).

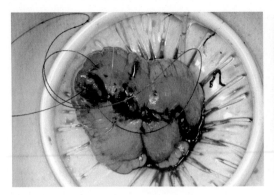

Fig. 15.42 The neobladder is inserted through the umbilicus. Two barbed V-Loc hemi-sutures and needles are left in place before insertion of the reservoir into the abdominal cavity that will facilitate the initiation of the urethroneovesical anastomosis

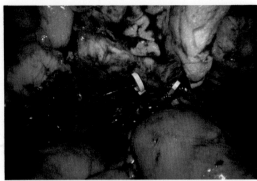

Fig. 15.44 The ends of V-Loc sutures are tied to the pubic bone with Hem-o-loks in the fashion of a urethropexy with the intention to facilitate continence recovery

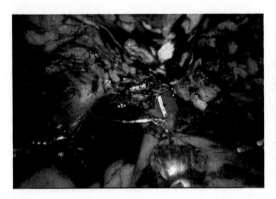

Fig. 15.43 Laparoendoscopic view of urethro-neovesical anastomosis. A marked suture is used to pull the neobladder and direct it appropriately into the pelvic cavity facing the urethral stump. A silicone urethral catheter is placed into the neobladder. The two barbed hemi-sutures starting at 6 o'clock position progress on each side to meet at 12 o'clock

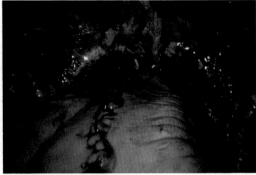

Fig. 15.45 The neobladder is filled with saline, and both the reservoir and the anastomosis are visually inspected to confirm integrity

A Blake drain (Johnson & Johnson) left on the pelvic operative field and both urinary diversion catheters are extracted from the 10-mm port with grasping forceps before it is definitely taken out. The umbilical wound is closed carefully with 3/0 Vicryl Rapide. The ureteric stents are extracted before admission after cystography on day 7, and the pelvic drainage is taken out the following day. In the absence of complications, the patient is discharged before day 10. Some weeks later the umbilical scar appears totally invisible, and the residual scar corresponding to the 10-mm port appears somewhat like a large freckle (Fig. 15.46).

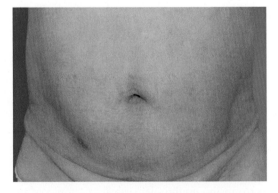

Fig. 15.46 External view at 3 months of a patient with LESS radical cystectomy, lymph node dissection, and Studer's neobladder. No incision can be seen and the patient is very satisfied and fully continent

Ileal Conduit

After specimen is retrieved if an ileal conduit is decided, the KeyPort is reintroduced, and a fixation stitch is placed to avoid gas leakage. Sometimes this stitch is not needed as enlargement of original umbilical incision may be very discrete or null in females after vaginal extraction. The marking intestinal suture is gently transferred from the 10-mm port to the umbilical incision, together with the distal end of both ureters. A 15-cm segment of ileum (Fig. 15.47) is isolated extracorporeally choosing a nice mesentery (Fig. 15.48). Bowel continuity is reestablished with latero-lateral mechanical suture using GIA surgical stapler and closure with TA stapler, confirming appropriate passage of intestinal content (Fig. 15.49). The excluded segment is used to perform an ileal conduit, to which stent

spatulated ureters are anastomosed separately following Nesbit's technique also extracorporeally (Fig. 15.50). Integrity of the conduit and ureteral anastomosis is confirmed by instillation of saline into the segment that will also have a cleaning effect (Fig. 15.51).

Finally the incision of the 10–12-mm port is widened and transformed into the orifice on right iliac fossa to which the stoma will be fit (Fig. 15.52). Fatty tissue is extracted and aponeurosis widened to allow the passage of the conduit. With the help of two Babcock clamps, the conduit is transferred from the umbilical incision to the cutaneous opening to complete construction of the intussuscepted end-to-end ileostomy.

A Blake drain (Johnson & Johnson) is inserted into the pelvis through the umbilical port and extracted out together with the reusable umbilical platform. The ureteral stents come out through

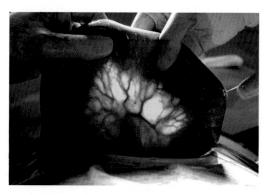

Fig. 15.47 The intestine and mesentery are inspected to choose the segment to construct the ileal conduit

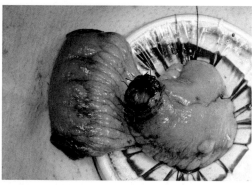

Fig. 15.49 Bowel continuity is reestablished with mechanical staples

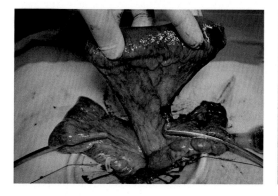

Fig. 15.48 A 15-cm intestinal segment is isolated outside the umbilicus

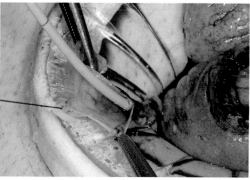

Fig. 15.50 The ureters are spatulated and stented for separate anastomosis to the ileal loop

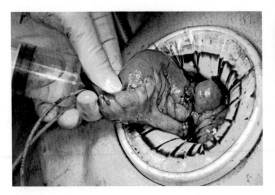

Fig. 15.51 Saline is instilled into the conduit to test integrity of proximal closure and ureteral anastomosis

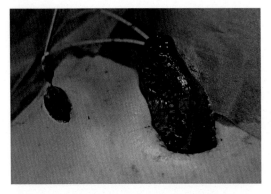

Fig. 15.52 The hole of the accessory 10–12-mm port is converted into the orifice to perform the cutaneous ileostomy. The ileal conduit will be introduced and transferred from the umbilicus to the orifice in right iliac fossa

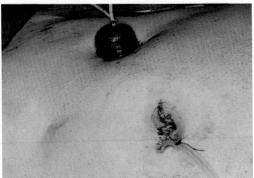

Fig. 15.53 The ileostomy is ended in an end-to-end intussuscepted nipple fashion to prevent retraction, and the umbilical wound is closed with a drain coming through the incision, thus avoiding another extra orifice for drainage

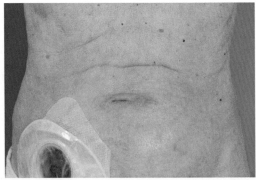

Fig. 15.54 External aspect of the abdomen of an elderly man with LESS radical cystectomy, pelvic lymph node dissection, and ileal conduit. No incision is visible and he is very satisfied with the procedure

the ileostomy. The umbilical wound is closed carefully with 3/0 Vicryl Rapide (Fig. 15.53). Some weeks later the umbilical scar appears totally invisible, and the patient shows the ileostomy with no apparent incision (Fig. 15.54).

Present and Future of LESS Radical Cystectomy

The dilemma of which is the best form of urinary diversion is not yet closed. An orthotopic bladder substitute must be offered whenever complete removal of any extravesical tumor extension and terminal ureteral disease is possible and also if there is no tumor at the edge of the urethral resection. We consider LESS-RC with orthotopic

neobladder is the least invasive form of possibly the most invasive urologic surgery. The appropriateness of lymph node dissection is crucial, not only to correctly evaluate the need of adjunct therapy but also for prognosis itself. Continence and potency are also important issues in these patients; however, the high mortality rate of the disease leaves cosmetics, patient recovery, and analgesic needs to a second or third stage of concern. First is life, second are continence and potency, and third come the rest. Taking this fact in mind, we believe that laparoendoscopic surgery should be equivalent to laparoscopy in terms of both oncological and functional results, possibly with better indemnity of the abdominal wall even than in laparoscopy. In fact, there are no case of evisceration in these patients and no case of wound infection or wound dehiscence, as sometimes presented in cases of laparoscopic or robot-assisted laparoscopic radical cystectomy when the diversion was performed extracorporeally through a 10-cm infraumbilical incision.

The median follow-up of these patients is presently 51 (IQR 20–79) weeks. Of course we do not have available data on bladder cancer survival, but we can say the positive margin rate is 3.3 %, and the median number of nodes removed is 19 (11–41). Incidental prostate cancer has been discovered in 20 % of the patients. Operative data also reveal this surgery is within the range of security that should be expected for a center of high standard of care, especially when it has been performed in a population with median age of 70 (64.3–77.8) yr and median Charlson index of 3 (2–4). Intraoperative and postoperative transfusion rates are 10 % and 20 %, respectively, and median differential hemoglobin is 2.1 (1.7–3.2) g/dL. Median total operative time is 330 (285–376) min. Median visual analogue pain scale on postoperative day 3 is 3 (2–4) and median hospital stay is 9.2 (8–13). The proportion of patients with complications according to Clavien-Dindo classification is 36.7 %, and the proportion of patients with major complications (grade III or above) is 10 %.

Both laparoscopic radical cystectomy and laparoscopic robot-assisted cystectomy are feasible competing alternatives. But the question is: how can LESS be better than laparoscopy? Single-port surgery is the progressive result of small steps based on minor adjustments of previous techniques, the same as the tuning of an instrument is carried out with minor adjustments, and the real value of each one is difficult to define. The result is that from the sum of all these small adjustments exquisite tuning is achieved. The initial impetus to promote minimally invasive surgery in the hands of laparoscopy focused on avoiding the morbidity of laparotomy. Improvements regarding less pain, less bleeding, better recovery of intestinal motility, and decreased need for analgesics are the main achievements of the laparoscopic approach [25–27] without any sacrifice in oncologic

safety [3]. The same but to a higher extent can be anticipated for LESS-RC.

The performance of LESS surgery through reusable platforms is very cost-effective. In the hands of experienced surgeons working in centers of excellence, this alternative is very attractive both for health supporters and patients. There is no doubt that the experience in this type of patients is still very limited even worldwide and that more casuistry must be accumulated in order to acknowledge the benefits of this procedure. Of course experience and specific training are mandatory to carry out a progressive learning to compensate for the laterality change [28]. The use of accessory trocars as hybrid LESS very much facilitates this approach [20, 29, 30].

In a close future, new platforms will be developed that further close the gap between reality and dreams to make LESS surgery even less invasive. Popularization of many present and future adjuncts such as organ retrieval systems, wound closing devices, hemostatic agents, adhesives, and sealants is also crucial in the field. On the other hand, quality of vision, together with precision, durability, and reliability of our instruments, is a reality for which we are in debt to producers, developers, and investigators in the direction to make surgery every day more satisfactory both for patients and doctor. The performance of radical surgery for bladder cancer through single-port systems, which can be coupled to the natural scar of the navel, both in male and female, and also can be transvaginal NOTES assisted in the female, is an excellent example of surgical development. Until more precise articulating instruments get developed to facilitate the difficult reconstructive steps of the surgery, the two-port technique we describe is at present the most secure, less time-consuming, and cheapest alternative available to perform, not only a high-quality oncologic procedure but also an elegant orthotopic urinary diversion with highest possibilities of good functional recovery.

Acknowledgments The authors acknowledge Mr. Jesús Arconada, Mr. José Domínguez, and surgical nurse Mrs. Ana Aparicio for their technical support and help in this experience.

References

1. Guey LT, García-Closas M, Murta-Nascimento C, et al. Genetic susceptibility to distinct bladder cancer phenotypes. Eur Urol. 2010;57:283–92.
2. Núñez-Mora C, García Mediero JM, Cabrera-Castillo PM, García-Tello A, González J, Angulo JC. Feasibility of lymphadenectomy in laparoscopic radical cystectomy. Urology. 2010;76:759–63.
3. Haber GP, Gill IS. Laparoscopic radical cystectomy for cancer: oncological outcomes at up to 5 years. BJU Int. 2007;100:137–42.
4. Haber G-P, Crouzet S, Gill IS. Laparoscopic and robotic assisted radical cystectomy for bladder cancer: a critical analysis. Eur Urol. 2008;54:54–64.
5. Guillotreau J, Gamé X, Mouzin M, et al. Radical cystectomy for bladder cancer: morbidity of laparoscopic versus open surgery. J Urol. 2009;181: 554–9.
6. Guillotreau J, Miocinovic R, Gamé X, et al. Outcomes of laparoscopic and robotic radical cystectomy in the elderly patients. Urology. 2012;79:585–90.
7. Snow-Lisy DC, Campbell SC, Gill IS, et al. Robotic and laparoscopic radical cystectomy for bladder cancer: long-term oncologic outcomes. Eur Urol. 2014; 55:193–200.
8. Khan MS, Elhage O, Challacombe B, Rimington P, Murphy D, Dasgupta P. Analysis of early complications of robotic-assisted radical cystectomy using a standardized reporting system. Urology. 2011;77: 357–62.
9. Treyer A, Saar M, Kopper B, Kamradt J, Siemer S, Stöckle M. Cistectomía radical laparoscópica asistida por robot: evaluación de los resultados funcionales y oncológicos. Actas Urol Esp. 2011;35:152–7.
10. Tyritzis SI, Hosseini A, Collins J, et al. Oncologic, functional, and complications outcomes of robot-assisted radical cystectomy with totally intracorporeal neobladder diversion. Eur Urol. 2013;64:734–41.
11. Kaouk JH, Autorino R, Kim FJ, et al. Laparoendoscopic-single-site surgery in urology: worldwide multi-institutional analysis of 1076 cases. Eur Urol. 2011;60:998–1005.
12. White MA, Haber G-P, Autorino R, et al. Robotic laparoendoscopic single-site radical prostatectomy: technique and early outcomes. Eur Urol. 2010;58: 544–50.
13. Cáceres F, Cabrera PM, García-Tello A, García-Mediero JM, Angulo JC. Safety study of umbilical single-port laparoscopic radical prostatectomy with a new DuoRotate system. Eur Urol. 2012;62:1143–9.
14. Angulo JC, Cáceres F, Arance I, Romero I, RamóndeFata F, Cabrera PM. Cistectomía radical laparoscópica con neovejiga ileal ortotópica a través de puerto único umbilical. Actas Urol Esp. 2012;36:554–61.
15. Kaouk JH, Autorino R. Comentario: Cistectomía radical laparoendoscópica con neovejiga ileal ortotópica a través de puerto único umbilical. Actas Urol Esp. 2012;36:562–3.
16. White WM, Haber G-P, Goel RK, Crouzet S, Stein RJ, Kaouk JH. Single-port urological surgery: single-center experience with the first 100 cases. Urology. 2009;74:801–4.
17. Kaouk JH, Goel RK, White MA, et al. Laparoendoscopic single-site radical cystectomy and pelvic lymph node dissection: initial experience and 2-year follow-up. Urology. 2010;76:857–61.
18. Liu CX, Xu AB, Chen BS, Zheng SB, Li HL, Xu YW. Laparoendoscopic single-site surgery radical cystectomy with orthotopic taenia myectomy sigmoid neobladder: initial report (in Chinese). Nan Fang Yi Ke Da Xue Xue Bao. 2010;30:1385–8.
19. Huang J, Lin TZ, Xu KW, et al. Application of modified single port laparoscopic radical cystoprostatectomy and orthotopic ileal neobladder (in Chinese). Zhonghua Yi Xue Za Zhi. 2010;90:1542–6.
20. Lin T, Huang J, Han J, et al. Hybrid laparoscopic endoscopic single-site surgery for radical cystoprostatectomy and orthotopic ileal neobladder: an initial experience of 12 cases. J Endourol. 2011;25: 57–63.
21. Ma L, Bi H, Hou X-F, et al. Laparoendoscopic single-site radical cystectomy and urinary diversión: initial experience in China using a homemade single-port device. J Endourol. 2012;26:355–9.
22. Horstmann M, Kugler M, Anastasiadis AG, Walcher U, Herrmann T, Nagele U. Laparoscopic radical cystectomy: initial experience using the single-incision triangulated umbilical surgery (SITUS) technique. World J Urol. 2012;30:619–24.
23. Leissner J, Ghoneim MA, Abol-Enein H, et al. Extended radical lymphadenectomy in patients with urothelial bladder cancer: results of a prospective multicenter study. J Urol. 2004;171:139–44.
24. Nuñez-Mora C, García-Mediero JM, Cabrera-Castillo PM, Pérez-Utrilla M, Angulo-Cuesta J. Results of simplified urethropexy in the recovery of continence after radical laparoscopic prostatectomy. J Endourol. 2011;25:1759–62.
25. Porpiglia F, Renard J, Billia M, et al. Open versus laparoscopy-assisted radical cystectomy: results of a prospective study. J Endourol. 2007;21:325–9.
26. Hemal AK, Kolla SB, Wadhwa P. Evaluation of laparoscopic radical cystectomy for loco-regionally advanced bladder cancer. World J Urol. 2008;26: 161–6.
27. Berger A, Aron M. Laparoscopic radical cystectomy: long-term outcomes. Curr Opin Urol. 2008;18: 167–72.
28. Cáceres F, Cabrera PM, Mateo E, Andrés G, Lista F, Angulo JC. Puesta en marcha de un programa de entrenamiento para laparoscopia. Actas Urol Esp. 2012;36:418–24.
29. Liatsikos E, Kyriazis I, Kallidonis P, Do M, Dietel A, Stolzenburg JU. Pure single-port laparoscopic surgery or mix of techniques? World J Urol. 2012;30:581–7.
30. García-Mediero JM, Cabrera PM, Cáceres F, Mateo E, García-Tello A, Angulo JC. Estado actual de la cirugía transumbilical por puerto único: retos y aplicaciones. Actas Urol Esp. 2013;37:106–13.

Laparoendoscopic Single-Site (LESS) Sacral Colpopexy

16

Wesley M. White, Ryan B. Pickens, and Robert F. Elder

Introduction

As the general population has aged yet remained active, the demand for correction of pelvic organ prolapse (POP) has progressively increased [1, 2]. Traditionally, management of POP has come in the form of cautious observation, pessary fitting and use, myriad vaginal repairs, and/or abdominal sacral colpopexy (ASC). The ideal treatment approach and/or type of operation should be based not only on the objective outcomes of the myriad procedures but also on the expectancies, desires, and risk factors of the individual and the proficiency and purview of the surgeon.

Among patients that desire, and are considered good candidates for, definitive surgical reconstruction, ASC is considered the "gold standard" technique owing to superior anatomical support of the vaginal apex [3–5]. Historically, open ASC was considered a disproportionately invasive procedure associated with prolonged convalescence and increased pain as compared to native-tissue and/or mesh-augmented vaginal repair. The application of laparoscopy and robotics during ASC has dramatically improved morbidity associated with the procedure while continuing to offer durable and satisfactory outcomes [5]. Coupled with the current climate of fear surrounding mesh-augmented vaginal repair, ASC has become the preferred corrective procedure for pelvic organ prolapse for many patients and providers.

Sacral Colpopexy would appear to be an ideal indication for LESS. Prior studies examining patient-driven factors for pursuing LESS include a benign surgical indication and female gender [6]. Moreover, from a purely technical standpoint, access to the vagina externally for manipulation alleviates some element of triangulation loss, a major criticism and impediment of LESS in general [7]. Results from a retrospective, matched cohort study demonstrated equivalent results between laparoscopic, robotic, and LESS ASC with improved cosmesis and high patient satisfaction in the LESS group [7].

Despite these seemingly ideal circumstances and promising early results, the major impediment to LESS ASC remains the significant amount of reconstruction required during the

W.M. White, MD (✉)
Department of Urology, Laparoscopic and Robotic Urologic Surgery, The University of Tennessee Medical Center, Knoxville, TN, USA
e-mail: WWhite@mc.utmck.edu

R.B. Pickens, MD
Division of Urology, Department of Surgery, University of Tennessee Medical Center, Knoxville, TN, USA
e-mail: rpickens@utmck.edu

R.F. Elder, MD
Women's and Children's Health, Obstetrics and Gynecology Surgery, University of Tennessee Medical Center, Knoxville, TN, USA
e-mail: redler@utmck.edu

© Springer Science+Business Media New York 2017
J.H. Kaouk et al. (eds.), *Atlas of Laparoscopic and Robotic Single Site Surgery*,
Current Clinical Urology, DOI 10.1007/978-1-4939-3575-8_16

procedure. Freehand intracorporeal suturing and knot-tying using an in-line approach are extraordinarily challenging even among laparoscopic experts. ASC demands precise mesh placement and suture fixation, and the ability to reproducibly place and secure sutures using LESS is demanding. As has been repeatedly demonstrated with other reconstructive indications, the da Vinci® platform greatly facilitates intracorporeal suturing and may likewise alleviate many of the limitations of conventional LESS ASC [8]. However, the existing robotic platform is not purpose-built for LESS and newer configurations are not yet FDA approved for ASC. This textbook chapter will describe our group's technique for reduced port robotic and LESS ASC using the existing da Vinci Si® platform and offer pearls of wisdom for patient selection, technical nuances, and troubleshooting.

Patient Selection and Evaluation

The indications for LESS ASC parallel those of standard multi-port ASC and include women with symptomatic stage II or greater anterior, apical, or posterior vaginal vault prolapse, those with recurrent prolapse following primary vaginal repair, those with primary prolapse with the need for concomitant abdominal surgery, and/or those women with severe multi-compartment prolapse with a significant apical component. Women with an in situ uterus may be considered for uterus-sparing sacro-hysteropexy or may elect to undergo concomitant supracervical hysterectomy at the time of Sacral Colpopexy (our preferred practice). Prior abdominal surgery is common among this patient population and is not considered a contraindication.

All patients should undergo a thorough history and physical examination, and a thorough attempt should be made to reconcile the patient's symptoms with their examination findings. Our center employs a multidisciplinary team of urologists and gynecologists to offer patients a complete range of diagnostic and therapeutic options. We find this cooperative approach is ideal for both our patient population and our providers.

The most common presenting symptoms include urinary, sexual, and bowel bother in addition to classic complaints of vaginal pressure or heaviness. Women with advanced prolapse may report the need for manual reduction and/or the ability to directly visualize the vaginal apex or uterus. Concomitant urinary incontinence may be mixed and particular attention should be paid to the presence of occult stress urinary incontinence. A voiding log and post-void residual measurement are recommended. Likewise, quality of life questionnaires are useful to establish a baseline for later reference. Multichannel urodynamics may be a useful adjunct in select circumstances, especially among women with high-grade prolapse. It is our belief that many of these women have an element of detrusor underactivity owing to prolonged relaxation. Patients should be counseled preoperatively on the possibility of persistent and/or de novo postoperative voiding dysfunction or hesitancy, especially in the setting of concomitant mid-urethral sling.

Physical examination should be systematic and thorough. The abdomen should be examined for the presence of prior surgical intervention. Again, although not a specific contraindication to ASC, the wisdom of performing LESS ASC in a hostile field must be questioned. A bimanual examination should be performed to assess for the presence and size of a uterus (if present) and the presence of adnexal pathology. A bivalve speculum should be inserted to assess the vaginal apex and/or cervix. The speculum should then be disarticulated to evaluate the anterior and posterior compartments. The presence and grade of prolapse in the anterior, apical, and posterior compartments should be quantified utilizing the pelvic organ prolapse quantification (POP-Q) system. Estrogen status and the integrity of the levator musculature and perineal body are likewise assessed.

A cough stress test or cotton swab test is typically employed to evaluate for urethral hypermobility/stress urinary incontinence. Although published studies suggest that women without existing complaints of stress incontinence may benefit from mid-urethral sling owing to the presence of occult leakage, our practice is to individualize our approach to sling placement including intraoperative Crede maneuver.

Preoperative preparation includes selective medical clearance and a thorough explanation of surgical risks including, but not limited to, injury to the bladder or ureters, inadvertent vaginal entry, mesh-related complications including erosion or extrusion, vaginal foreshortening, dyspareunia, postoperative voiding dysfunction including retention, and other imponderables. A type and screen are not needed. Venous thromboembolism prophylaxis is employed with either sequential compression devices or subcutaneous heparin. Two large-bore IV lines are placed and the patient is administered a perioperative dose of a first- or second-generation cephalosporin.

Surgical Technique: Reduced Port Sacral Colpopexy

Given the inherent aforementioned challenges associated with pure LESS ASC, many surgeons will prefer a stepwise approach to the technique. In this circumstance, reduced port ASC is considered a safe yet educational transition. Surgeons may prefer to eliminate the accessory robotic trocar first and then the assistant port as able. Port size reduction from 8 mm standard robotic trocars to 5 mm low-profile "pediatric" trocars then follows. Ideally, reduced port robotic ASC employs the umbilicus and two very concealable 5 mm incisions. This configuration, in our experience, provides consistent triangulation but without the laterally oriented trocars that tend to be the most painful. Moreover, reduced port ASC provides valuable insight into the advantages and nuances of pure LESS ASC.

The patient is brought to the operating room and placed in the supine position. General endotracheal anesthesia is administered and the patient is subsequently converted to the low lithotomy position in Allen stirrups. We prefer to tuck the patient's arms and use a foam back pad to prevent movement of the patient. It is important for the patient's perineum to approach the edge of

the bed to facilitate external manipulation of the vagina during the case as well as access to the vagina for subsequent mid-urethral sling and/or distal rectocele repair, as needed. The abdomen, vagina, and perineum are widely prepped with Betadine or chlorhexidine solution and the entire field draped into a sterile field. Our preference is used to employ a laparoscopic one-piece gynecology drape (prefabricated service pockets and Velcro straps) that affords dual access to both the abdomen and vagina. A Foley catheter and vaginal manipulator are placed.

The relevant pelvic landmarks are identified and an approximate 12 mm incision is made in a periumbilical fashion (Fig. 16.1). A Veress needle is inserted into the peritoneal cavity and confirmation of access achieved with use of a saline drop test. The abdomen is insufflated with CO_2 gas to a maximum pressure of 15 mmHg. The Veress needle is removed and a standard 12 mm operative trocar is placed. In some circumstances, it is very helpful to employ a balloon-tipped trocar to prevent inadvertent slippage of the trocar. The robotic 0° camera is introduced through this trocar and the abdomen widely inspected. The patient is then placed in steep Trendelenburg position and the table is maximally lowered. Under direct vision, two additional 5 mm trocars are then placed approximately 9 cm lateral and just caudad to the umbilicus (Fig. 16.2). The da Vinci robot is then positioned with its base either between the patient's legs (standard docking) or at an acute perpendicular angle near the base of the operative

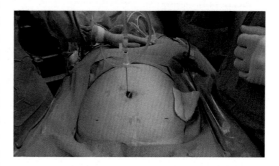

Fig. 16.1 Intraoperative photograph demonstrating initial periumbilical incision employed during reduced port and LESS ASC

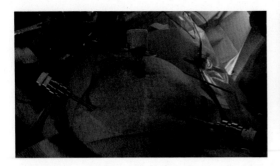

Fig. 16.2 Intraoperative photograph demonstrating port configuration for reduced port ASC. A 12 mm periumbilical port and two low-profile 5 mm robotic trocars have been placed

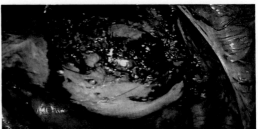

Fig. 16.4 Following initial dissection of the peritoneum over the vaginal apex, a plane is created anteriorly between the anterior aspect of the vaginal wall and the posterior aspect of the bladder

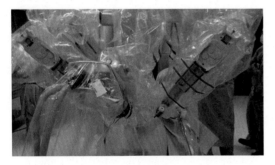

Fig. 16.3 Intraoperative photograph demonstrating docked position of robot for reduced port ASC

table (side dock). Many urologists will feel more comfortable with a standard docking approach given its ubiquity during male pelvic surgery (Fig. 16.3). However, side docking, commonly employed during benign gynecologic procedures, offers several distinct advantages during ASC including unfettered access to the vagina for manipulation and anatomic guidance. With a reduced port approach, side docking does not compromise ergonomics including instrument clashing and access to the deep pelvis. However, our experience with side docking during pure LESS ASC has been riddled with unique ergonomic challenges beyond those typically seen with the reduced port technique. We strongly advocate standard docking with pure LESS ASC.

Once the robot has been docked, we insert a "right-handed" 5 mm monopolar "paddle" and a "left-handed" grasping forceps. Identification of relevant pelvic anatomy ensues including the elimination of often-inevitable pelvic adhesions.

The Foley catheter is manipulated to clearly demarcate the limits of the bladder and the vaginal manipulator is employed to define the apex of the vagina. The sigmoid colon is reflected to the left side of the patient to accentuate the sacral promontory. To facilitate lateral traction on the sigmoid colon, we prefer to use a percutaneously placed 0-silk suture that is placed judiciously in a figure-of-eight fashion through the pedunculated fat of the sigmoid colon or taenia coli.

Dissection is carried onto the anterior surface of the vagina following hysterectomy. Thus far, we have not been able to perform concomitant supracervical hysterectomy with a reduced port approach given limitations associated with exclusive use of 5 mm instruments (tissue-sealing devices/clip appliers). In general, blunt dissection with pinpoint cautery nicely sweeps the bladder anteriorly off the surface of the vagina. This dissection is carried down to the approximate level of the trigone (Fig. 16.4). Again, manipulation of the Foley catheter can help reconcile these landmarks. The posterior peritoneum is then dissected off the cervical stump/posterior vagina and carried distally toward to the rectovaginal pouch. In general, the initial dissection can be very indistinct, but with further progress, a very nice areolar plane avails itself down to the presumed level of the perineal body. Again, a savvy bedside assistant can help confirm the approximate level of posterior dissection.

The sacral promontory is then palpated and the retroperitoneum opened at the level of its "drop-off." Typically, the promontory is readily

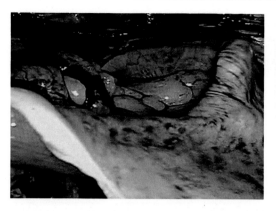

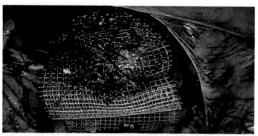

Fig. 16.6 A Y-shaped polypropylene mesh is affixed to the anterior and posterior aspects of the vagina using interrupted 0-Vicryl suture. Sutures are thrown in a full-thickness manner

Fig. 16.5 The retroperitoneum over the sacral promontory is incised and the anterior longitudinal ligament exposed. A retroperitoneal tunnel is created from the level of the sacral promontory down to the posterior aspect of the vagina

apparent in all but the most obese of patients. A bedside assistant can remove a 5 mm robotic instrument and temporarily place a conventional laparoscopic instrument to definitively palpate the sacral promontory. In our experience, however, "learned tactile feedback" with the robot makes identification straightforward. The anterior longitudinal ligament is clearly defined and a retroperitoneal tunnel created from the level of the sacral promontory down the length of the posterior cul-de-sac to meet with the previously created peritoneotomy over the posterior aspect of the vagina (Fig. 16.5). Alternatively, the retroperitoneum can be opened down the length of the posterior pelvis. While creating a retroperitoneal tunnel hastens reconstruction later in the case, its development in a reduced port or LESS fashion can be frustrating. Moreover, with the availability of barbed suture, the reconstruction of the incised peritoneum can be performed quickly. If a tunnel is not created, one must be cognizant of the right ureter and must avoid its entrapment during closure.

The robotic camera is then temporarily removed and a prefashioned Y-shaped polypropylene mesh introduced in a direct but blinded fashion. We typically trim our mesh to 6–7 cm anteriorly and posteriorly, but this is highly dependent on patient-specific anatomy. The mesh is introduced and subsequently affixed to the anterior and posterior aspects of the vagina using a series of 0-Vicryl sutures (Fig. 16.6). Typically, six sutures are placed both anteriorly and posteriorly in three rows of two sutures each. Using a reduced port configuration without an assistant port can make this step of the procedure very tedious in that the camera must be exchanged for sutures and the right-handed needle driver must be exchanged for scissors. Likewise, needle retrieval can be tedious and has, at times, required use of a standard laparoscopic 5 mm camera or flexible-tipped fiber-optic scope such that needles may be safely extracted. One may also consider fixing the graft to the vagina using a barbed suture in a "switchback" fashion. The flexibility of the barbed suture obviates repetitive suture exchange.

Following mesh fixation to the cervical stump/vagina, the tail of the graft is brought out through the previously created retroperitoneal tunnel (or up to the level of the promontory if the retroperitoneum was split). The tail of the graft is affixed to the anterior longitudinal ligament using two interrupted 0-Ethibond sutures. Care must be taken to apply appropriate but not undue tension when reducing the vaginal apex externally. Overtightening of the graft fails to account for inevitable mesh contracture and potential vaginal foreshortening.

Once the graft has been adequately positioned, the retroperitoneum is closed over the vagina and sacrum using a running barbed suture of choice (Figs. 16.7 and 16.8). We find this technique again provides secure coverage of the graft with a modicum of frustration.

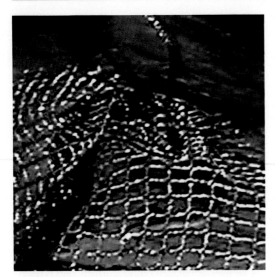

Fig. 16.7 The retroperitoneum is closed to exclude the graft entirely from the peritoneal cavity

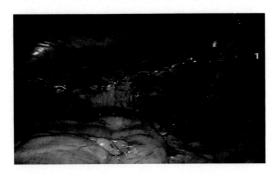

Fig. 16.8 Using a barbed suture, the anterior and posterior vaginal flaps are closed to fully cover and re-retroperitonealize the Y-shaped graft

Ports are removed under direct vision following release of the colonic traction suture. The midline 12 mm incision is closed using a 0-Vicryl suture in a meticulous fashion. Skin incisions are then closed in a subcuticular fashion.

The patient is then converted to the exaggerated lithotomy position and a thorough vaginal examination performed to assess for apical support. Often, a distal rectocele will be inadequately addressed abdominally and will require primary vaginal repair at this stage. Cystoscopy is likewise performed to ensure ureteral efflux and integrity of the bladder. If mid-urethral sling is planned, this is performed at this time. A Foley catheter is replaced as well as an estrogen-soaked vaginal pack.

The patient is admitted to the hospital for a 23-h observation and ambulated that evening. A regular diet is ordered. Laboratory testing is unnecessary. The vaginal pack and catheter are removed the next morning and the patient is discharged home by noon the following day. Patients are instructed to avoid heavy lifting (>15 lb) and sexual intercourse for a minimum of 4 weeks. A stool softener is prescribed to avoid postoperative constipation.

Surgical Technique: LESS Sacral Colpopexy

In many respects, LESS ASC mimics the aforementioned surgical steps of reduced port ASC. As previously stated, some aspects of ASC are made easier by employing a multichannel port with more flexibility as opposed to 5 mm trocars alone. These advantages are most readily apparent when and if supracervical hysterectomy is performed. Suture exchange, in particular, is significantly easier using a multichannel port platform. The obvious and unavoidable pitfall with LESS ASC then becomes the disproportionate amount of reconstruction/suturing required in an in-line fashion. Fortunately, the bedside assistant can often manipulate the vagina toward the instruments to ease instrument clashing and facilitate precise needle placement.

Patient preparation and positioning are identical to that previously described. An approximate 12 mm incision is made on the inner curve of the umbilicus and dissection carried down to the rectus fascia. The fascia is scored with electrocautery and the peritoneum directly entered. Depending on the multichannel platform chosen, the fasciotomy is extended to accommodate port placement. In general, we prefer to use a low-profile multichannel port for pure LESS ASC without supracervical hysterectomy and the larger-profile GelPoint when supracervical hysterectomy is planned (given the need for specimen extraction). Often, postmenopausal women will have a relatively small uterus that can still be extracted through a lower-profile fascial opening.

Once the port has been positioned, the robot is docked between the patient's legs and a standard 30-degree robotic trocar placed through the larger and more "superiorly" positioned channel. A combination of 5 mm and possibly 8 mm robotic instruments can be inserted depending on surgeon preference. We have likewise previously placed an additional 5 mm or 8 mm trocar adjacent to the multichannel port through a separate fascial stab incision to re-create an element of triangulation.

Similar to reduced port ASC, restoration and identification of normal anatomy represent the first step. Likewise, a percutaneously placed retraction suture is placed to expose the sacral promontory. The steps of the operation thereafter follow those as described above. Unique to pure LESS ASC include easier suture and mesh delivery into the abdomen and particular difficulty in accurate suture placement at the level of the sacral promontory. Unlike the vagina that can be manipulated into the operative field, the sacrum remains fixed and precise suture placement in a longitudinal fashion can be tedious. Likewise, knot-tying at the sacrum with an easily frayed Ethibond suture can be frustrating.

Conclusions

The volume of patients with symptomatic pelvic organ prolapse is growing and the demand for durable surgical correction is likewise expected to grow. ASC represents the surgical approach with the highest degree of durability and its popularity is expected to grow given recent fear regarding the vaginal placement of synthetic mesh. Laparoscopic and robotic ASC are now considered the preferred treatment options for women with high-grade and/or apical relaxation. Those surgeons comfortable with these techniques should confidently consider reduced port and LESS ASC in select patients to further minimize the morbidity of these procedures and to further optimize cosmesis.

References

1. Maher C, Baessler K, Glazener CM, et al. Surgical management of pelvic organ prolapse in women. Cochrane Database Syst Rev. 2007;(3);CD004014.
2. Nygaard IE, McCreery R, Brubaker L, et al. Abdominal sacrocolpopexy: a comprehensive review. Obstet Gynecol. 2004;104:805–23.
3. Geller EJ, Siddiqui NY, Wu JM, et al. Short-term outcomes of robotic sacrocolpopexy compared with abdominal sacrocolpopexy. Obstet Gynecol. 2008;112:1201–6.
4. McDermott CD, Hale DS. Abdominal, laparoscopic, and robotic surgery for pelvic organ prolapse. Obstet Gynecol Clin N Am. 2009;36:585–614.
5. Pollard ME, Eilber KS, Anger JT. Abdominal approaches to pelvic organ prolapse repairs. Curr Opin Urol. 2013;23:306–11.
6. Autorino R, White WM, Gettman MT, et al. Public perception of "scarless" surgery: a critical analysis of the literature. Urology. 2012;80:495–502.
7. White WM, Goel RK, Swartz MA, Moore C, Rackley RR, Kaouk JH. Single-port laparoscopic abdominal sacral colpopexy: initial experience and comparative outcomes. Urology. 2009;74:1008–12.
8. Kaouk JH, Autorino R, Kim FJ, Han DH, Lee SW, et al. Laparoendoscopic single-site urologic surgery in urology: worldwide multi-institutional analysis of 1076 cases. Eur Urol. 2011;60:998–1005.

Transvesical LESS Applications

17

Rene J. Sotelo Noguera,
Luciano A. Nuñez Bragayrac,
and Marino Cabrera Fierro

Introduction

Since its first description in 2007 by Rane et al. [1], laparoendoscopic single site surgery (LESS) has evolved, from the initial concept to the design of many new technologies and instruments. LESS access can be obtained either by performing a single skin and fascial incision through which a single multichannel access platform is placed (single port) or by placing several low-profile ports through separate fascial incisions (single site). Nowadays LESS in the urological field can be performed in any of the organ systems that we manage surgically including the kidney, ureter, bladder, and prostate.

In 2003, Olsen et al. [2] performed a pilot animal model in pigs and found that under carbon dioxide insufflation of the bladder at around 10 mmHg pressure, a large potential working space was obtained that allows various intravesi-

cal procedures. This was named "pneumovesicum." They performed a Cohen cross-trigonal ureteral reimplantation, using standard laparoscopic instruments.

Two years later, Yeung et al. [3], based on the work of Olsen, reported a novel technique of ureteral reimplantation in ten boys and six girls with vesicoureteral reflux (VUR), after the creation of pneumovesicum with Cohen's technique. The procedure was preceded by distention of the bladder with saline and insertion of a 5-mm Step port over the bladder dome under cystoscopic guidance. The bladder was then drained and insufflated with CO_2 to 10–12 mmHg pressure with a suction catheter inserted per urethra to occlude the internal urethral meatus. A 5-mm 30° endoscope was used to provide intravesical vision. Two more 3- to 5-mm working ports with balloons at the tip were inserted on the lateral bladder wall on either side, with the disadvantage of leaving multiple open holes after the surgery. At follow-up they reported a success rate of 96 % and the only complication was subcutaneous pelvic emphysema in two boys that resolved spontaneously. In this first clinical experience, the investigators used the bladder as a potential working space with the creation of the "pneumovesicum" and minimally invasive surgical techniques.

In this chapter we will describe the transvesical LESS approach to different pathologies, including some initial reports. In 2008, Desai

R.J. Sotelo Noguera, MD (✉)
Robotics and Minimal Invasive Surgery, Urology
Department, Instituto Medico La Floresta, Caracas,
Venezuela
e-mail: renesotelo@mac.com

L.A. Nuñez Bragayrac, MD • M. Cabrera Fierro, MD
Robotics and Minimal Invasive Surgery,
Urology Department, Instituto Medico La Floresta,
Caracas, Venezuela
e-mail: lucianonb@yahoo.com;
cabreramarino@gmail.com

© Springer Science+Business Media New York 2017
J.H. Kaouk et al. (eds.), *Atlas of Laparoscopic and Robotic Single Site Surgery*,
Current Clinical Urology, DOI 10.1007/978-1-4939-3575-8_17

et al. [4] described for the first time the use of this approach in three patients with benign prostatic hyperplasia. In the so-called single-port transvesical enucleation of the prostate (STEP), the R-Port device was introduced percutaneously into the bladder through a 2.5-cm incision. After establishing pneumovesicum, the adenoma was enucleated in its entirety transvesically and was extracted through a single incision in the bladder and skin. This represents an important evolution from the technique initially reported in 2003, which was limited by the fact that multiple punctures were left open. This new approach reported in 2008 allowed one single-site incision and the possibility to work in combination with a transurethral instrument.

After this pioneering report, several other publications reported on successful transvesical procedures. In 2009 Desai et al. [5] updated their previous work with a multiinstitutional series of 34 patients, and all were technically successful in achieving complete enucleation of the adenoma using STEP. Digital assistance to complete adenoma enucleation was used in 19 (55 %) patients, and a suprapubic tube was inserted in 20 (57 %). There were complications during STEP in three patients (one death in a Jehovah's Witness who refused blood transfusion, one enterotomy, and one bleeding), as well as five late complications after STEP (four bleeding, one UTI).

Ingber et al. [6] presented two cases of female patients with lower urinary tract symptoms with eroded mesh into the bladder. They used a TriPort® single-site access system that was placed transvesically and carbon dioxide was used for insufflation of the bladder. A combination of straight and articulating laparoscopic instruments was used to dissect the mesh away from the bladder mucosa and transect each end for complete removal of the foreign body.

Sotelo et al. [7] described a case of an 80-year-old male patient with transitional cell carcinoma in the left renal pelvis, in whom we performed a radical nephroureterectomy with transvesical LESS mobilization of the distal ureter. The defect was closed with intracorporeal suturing with an extracorporeal knot, and there were no complications.

Roslan et al. [8] reported a left transvesical LESS ureteroneocystostomy in a 39-year-old female patient with grade V bilateral VUR, after a previous successful right extravesical Lich-Gregoire using laparoscopic technique. After creating pneumovesicum, they used a TriPort access system with a single incision. After the procedure, the left hydronephrosis was decreased significantly, and diuretic renography revealed no reflux or obstruction. At 16-month follow-up, the ultrasound showed no hydronephrosis. This was the first report of VUR treatment using transvesical LESS in an adult.

Using the same technique, Roslan [9] reported the case of a 72-year-old woman with a previous hysterectomy for benign disease. Physical exam showed a 3-mm wide fistula between the bladder trigone and the upper part of vaginal vault. After establishing pneumovesicum, they used a TriPort+® access system to repair the vesicovaginal fistulae (VVF). During 4 months' follow-up, they reported no recurrence of the fistula.

Roslan [10] also explored the transvesical LESS technique for diverticulectomy in two male patients with recurrent UTIs and one male patient with a noninvasive low-grade urothelial tumor within a diverticulum following a previous unsuccessful attempt at transurethral resection. Interestingly, when they dissected the diverticular wall and had difficulty getting sufficient traction on it, they introduced a grasper transurethrally to help with the traction. This did not result in any gas leak and no other complications were reported.

Following the STEP procedure of Desai, this group [11] reported the feasibility of robotic LESS (R-LESS) using a transvesical approach in two cadavers, one with multiple ports and another one with a single port. Fareed et al. [12] described their first experience of robotic STEP (R-STEP). In their nine cases, a modification of the original STEP technique was made. First, a transurethral incision of the prostatic urethra was performed cystoscopically at the apex using a Collin's knife. Second, a Gelport was used instead of a TriPort access system. A 12-mm trocar and two 5-mm trocars were placed, the pneumovesicum was created with CO2 set to 20 mmHg, and the DaVinci surgical system was docked. The rest of

Table 17.1 Transvesical LESS procedures

Author	Year	Procedure	# of patient(s)	Single-port device	Complications
Desai	2008	Adenomectomy	03	R-Port	Bowel injury (01)
Desai	2009	Adenomectomy	34	TriPort (30)/ QuadPort (4)	Death (01), bowel injury (01), hemorrhage (01)
Sotelo	2010	Bladder cuff	01	R-Port	–
Roslan	2012	Ureteroneocystostomy	01	TriPort	–
Roslan	2012	Vesicovaginal fistulae	01	TriPort	–
Roslan	2012	Diverticulectomy	02	TriPort	–
Fareed	2012	Robotic adenomectomy	09	GelPort	Hemorrhage (02), DVT (01), UTI (01), MI (01)
Gao	2013	Radical prostatectomy	16	QuaPort	–

DVT deep venous thrombosis, *UTI* urinary tract infection, *MI* myocardial infarction

the procedure was similar to the previous work. Despite being technically feasible and providing adequate relief of bladder outlet obstruction, the procedure was associated with a high risk of complications including gross hematuria requiring blood transfusion, UTI, and myocardial infarction with ICU admission.

More recently, Gao et al. [13] described 16 patients with organ-confined prostate cancer in whom they performed transvesical LESS radical prostatectomy in an anterograde fashion with no intraoperative complications. With a follow-up of 24 months, they reported no biochemical recurrences, as well as good sexual function in 75 % of patients, and total continence in all patients after 3 months. Their technique of pneumovesicum creation was similar to other authors' work.

In the next chapter, we will focus on the pneumovesicum development, bladder cuff excision for radical nephroureterectomy, and adenomectomy (see Table 17.1 for a summary of published series).

Indications

In selected patients such as those with previous surgery, a transvesical approach may be beneficial because of its minimally invasive nature by entering directly into the organ (the bladder), thereby avoiding adhesions and inadvertent

injuries. Many types of procedures can be performed transvesically ranging from simple prostatectomy to bladder cuff excision, ureteroneocystostomy, diverticulotomy, fistulae repair, and radical prostatectomy, although it is imperative for the surgeon to have expertise in this approach.

Contraindications

- Anticoagulation therapy
- Anesthetic contraindication
- Urethral stenosis
- Previous radiotherapy
- Contraindications for each individual surgery: bladder tumor for management of the distal ureter

Pneumovesicum Creation

Step 1: Patient Positioning and Multiport Insertion (Fig. 17.1)

First the patient is placed in supine position, with the legs together or abducted. The type of cystoscope (flexible or rigid) and position of the surgical team depend on the procedure being performed. Flexible cystoscopy may be performed up front to evaluate the urethra, bladder,

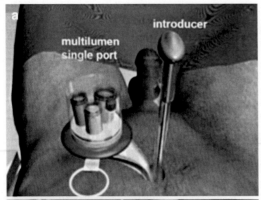

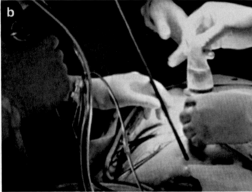

Fig. 17.1 (**a**) View of the TriPort with introducer. (**b**) Surgeon showing the outer ring of the TriPort (From Laparoscopic and Robot-Assisted Surgery in Urology: Atlas of Standard Procedures, Chapter 3 Urinary Bladder and Prostate, 2011, p. 294, René Sotelo, Camilo Giedelman, Mihir Desai; Fig. Step2. With kind permission of Springer Science+Business Media)

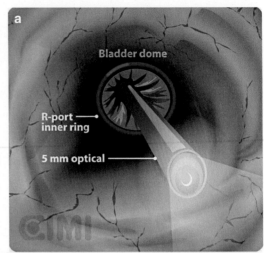

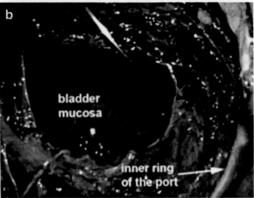

Fig. 17.2 (**a**) Inside view from the bladder of the TriPort at the bladder dome. (**b**) Outside view of the TriPort's ring (From Laparoscopic and Robot-Assisted Surgery in Urology: Atlas of Standard Procedures, Chapter 3 Urinary Bladder and Prostate, 2011, p. 295, René Sotelo, Camilo Giedelman, Mihir Desai; Fig. Step3b. With kind permission of Springer Science+Business Media)

and possible point of insertion of the multiport. The bladder is then filled with 400 cc of normal saline through a cystoscope or a urethral catheter, enough to elevate the bladder dome into the space of Retzius. A 2.5-cm skin incision is made just above the pubis down to the rectus fascia muscle; the bladder is identified and cleared of perivesical fat (Fig. 17.1a). The inner ring of the multiport is preloaded onto an introducer, which is then inserted into the bladder under cystoscopic assistance. We recommend placing two stitches before insertion of the multiport into the bladder to help with countertraction (Fig. 17.1b). Despite our experience with a different multiport, we recommend using either the TriPort®, QuadPort®, or GelPoint®.

Step 2: Creation of the Pneumovesicum (Fig. 17.2)

After the inner ring is introduced into the bladder, excess saline is suctioned out. The inner and outer rings are approximated by removing the slack on the plastic sleeve, thus cinching the abdominal and bladder wall between the rings of the R-Port in an airtight seal (Fig. 17.2). The valve of the multiport is inserted, and the bladder is insufflated with carbon dioxide to a pressure of 15 mmHg to create the pneumovesicum. The previously placed sutures can be used to close the defect at the end of the procedure and facilitate the introduction of the multiport.

Bladder Cuff Management

Step 3: Identification and Incision of Ureteral Meatus (Fig. 17.3)

After the multiport is placed in supine position, the patients are repositioned to a lateral decubitus position, which is important because the bleeding, the irrigation, and the urine would be kept at the opposite, without vision obstruction of the worked ureter; pneumovesicum is established and a 5-mm deflectable EndoEye® is introduced into the bladder through the multiport. The ureteral opening is identified, and we mark the bladder cuff with monopolar electrocautery (Figs. 17.3a, b). The next step is full-thickness bladder cuff incision, and proceeding with progressive mobilization of the distal ureter into the bladder with a grasper (Fig. 17.3c), a 5-mm Hem-o-lok is used to close the ureter.

Step 4: Sealing of the Bladder Defect (Fig. 17.4)

Then, we seal the bladder defect using intracorporeal suturing with extracorporeal knot ligation. An alternative to seal the bladder defect is to use a V-Loc™ closure suture in a running fashion: with the first stitch, the suture loop is extracorporeal; the needle is exteriorized and passed into the loop which is used as an anchor into the bladder. With one hand, we maintain extracorporeal traction and continue up with the stitch (Fig. 17.4). At this point, after checking for any bleeding or leaks, we remove the multiport, and close the bladder defect with the previously placed stitches, and continue with radical nephroureterectomy using standard laparoscopy.

Adenomectomy

Step 3: Incision of Bladder Mucosa (Fig. 17.3d)

After the pneumovesicum is established, careful observation of the ureteral orifices is done before bladder incision. With a monopolar hook, a U-shaped incision is made over the adenoma between the 3 o'clock and 9 o'clock position (Fig. 17.3d). Dissection is done until a whitish prostatic adenoma is observed. The correct dissection plane can be created with monopolar or ultrasonic scalpel and suction cannula movements.

The adenoma can be mobilized via a medial incision. This maneuver provides superior visualization of the adenoma.

Step 4: Enucleation of the Adenoma (Sotelo Prostatotomy Device) (Fig. 17.5)

The Sotelo prostatotomy laparoscopic device is used to facilitate the enucleation, mimicking finger or digital enucleation (Fig. 17.5a). This device is similar to a curette or an osteotome. The metallic curvilinear tip has a sharp cold knife on the distal side used to dissect the margin between the adenoma and the capsule (Fig. 17.5b). This instrument provides efficient and precise dissection of the adenoma. It is important to put a stitch on the adenoma or median lobe, which could be exteriorized, to create countertraction and facilitate mobilization of the adenoma.

Step 4.1: Finger Enucleation of the Adenoma and Transurethral Apical Incision

This method permits the insertion of the right index finger through the port. The multiport valve must be removed. This maneuver permits enucleation of the distal part of prostate. The left index finger is placed into the rectum to elevate the prostate.

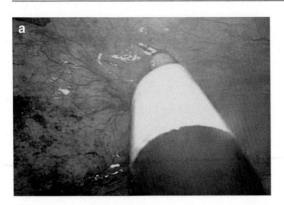

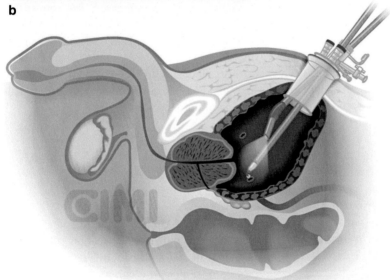

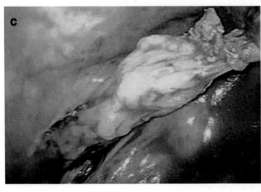

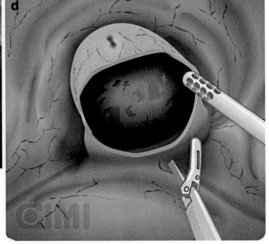

Fig. 17.3 (**a**) Bladder mucosa marked with electrocautery around ureteral orifice. (**b**) Bladder mucosa marked with electrocautery around ureteral orifice. (**c**) Mobilization of distal ureter inside the bladder. (**d**) Dissection of adenoma with suction

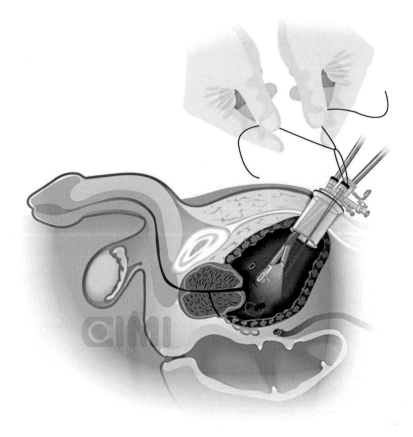

Fig. 17.4 Sealing the bladder defect with braided suture

Finally the multiport valve is reattached and the pneumovesicum is reestablished. The procedure finishes with the dissection of the urethra at the prostatic apex. In order to facilitate the incision of the urethra, a bipolar resectoscope can be used before any dissection from the cephalic direction.

Step 5: Hemostasis (Fig. 17.6)

Obtaining good hemostasis is the most important step after removal of the adenoma (Fig. 17.6a), which can be done with an extracorporeal knot or barber suture. The stiches are made at the 4 and 8 o'clock positions of the prostatic capsule in order to control the main prostatic arteries and vessels (Fig. 17.6b). The best maneuver for minor bleeding is identifying the correct dissection plane. During the initial learning curve, we recommended checking the lateral pedicles and decreas-

ing the pressure of pneumovesicum to confirm there is no active bleeding. Minor bleeding of the capsule can be controlled with monopolar hook or bipolar cautery.

Step 6: Trigonization and Closure of the Bladder (Fig. 17.7)

Extraction of prostatic adenoma is done prior to trigonization through the multiport device ring, and manual morcellation with Allis forceps can help to reduce the size of the prostatic adenoma (Fig. 17.7a).

Trigonization of the prostatic fossa is performed with running sutures from the posterior segment of the bladder neck stump to the apex of the prostatic fossa. Before trigonization, it is important to confirm that hemostasis is adequate (Fig. 17.7b). Extracorporeal knots can be used, and we recommend barbed suture 2/0.

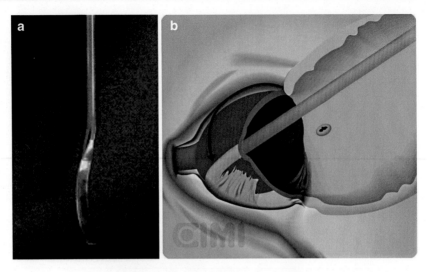

Fig. 17.5 (a) "Sotelo protostome" (From Laparoscopic and Robot-Assisted Surgery in Urology: Atlas of Standard Procedures, Chapter 3 Urinary Bladder and Prostate, 2011, p. 296, René Sotelo, Camilo Giedelman, Mihir Desai; Fig. Step5a. With kind permission of Springer Science+Business Media). (b) Dissection of adenoma with Sotelo protostome

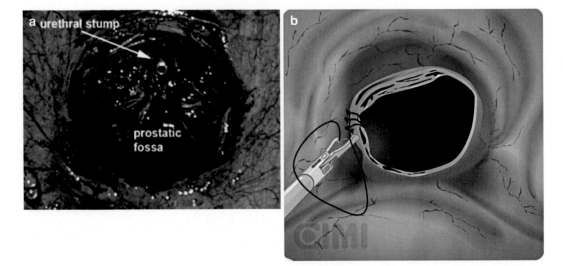

Fig. 17.6 (a) View of the prostate fossa previous "trigonization" (From Laparoscopic and Robot-Assisted Surgery in Urology: Atlas of Standard Procedures, Chapter 3 Urinary Bladder and Prostate, 2011, p. 296, René Sotelo, Camilo Giedelman, Mihir Desai; Fig. Step6a. With kind permission of Springer Science+Business Media). (b).Hemostasis with extracorporeal knot pusher

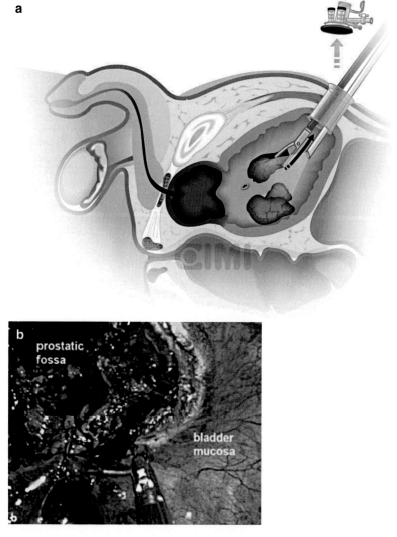

Fig. 17.7 (**a**) Extraction of adenoma through the TriPort. (**b**) Trigonization of the bladder inside the prostate fossa (From Laparoscopic and Robot-Assisted Surgery in Urology: Atlas of Standard Procedures, Chapter 3 Urinary Bladder and Prostate, 2011, p. 297, René Sotelo, Camilo Giedelman, Mihir Desai; Fig. Step8b. With kind permission of Springer Science+Business Media)

Step 7: Suprapubic and Urethral Catheter Insertion (Fig. 17.8)

Before bladder closure, place a 14 French drain laterally through the inner ring of the multiport device, or a suprapubic catheter can be inserted through the inner ring of the TriPort (Fig. 17.8a). The balloon should be inflated before the TriPort is removed. The ring of the TriPort is large enough to pass the distal part of the catheter. An indwelling 20 French 3-way catheter is also placed (Fig. 17.8b). Prior to removing the internal ring of the multiport device, it is important to ensure the correct placement of the catheter inside the bladder. Stay sutures of the bladder wall can be tied along with additional absorbable sutures, providing a watertight closure. The rectus fascia and skin are then closed in a standard fashion.

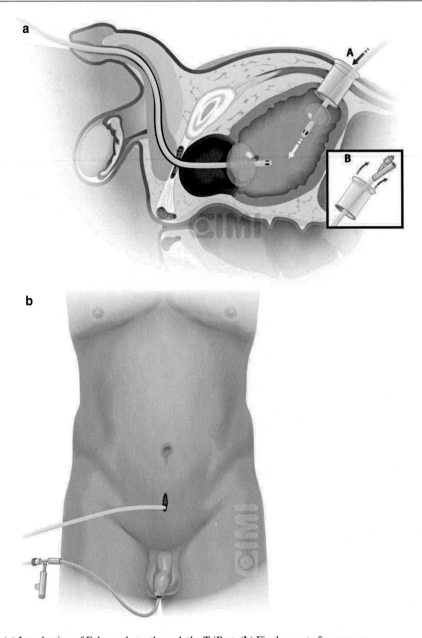

Fig. 17.8 (**a**) Introduction of Foley catheter through the TriPort. (**b**) Final aspect after surgery

Conclusion

Laparoendoscopic single-site transvesical surgery has many applications in urology. In the last few years, many different procedures have been reported using this technique: prostatic adenomectomy, radical prostatec-tomy, diverticulectomy, vesicovaginal repair, etc. However, most of these studies are case reports and the expertise of the surgeon is a critical factor. Additional studies are necessary with more subjects and with further follow-up.

References

1. Rane A, Kommu S, Eddy B, et al. Clinical evaluation of a novel laparoscopic port (R-port) and evolution of the single laparoscopic port procedure (SLiPP). J Endourol. 2007;21 Suppl 1:A22–3.
2. Olsen LH, Deding D, Yeung CK, Jorgensen TM. Computer assisted laparoscopic pneumovesical ureter reimplantation a.m. Cohen: initial experience in a pig model. APMIS. 2003;Suppl 109:23–25.
3. Yeung C, Sihoe J, Borzi P. Endoscopic cross-trigonal reimplantation under carbon dioxide bladder insufflation: a novel technique. J Endourol. 2005;19(3):295–9.
4. Desai M, Aron M, Canes D, et al. Single-port transvesical simple prostatectomy: initial clinical report. Urology. 2008;72:960–5.
5. Desai M, Fareed K, Berger A, et al. Single-port transvesical enucleation of the prostate: a clinical report of 34 cases. BJU Int. 2010;105(9):1296–300.
6. Ingber M, Stein R, Rackley R, et al. Single-port transvesical excision of foreign body in the bladder. Urology. 2009;74(6):1347–50.
7. Sotelo R, Ramirez D, Carmona O, et al. A novel technique for distal ureterectomy and bladder cuff excision. Actas Urol Esp. 2011;35(3):168–74.
8. Roslan M, Markuszewski MM, Kłącz J, et al. Laparoendoscopic single-site transvesical ureteroneocystostomy for vesicoureteral reflux in an adult: a one year follow-up. Urology. 2012;80(3):719–23.
9. Roslan M, Markuszewski MM, Baginska J, et al. Suprapubic transvesical laparoendoscopic single-site surgery for vesicovaginal fistula repair: a case report. Videosurgery Miniinv. 2012;7(4):307–10.
10. Roslan M, Markuszewski MM, Kłącz J, et al. Laparoendoscopic single-port transvesical diverticulectomy: preliminary clinical experience. J Endourol. 2012;26(8):975–9.
11. Desai M, Aron M, Berger A, et al. Transvesical robotic radical prostatectomy. BJU Int. 2008;102(11):1666–9.
12. Fareed K, Zaytoun OM, Autorino R, et al. Robotic single port suprapubic transvesical enucleation of the prostate (R-STEP): initial experience. BJU Int. 2012;110(5):732–7.
13. Gao X, Pang J, Si-tu J, et al. Single-port transvesical laparoscopic radical prostatectomy for organ-confined prostate cancer: techniques and outcomes. BJU Int. 2013;112(7):944–52.

Mini-Laparoscopic Surgery and Hybrid LESS

Francesco Porpiglia and Cristian Fiori

Introduction

In the last years, the availability of instruments equal or less than 3 mm in size and the development of mini-scopes have boosted the "rediscovery" of mini-laparoscopic and needlescopic surgery [1, 2]. These instruments represent the evolution and sophistication of conventional laparoscopy towards the minimisation of trauma-related access and, theoretically, towards decreasing of surgical morbidity.

It is with the same purpose that other innovative laparoscopic techniques such as NOTES (natural orifice transluminal endoscopic surgery) and LESS (laparo-endoscopic single-site surgery) have been proposed [3, 4]. Whilst NOTES procedures are still having a limited impact in clinical practice [5, 6], LESS procedures have been more often adopted in tertiary care centres [7, 8]. However, the LESS approach is difficult and time-consuming so that additional ports are frequently required [9].

In this chapter, we describe the most commonly performed mini-laparoscopic procedures, and we discuss the role of mini-laparoscopy as an adjunct to LESS (i.e. mini hybrid LESS).

Definition

Unfortunately, there has been limited consensus on what terminology should be used, and it has not been determined which number or combination of these miniaturised instruments is required to qualify a procedure as "mini-laparoscopic".

In this chapter, we define "mini-laparoscopic" instruments as being 3 mm in size and needlescopic instruments as those less than 3 mm in size (2-mm instruments are the most commonly used). Thus, we define as "mini-laparoscopic" a procedure in which all the operative ports allocate 3-mm instruments and one standard (5- or 10-mm) port allocates scope or standard instruments whenever necessary. Moreover, this port allows an improvement of carbon dioxide insufflation. When possible, in case of transperitoneal procedure, this last port is placed at the level of umbilicus in order to maintain the ideal concept of "scarless surgery" without compromising the safety of the procedures.

Moreover, we defined "mini hybrid LESS", a procedure in which a multiport device and two or more planned mini-ports are used.

F. Porpiglia, MD (✉) • C. Fiori
Division of Urology, Department of Oncology,
School of Medicine-University of Turin,
"San Luigi" Hospital, Regione Gonzole 10,
Orbassano, Turin 10043, Italy
e-mail: porpiglia@libero.it

© Springer Science+Business Media New York 2017
J.H. Kaouk et al. (eds.), *Atlas of Laparoscopic and Robotic Single Site Surgery*,
Current Clinical Urology, DOI 10.1007/978-1-4939-3575-8_18

Patient Selection

In general, beyond the indications related to the urological disease, we retain that the safety and the effectiveness of a given mini-laparoscopic procedure can be maximised by treating non-morbidly obese patients who did not previously undergo significant abdominal surgery.

Ports and Surgical Instruments

We routinely use Storz instrumentation (Karl Storz®, Tuttlingen, Germany). Alternative mini-laparoscopic and needlescopic sets are manufactured and commercially available. Our basic sets of mini-laparoscopic instruments and ports are illustrated in Figs. 18.1, 18.2 and18.3.

Ports 3.5-mm (inner diameter) ports 10 or 15 cm in length to use on the basis of patient habitus. All ports have a Luer-Lock connector for insufflation and a reusable silicone leaflet valve.

Scopes Straight Forward telescope 0°, enlarged view, diameter 3.3 mm, length 25 cm for retroperitoneoscopic procedures, and Forward-Oblique telescope 30°, enlarged view, diameter 3.3 mm, length 25 cm for transperitoneal procedures. A specific adaptor for scopes allows for telescope changing under sterile conditions.

Instruments All instruments are 3 mm in size and 36 cm in length. Basic set includes at least the following:

- Kelly dissecting and grasping forceps, with long, double-action jaws
- Grasping forceps, with fine atraumatic serration and fenestrated, single-action jaws
- Scissors, serrated, curved and conical, with irrigation connection for cleaning, double-action jaws
- Bipolar coagulating forceps
- Ultramicro needle holder, straight handle
- Suction and irrigation device with two-way stopcock connector

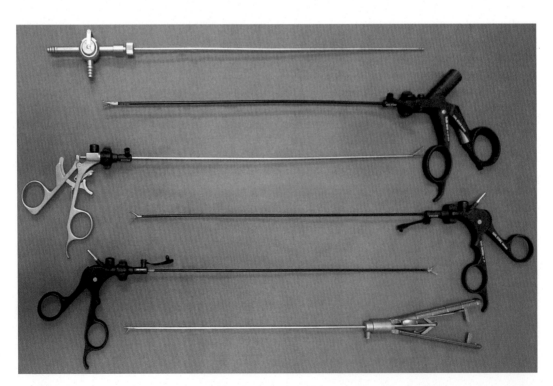

Fig. 18.1 3-mm instruments. From the *top* of the figure: suction device, bipolar forceps, grasping forceps and Kelly dissection forceps, scissors, and needle holder

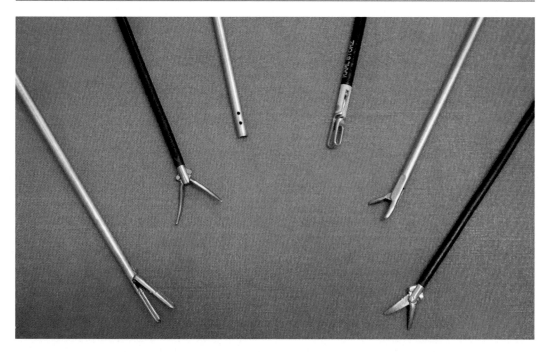

Fig. 18.2 Tips of 3-mm instruments. From the *left* of the figure: grasping forceps and Kelly dissection forceps, suction device, bipolar forceps, needle holder and scissors

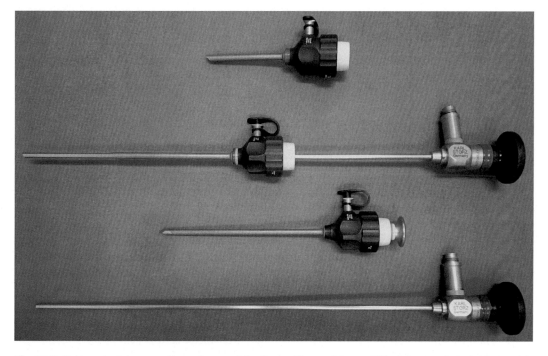

Fig. 18.3 Ports and mini-scopes. From the *top* of the figure: 10-cm mini-port, 30° mini-scope through 15-cm mini-port, 15-cm mini-port and trocar with pyramidal tip, 0° mini-scope

Many other instruments are available for specific surgical situations and according to surgeon's preferences.

Current Indications: Review of the Literature

Reconstructive Surgery

A few papers have been reported on mini-laparoscopic or needlescopic reconstructive surgery. In a retrospective analysis, Tsai et al. described a technique for ureteral reimplantation in patients with vesicoureteral reflux using a 3-mm port [10]. Nine patients were treated with mini-laparoscopic nerve-sparing extravesical ureteral reimplantation. The authors concluded that this approach was an effective and safe technique for primary vesicoureteral reflux, with a better cosmetic result (three 3.5-mm incisions) and faster recovery in comparison to the open surgical technique.

In a "milestone" paper on needlescopy, Gill and Soble reported on orchiopexy [11]. They treated five patients with cryptorchidism, all of the procedures were uneventful, and the patients were discharged on the same day of surgery.

An interesting field of application of mini-laparoscopy is pyeloplasty. Mini laparoscopic pyeloplasty has been studied in children by Tan who reported his experience using a 3-mm laparoscopic port and concluded that mL significantly enhances the ability to perform pyelo-ureteric "microanastomosis", reduces the postoperative pain and results in a "spectacular" postoperative cosmetic appearance [12].

More recently, Pini et al. presented their experience with small-incision access retroperitoneoscopic technique (SMART) pyeloplasty (p). The authors created the retroperitoneal space with a home-made 6-mm balloon trocar and used a 5-mm scope and two 3-mm instruments to perform pyeloplasty. They concluded that SMARTp is a safe procedure in experienced hands, providing better cosmetic results and faster drain removal and discharge compared to standard laparoscopic approach [13].

Extirpative Surgery

Different extirpative procedures have been performed with a mini-laparoscopic or needlescopic approach. In the previously cited paper [11], Soble and Gill reported five cases of nephrectomy, four cases of nephroureterectomy, five cases of orchiectomy in patients with cryptorchidism, three cases of pelvic lymph node dissection (LND), three cases of lymphocele and two cases of renal cyst marsupialisation. Conversion to conventional laparoscopy was recorded in only two cases, whilst conversion to open surgery was recorded in one case (pelvic LND) due to small bowel injury. The authors concluded that needlescopy is feasible and safe and may reduce postoperative pain, hospital stays and recovery time and may improve cosmesis.

Among the mini-laparoscopic or needlescopic extirpative procedures, adrenalectomy is the most frequently performed [2, 14, 15]. Recently, Liao et al. published the results of an interesting retrospective study that involved patients treated with transperitoneal needlescopic adrenalectomy for presumptively benign adrenal tumours <5 cm in size [16].

Surgical Interventions

Mini-Laparoscopic Transperitoneal Pyeloplasty (mLP)

Laparoscopic pyeloplasty (LP), a minimally invasive procedure with excellent functional results, has become the standard of care for ureteropelvic junction (UPJ) obstruction (UPJO) in centres with advanced laparoscopic expertise. We have already investigated the feasibility, the safety and the effectiveness of mLP in an adult population [17]; moreover, we have compared the results of standard and mLP concluding that mini-laparoscopy seems to improve postoperative outcomes and to allow better cosmetic results [18].

Herein, we describe left Anderson-Hynes mLP by using the transperitoneal approach.

- Standard indications: primary UPJ obstruction in young patient.
- Limits/contraindications: BMI >35; significant, previous abdominal surgery; multiple kidney stones; and narrow renal pelvis.
- Preoperative preparation is the same of standard laparoscopic procedure.

Instruments

Basic mini-laparoscopic set (as previously described) and standard laparoscopic set. Even if we do not do it routinely, consider two camera and laparoscopic vision systems, the first one for mini-scope and the second one for standard scope.

Surgical Technique

Patient Position and Placement of Ureteral Catheter

The patient is placed on flank position at a 45° angle towards the edge of the operative room table facing the surgeons. The legs are separated and protected with either pillow or foam mat; in women, the lower limb of the same side of the UPJ which is to be treated has to remain abducted to enable easier access to the vaginal vestibulum. The head and the neck are kept in neutral position whilst both arms are supported appropriately with armrests. The patient's thoracic and lumbar areas are supported in lateral position, and all pressure points are protected by foam mat. The table is broken at the level of the umbilicus by approximately 10–15°. Finally, light cohesive retention bandage is used to fix the patient to the table. Operating field includes the genitals.

Preliminary cystoscopy is carried out using a 17-Fr flexible cystoscope. Ureteral meatus is identified, a 0035″ guidewire is inserted up along the ureter and the cystoscope is then withdrawn.

Subsequently, a 6-Fr ureteral open-end stent is slid upwards along the guidewire for 15–20 cm. The wire is withdrawn, and a Foley catheter is positioned in the bladder to which the ureteral catheter is fixed. By this way, surgeon has a retrograde access to the excretory system during the intervention. Alternatively, pneumocystoscopy can be performed as previously described [19].

Port Placement

The pneumoperitoneum is induced using a Veress needle, and then the first port for the scope is positioned at the umbilicus to maximise cosmetic results. We routinely use a mini-port performing a "pure" mini-laparoscopic procedure; nevertheless, a 5-mm or 10-mm port can be placed at this level without compromising the cosmetic results. This standard port is very helpful to improve the insufflation flow and the quality of the laparoscopic vision. Moreover, this port, if necessary, can be used for placing Hem-o-lok clips (Weck Closure Systems, Research Triangle Park, North Carolina, USA) using a 3-mm scope through the mini-ports.

A standard port is placed at the umbilicus for 10-mm 30° scope. Two mini-ports are placed under direct vision along the hemiclavear line on the left and on the right of the mini-scope; the disposition of the three ports should form a triangle (Fig. 18.4).

Access to the Retroperitoneum

We describe a transmesocolic access [20]. The small bowel is pushed medially with caution and the left colonic flexure is lifted upwards. By this way, the left mesentero-colic space is exposed, becoming the operative field. This space is limited medially by the inferior mesenteric vein and laterally by the medial margin of the descending colon (Fig. 18.5). Sometimes, in thin patients, the ureter can be visualised through the peritoneum thanks to its peristalsis

Fig. 18.4 Patient position and ports' placement during left mLP. Note the ureteral catheter that allows a retrograde access to excretory system

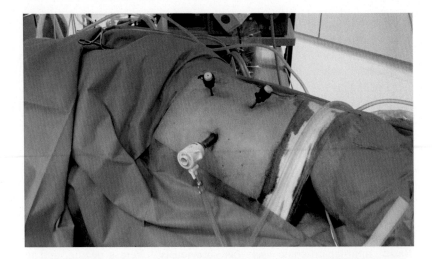

Fig. 18.5 Operative field in the initial step of mLP. *IMV* inferior mesenteric vein, *GV* gonadal vein, *DC* descending colon

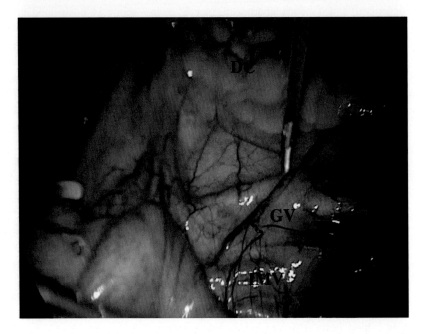

in this space; anyway, the most important landmark is represented by gonadal vein (Fig. 18.6). A 5-cm incision of the descending mesocolon is then made longitudinally, along the lateral border of the gonadal vein (Fig. 18.7). If the incision is performed at the level of the lumbar ureter, the gonadal vein and ureter run in a parallel fashion and close together (Fig. 18.8); when the incision is made more cranially, the ureter can be in a different direction, and the

identification of the ureter can be more difficult. Usually gonadal vein is respected but when limits operative field it can be coagulated with bipolar forceps (or secured and sectioned). Then, the incision can be cranially extended to create a peritoneal window allowing a direct access to the renal pelvis. In this phase, the left colic artery (or a branch of this) is visualised; sometimes, it makes difficult the dissection of the ureter but it should be preserved (Fig. 18.9).

Fig. 18.6 Operative field in the initial step of mLP, in a thin patient. *IMV* inferior mesenteric vein, *GV* gonadal vein, *DC* descending colon, *U* ureter

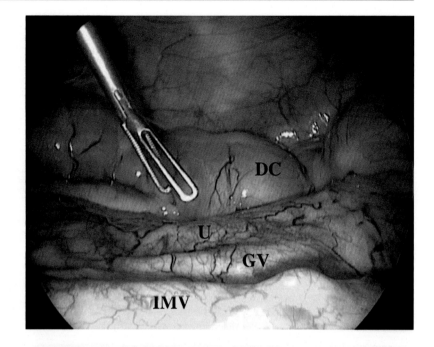

Fig. 18.7 Mesocolon incision is performed along the lateral margin of the gonadal vein. In this case, Hem-o-lok clip is used to displace the bowel. Hem-o-lok clips are placed through the umbilical port after the exchange of the scope (10–3 mm) and are removed at the end of the procedure

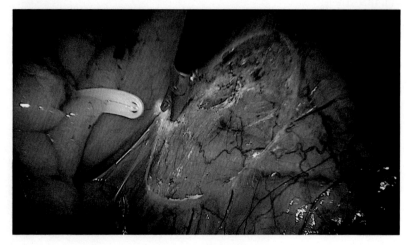

UPJ Dissection

UPJ is gently dissected from adherent tissues by blunt and sharp dissection avoiding energy source near the ureter (Fig. 18.10). In this phase, mini-laparoscopic technique requires a careful dissection and coagulation of all small vessels to prevent bleeding because a mini suction device is somewhat inefficient in case of significant bleeding.

Sometimes, an adjunctive mini-port placed just below the xyphoid is required to improve the quality of UPJ exposition. This manoeuvre allows a better visualisation of the UPJ and facilitates the UPJ dissection and further steps of the procedure (Fig. 18.11).

UPJ Resection and Spatulation of the Ureter

The UPJ is incised (Fig. 18.12) by using cold scissors. The ureter is spatulated laterally for 1–1.5 cm (depending on the pelvis incision) by using cold

Fig. 18.8 Mesocolon incision is extended cranially and retroperitoneum is reached. Note that at this level, ureter (*U*) and gonadal vein (*GV*) run in parallel fashion and close together

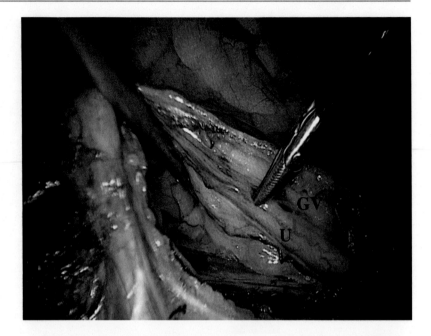

Fig. 18.9 The left colic artery (*CA*) is identified. It lies on the operative field and it should be preserved. Note that cranially to this artery, ureter and gonadal vein have different directions

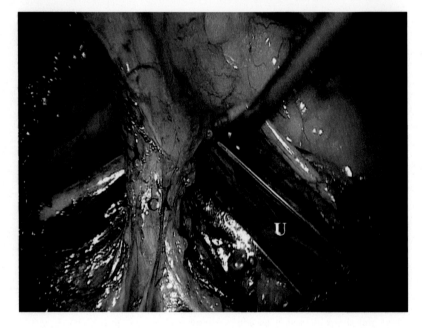

scissors (Fig. 18.13). Retrograde irrigation through the ureteral catheter can facilitate this step. Note that 3-mm scissors are more flexible than the other 3-mm instruments, and this makes sectioning and spatulating the ureter more difficult. Moreover, the quality of cutting of 3-mm scissors declines after a few procedures. In this phase, the UPJ can be left in place and it is manip-ulated with the forceps; by this way, neither the ureter nor the pelvis is grasped (Fig. 18.14).

Placement of First Stitch and Ureteropelvic Anastomosis

The anastomosis between pelvis and ureter is performed with a standard technique. The 3-mm needle holders are very efficient and

Fig. 18.10 UPJ and pelvis are gently dissected

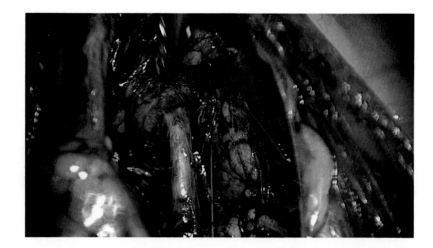

Fig. 18.11 The lower pole of the kidney is lifted up by a forceps that is introduced through an adjunctive mini-port (*). This manoeuvre allows a better visualisation of the UPJ and facilitates the next steps of the procedure

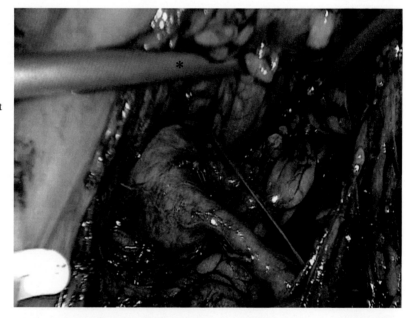

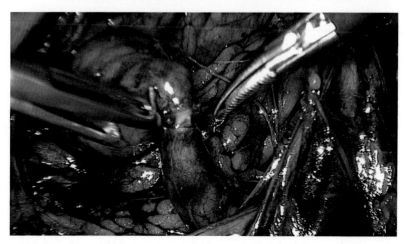

Fig. 18.12 UPJ is incised by using cold scissors

Fig. 18.13 Ureter is spatulated by using cold scissors. Note that in this phase, the UPJ is not resected; this trick prevents the retraction of the ureter and allows the manipulation without grasping of the pelvis and the ureter because the surgeon can grasp only the tissue of UPJ

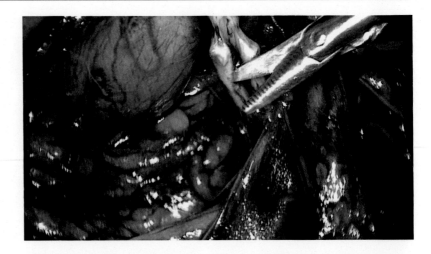

Fig. 18.14 Pelvis (*P*), spatulated ureter (*SU*) and UPJ incised but left in place are clearly shown

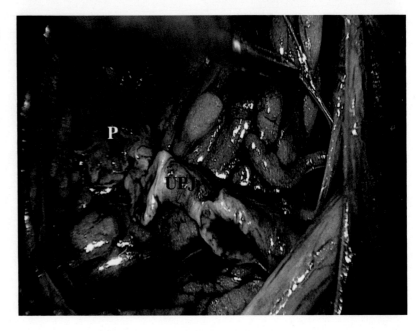

similar to standard instruments in terms of stiffness and grasp of the needle.

The first stitch is usually passed from the lowest point of the V-shaped spatulated ureter to the lowest point of the pelvis incision (Fig. 18.15). We use a 4/0 or 5/0 monofilament suture (4/8 needle) that is inserted through a mini-port. As this stitch is crucial, it is carefully tied and tension between pelvis and ureter has to be checked in this phase. After the placement of the first stitch, sometimes the suspension of the pelvis (or peripyelic tissue) to the abdominal wall using a straight needle is helpful to facilitate the suturing (Fig. 18.16).

The posterior portion of anastomosis is performed with a 5/0 monofilament, running suture. After completing the posterior portion of anastomosis, the UPJ is resected and removed through one of the mini-ports (Fig. 18.17), and a guidewire is inserted through the ureteral catheter and it is held in to the pelvis by a forceps (Fig. 18.18). Then ureteral catheter is removed and a double J stent is placed in a retrograde fashion. Proximal curl of the stent is placed in the pelvis, whilst the distal curl is checked by the assistant surgeon with a flexible cystoscopy [19].

Finally, the anterior wall of the anastomosis is completed with a running suture beginning at the

Fig. 18.15 The first stitch of ureteropelvic anastomosis is passed from the lowest point of the V-shaped spatulated ureter to the lowest point of the pelvis incision. Note the forceps of the assistant that allows a good visualisation of the ureter. In this case, we used a 5–0 Ethicon-Vicryl® suture; now we use 5/0 monofilament suture

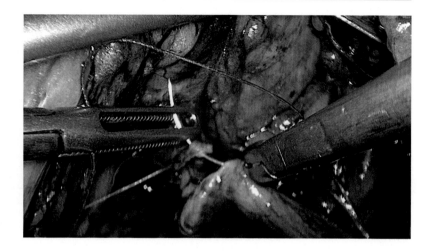

Fig. 18.16 The pelvis is suspended to the abdominal wall. This allows a good visualisation of the suture's margins

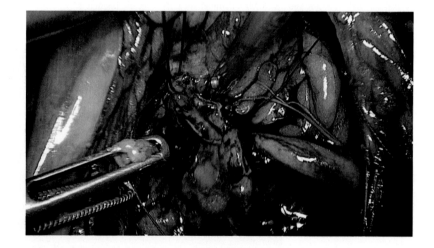

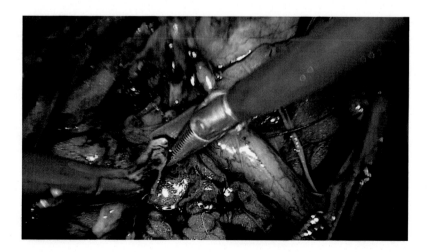

Fig. 18.17 UPJ resection by using cold scissors

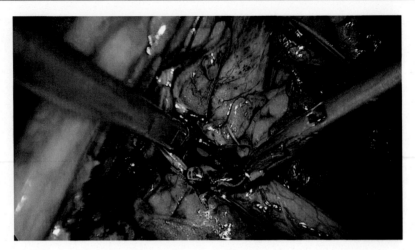

Fig. 18.18 The posterior wall of anastomosis is completed. A guidewire is placed into the ureter in a retrograde fashion, through the ureteral catheter. The guidewire is then held by a forceps, and the ureteral catheter is easily exchanged with a double J stent in a retrograde fashion. Alternatively, guidewire and stent can be introduced through the assistant mini-port and placed in an anterograde fashion

Fig. 18.19 Anterior wall of anastomosis is completed; suspension and assistant's forceps are removed

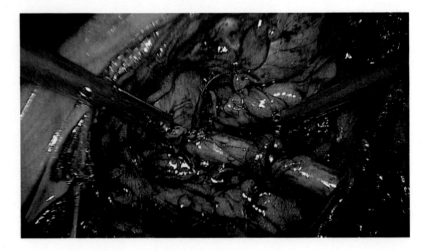

cranial point (Fig. 18.19). Then, bladder can be filled with saline solution until the pelvis distends to check fluid leakage.

The reconstruction of mesocolon is usually performed by using running suture (Fig. 18.20). The extraction of needles through the mini-ports requires particular care. We use to reduce the bending of the needle with the needle holders before the extraction.

A small drain is placed through the right mini incision (Fig. 18.21). Mini-laparoscopic port sites require no suture closure; a single small adhesive strip is applied to approximate the skin edges.

The right UPJ is reached through an incision in the posterior peritoneum and, if necessary, via a right colon flexure-reflecting approach. The remnant steps of the procedures are the same.

Postoperative Management

- Start light diet in postoperative day (POD) 1 and early mobilisation (POD 1 or 2).
- Remove drain POD 2.
- Remove catheter POD 3 or 4.
- Remove double J stent after 4–6 weeks.

Fig. 18.20 Although not mandatory, we usually perform a mesocolon reconstruction (same case as in Fig. 18.6)

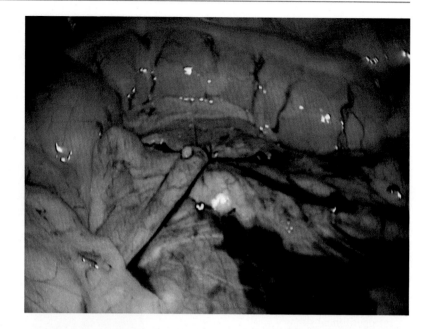

Fig. 18.21 A small drain is left in place. Note that the tip of this drain is placed through the suture in the retroperitoneum (same case as in Figs. 18.6 and 18.20)

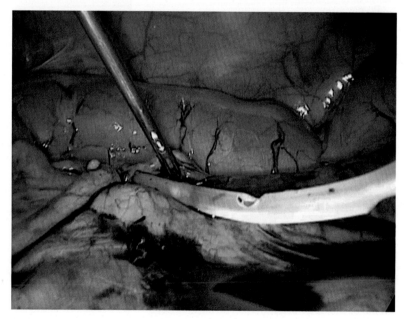

Retroperitoneoscopic Adrenalectomy (Mini-rA)

Among the extirpative procedures, adrenalectomy by using small instruments is the most frequently performed [13–15]. More than 10 years ago, Gill et al. reported the Cleveland experience with "needlescopy" to treat adrenal disease [14]. More recently, Liao et al. published the results of

the first large series of patients (112) treated with transperitoneal needlescopic adrenalectomy for small adrenal tumours [16]. The authors concluded that needlescopic adrenalectomy is safe and effective for most adrenal tumours less than 5 cm in size and has acceptable operative times, although patients with previous upper midline or ipsilateral upper quadrant open surgeries might not be suitable candidates for such a technique.

On the contrary, there is a lack of data about mini-laparoscopic retroperitoneal adrenalectomy. Retroperitoneoscopy is a good alternative to transperitoneal procedures, it can be safely performed in patients who had previous abdominal surgery too, it provides direct access to the adrenal gland, it avoids handling and the potential injuries of the bowel and it takes advantage of naturally existing anatomical planes. We have recently presented our experience about 50 cases of mini-rA [21].

Herein, we present our technique for right mini-rA.

- Standard indications: benign adrenal lesion.
- Limits/contraindications: large masses (>6 cm); uncontrolled pheochromocytoma. BMI >35 (relative); and significant, previous retroperitoneal surgery.
- Preparation is the same of standard procedure.

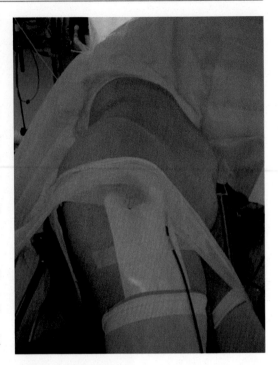

Fig. 18.22 Patient position for a right retroperitoneoscopy. Note the light cohesive retention bandage that we use routinely to fix the patient to the table

Instruments

Basic mini-laparoscopic set (as previously described) and standard laparoscopic set. Even if we do not do it routinely, consider two camera and laparoscopic vision systems.

Surgical Technique

Patient's Position

A Foley catheter is placed. The patient is placed on fully flank position, on the table towards the edge of the table facing the surgeons, who stand on the backside of the patient. The legs are separated and protected with either pillow or foam mat. The head and neck are maintained in neutral position whilst both arms are appropriately supported with armrests. The patient's thoracic and lumbar areas are supported in lateral position, and all pressure points are protected by foam mat. The table is broken at the level of the umbilicus by approximately 15–20°. Finally, light cohesive retention bandage is used to fix the patient to the table (Fig. 18.22).

Gaining Access to the Retroperitoneum

Initially, a 12–15-mm transverse incision is made 1–2 cm just above the iliac crest, at the level of the Petit triangle. The abdominal wall and the transversalis fascia are incised with scissors. Once the retroperitoneum is reached, the space is dissected with the finger and expanded by using a dilatation balloon under direct vision. Subsequently, two mini-ports are inserted under digital guidance at the level of the anterior and posterior axillary line; then the third mini-port is placed at the level of the tip of 12th rib. Finally, a ten (12-mm) standard port is placed at the level of the first incision. The ports form a "diamond" shape (Fig. 18.23). Retropneumoperitoneum is inducted by carbon dioxide pressure, fixed at 12 mmHg.

Dissection of the Retroperitoneal Space and Dissection of the Adrenal "Space"

The most important landmark of retroperitoneoscopic procedure is the psoas muscle (Fig. 18.24). The dissection of the retroperitoneal space is

Fig. 18.23 Port placement for mini-rA. Three mini- and one 12-mm ports are placed in a diamond shape. Retropneumoperitoneum is inducted through the standard port. *A* abdomen and *H* head

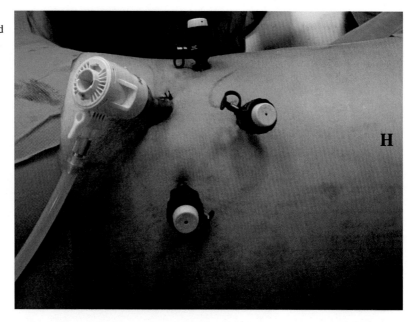

Fig. 18.24 The psoas muscle is the most important landmark of the retroperitoneoscopic procedure. Once identified, it leads to the dissection of the renal and adrenal space

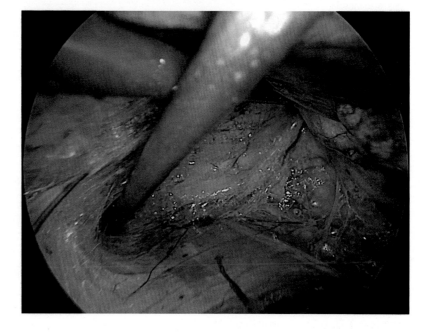

done in cranial direction on the top of the psoas muscle until the quadrate lumbar muscle. The dissection involves the upper pole of the kidney, perirenal fat and adrenal gland. This dissection should be performed en bloc; there is no need to identify the adrenal gland at this moment (Fig. 18.25).

Then the adrenal space together with the upper pole of the kidney and surrounding fat tissue are dissected from the transverse muscle (lateral side), diaphragm (upper side), psoas muscle (posterior side) and liver (Fig. 18.26). At the separation of the adrenal space from the diaphragm, small adrenal vessels are identified. Usually,

Fig. 18.25 The dissection of the retroperitoneal space is until the quadrate lumbar muscle

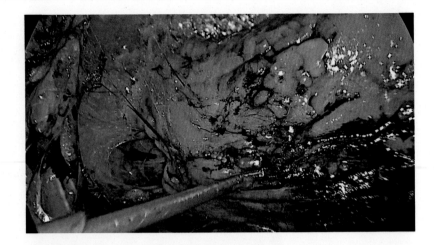

Fig. 18.26 The adrenal space together with the upper pole of the kidney and surrounding fat tissue is dissected from the transverse muscle, diaphragm (*D*), psoas muscle (*PM*) and liver (*L*). In this phase, there is no need of identification of the gland

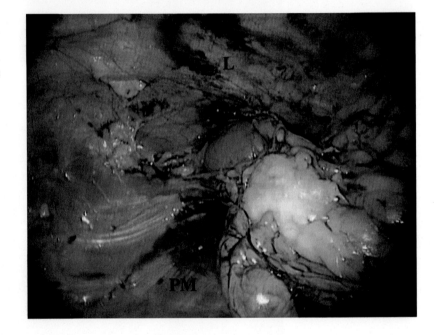

careful coagulation by using bipolar forceps is enough to prevent bleeding.

Dissection Between the Adrenal Gland and Upper Pole of the Kidney

After en bloc dissection, perirenal fat between the upper pole and adrenal gland has to be divided. Fatty tissue is dissected along the surface (upper pole) of the kidney; by this way, the adrenal space lies separately from the kidney (Fig. 18.27).

Management of the Adrenal Pedicles

With a forceps, the assistant reflects the upper pole of the kidney downwardly; then the adrenal gland is lifted up by grasping the surrounding fat. This manoeuvre allows the identification of inferior and posterior vessels that are located at the lower median site of the adrenal gland (Fig. 18.28). These vessels are carefully coagulated by using bipolar forceps and divided.

Then, dissection of the adrenal gland can be performed both with ascending and with descending direction, depending on surgeon's preference.

Fig. 18.27
Identification of the
dissection plane
between the perirenal
fat and adrenal space.
Sometimes, this step
can be challenging,
especially in case of
large amount of fat
tissue. The
identification of the
upper pole of the
parenchyma of the
upper pole of the
kidney may help the
dissection

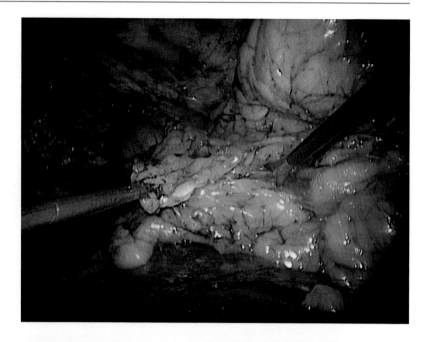

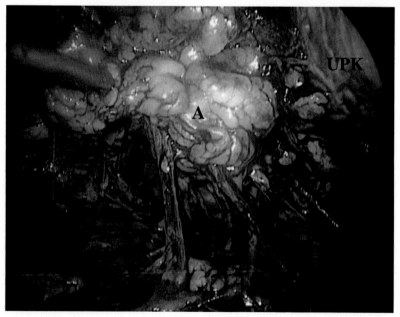

Fig. 18.28   Then adrenal gland (*A*) is lifted up by using a forceps, whilst the assistant reflects the upper pole of the kidney (*UPK*) downwardly. By this way, posterior adrenal vessels are identified and dissected. We use to coagulate carefully these vessels by using a bipolar forceps. When needed an alternative step that is possible. The standard scope is removed and a mini-scope is introduced through one of the mini-ports. Hem-o-lok clip applier is introduced through the standard port and vessels are secured with Hem-o-lok

After the transection of the inferior and posterior adrenal vessels, the fat around the adrenal vein is carefully dissected. The adrenal vein and the vena cava are clearly exposed and dissected (Fig. 18.29). The 10-mm laparoscope is then removed, and the 3-mm mini-scope is introduced

Fig. 18.29 After the section of posterior and inferior adrenal vessels, the main adrenal vein (*AV*) and the cava vein (*CV*) are identified and dissected

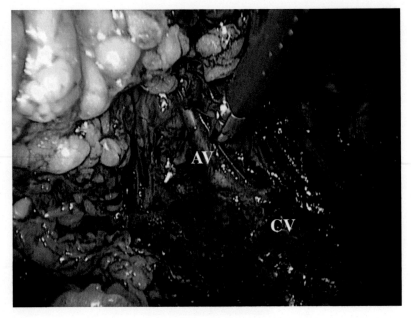

through the right mini-port. The vein is then secured with Hem-o-lok (through the 10-mm port) (Fig. 18.30) and sectioned.

Finally, the remaining inner part of the adrenal gland is completely freed. At the end of the adrenal dissection, the adrenal space is correctly visualised (Fig. 18.31).

Specimen Entrapment

The specimen is placed in a retrieval bag that is inserted through the 10-mm port; this step is controlled by a 3-mm scope inserted through one of the mini-ports. Before the specimen extraction, haemostasis is carefully controlled after the interruption of carbon dioxide insufflation. A drain is left through the port at the level of the posterior axillary line, and ports are removed under direct vision.

In case of left adrenalectomy, patient's position and port's disposition are shown in Fig. 18.32. The main steps of the procedure are the same; adrenal vein can be carefully coagulated with bipolar forceps for a long segment. The vein is then transected close to the adrenal gland, leaving the coagulated stump at the renal vein as long as possible. Thus, in these cases, the procedure is completely clip-less.

Postoperative Management

- Start diet on postoperative day (POD) 1 and early mobilisation on POD 1.
- Remove catheter and drain on POD 1 (when minimal output).

In case of functional lesion, repeated controls of electrolytes and blood pressure are needed; consider hydrocortisone replacement if needed; and involve endocrinologists in this phase.

Retroperitoneoscopic Mini Partial Nephrectomy (Mini-rPN)

Partial nephrectomy (PN) emerged as a gold standard approach for T1 RCC [22]. The rationale for PN is twofold: first, PN has the same oncological outcomes than radical nephrectomy (RN); second, it has been clearly reported that radical nephrectomy (RN) is associated with higher mortality and more renal failure [22]. Laparoscopic PN (LPN) and more recently robotic PN have gained widespread acceptance, at least in tertiary care centres, thanks to well-known benefits of mini invasiveness [23].

Fig. 18.30 The adrenal vein is secured by using Hem-o-lok clips, and this step is controlled by 3-mm scope

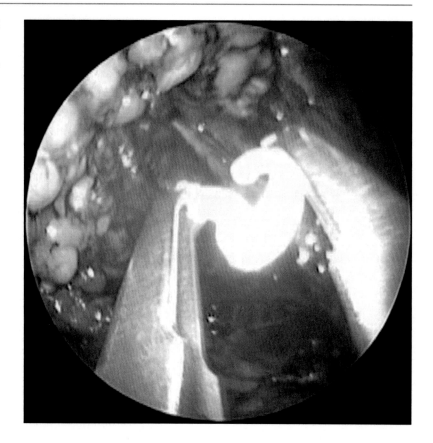

Fig. 18.31 The adrenal space is clearly identified. Note the Hem-o-lok clips that secure the stump of the adrenal vein. The whole intervention is performed by using the natural existing dissection planes

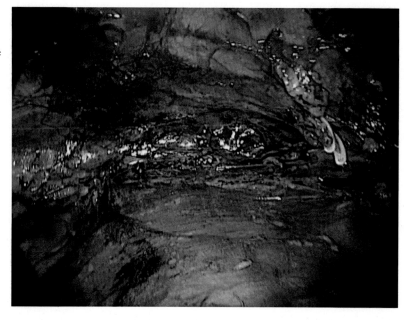

To date, no data about LPN performed with mini-instruments are available in literature.

Recently, based on our positive experience with mini-laparoscopy, we introduced mini-LPN with retroperitoneoscopic approach in "highly selected" cases at our institution. Although still unpublished, our initial results are encouraging.

Herein, we describe our technique for right mini-rPN.

- Standard indication: small, exophytic, posterior renal tumours.
- Limits/contraindications: BMI >35 and significant, previous retroperitoneal surgery.
- Preoperative preparation is the same of standard procedure.

Instruments

Basic mini-laparoscopic set (as previously described) and standard laparoscopic set. Even if we do not do it routinely, consider two camera and laparoscopic vision systems.

Surgical Technique

Patient's position, ports' disposition (see Fig. 18.32) and retroperitoneal space dissection are the same of mini-rA (see also Figs. 18.22, 18.23 and 18.24).

Dissection of Renal Artery

The psoas muscle is freed completely, leaving the perirenal fat untouched. Identification of the hilar vessels is basic to control bleeding in case of haemorrhage. Usually, the identification of the renal artery by using retroperitoneal approach is easy, but it can be difficult in cases of abundant renal hilar fatty tissue. In this phase, kidney and perirenal fat are lifted up with a 3-mm forceps, as in standard procedure (Fig. 18.33).

Identification of the Tumour

Full or partial mobilisation of the kidney is performed depending on the tumour location. When possible, targeted dissection of perirenal fat is performed. Sometimes, the identification of the tumour is more difficult and a more extensive dissection of the fat is required. In these cases, intra-operative laparoscopic ultrasonography can also be used to delineate tumour location and characteristics. When necessary, the 10-mm laparoscope is removed, and the 3-mm mini-scope is introduced through the right mini-port. The probe is then used through the 10-mm port.

Clamping of the Renal Artery

Seeing as we treated with this technique highly selected patients (small, exophytic tumours; see "Indication" section), usually, we perform a "clampless" procedure. Nevertheless, based on the surgeon preferences and tumour characteristics, renal artery can be occluded by using a bulldog clamp introduced through the 10-mm port. In these cases, the use of mini-scope through a 3-mm port is basic.

Tumour Resection

To increase the working space in this phase, the assistant lifts up the peritoneum with a forceps introduced through the cranial mini-port. The renal parenchyma around the tumour can be demarcated circumferentially, with monopolar scissors. Carbon dioxide pressure is raised up until 18–20-mmHg. Then, renal parenchyma is incised, the peri-tumoural fat is gently grasped with a forceps (Fig. 18.34) and the correct plane between tumour and healthy tissue is reached. If it is possible, the tumour is excised along the pseudocapsule by blunt dissection by using suction device and bipolar forceps (Fig. 18.35). Vessels of the resection bed are coagulated with bipolar forceps. In some cases, sharp dissection or healthy tissue excision is needed.

Usually, we use 3-mm instruments during this phase. When bleeding occurs and 3-mm device does not allow an efficient suction, 10-mm scope is exchanged with a mini-scope introduced through one of the mini-ports (we usually use the right one). By this way, standard suction device and 5-mm instruments can be used, and when needed, on demand clamping of the artery can be done.

Fig. 18.32 Ports' disposition in case of left mini-rA. Note that this disposition of the ports is the same as of the right side. Black X identifies the side of the intervention (per protocol at our institution). *A* abdomen and *H* head

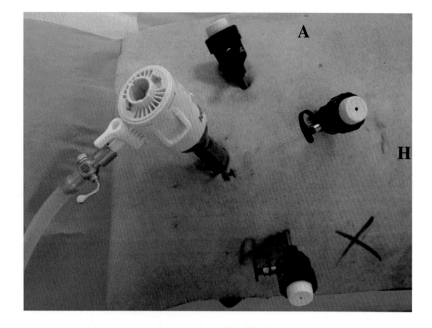

Fig. 18.33 Right mini-rPN. Dissection of the renal artery is one of the first steps of the procedure. Even we usually do not clamp the artery during this intervention; we prefer to dissect it with 3-mm forceps and suction device in case urgent clamping is required. *RA* renal artery, *b* branch of RA, *K* kidney, *v* venous vessels that lay across RA

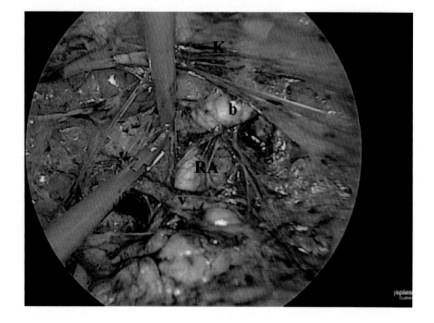

Renorrhaphy

The 10-mm scope is exchanged with the mini-scope placed through the right (anterior) mini-port. By this way, the surgeon works with the right hand through the 10 mm and with the left hand through a mini-port. Obviously, by this way, the working angle between the needle holders is closer than usual, but the triangulation of the instruments is enough to perform a suture which is comparable to that performed during a standard procedure. A 15-cm 2/0 monofilament suture with a Lapra-TY absorbable clip (Ethicon Endo-Surgery Inc., Cincinnati, Ohio, USA) placed at the end is introduced through the 10-mm port, and the renorrhaphy is performed. Hem-o-lok clips can be placed through the

Fig. 18.34 Incision of the renal parenchyma at the level of the border between tumour and healthy tissue. The fat around the tumour is gently grasped with a forceps to facilitate the incision. Note that the tumour is small and exophytic

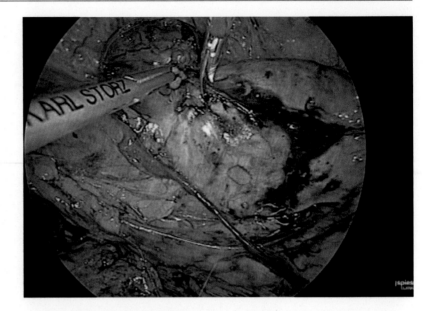

Fig. 18.35 The tumour is excised with blunt dissection along its pseudocapsule. In this phase, surgeon uses suction device with the left hand to improve the vision of the resection bed and bipolar forceps with the right hand to control bleeding. When possible, the use of scissors during enucleation is very limited

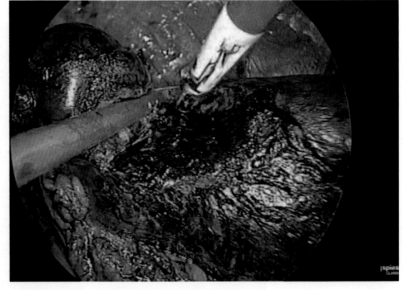

standard port, and suture is done as during a standard procedure (Figs. 18.36 and 18.37). Finally, haemostatic agents can be used.

A retrieval bag is introduced through a 10-mm port and this step is controlled by 3-mm scope. Before the specimen extraction, haemostasis is carefully controlled after the interruption of carbon dioxide insufflation, and a drain is put in place. The specimen is then removed through the 10-mm incision that is then sutured in two layers. Mini-laparoscopic port sites require no suture closure; a single small adhesive strip is applied to approximate the skin edges.

Postoperative Management

- Start diet on postoperative day (POD) 1 and early mobilisation on POD 1 or 2.
- Remove catheter and drain on POD 1 (when minimal output).

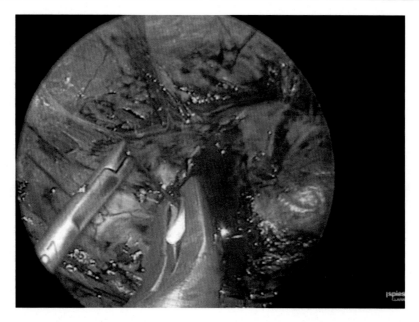

Fig. 18.36 Renorrhaphy. In this phase, surgeon uses 10-mm Hem-o-lok applier through the 10-mm port with the right hand and 3-mm needle holder with the left hand. The suture is directed through the depths of parenchymal defect on one side and exits on the opposite side of the defect. Hem-o-lok clips are used to secure the suture under moderate tension. Note that the angle between the two instruments is closer than in the standard procedure. This entire phase is controlled by 3-mm scope through the right mini-port. Note that the quality of vision is higher than usual thanks to SPIES system technology (Storz Medical System, Tuttlingen, Germany)

Fig. 18.37 Final view of the suture

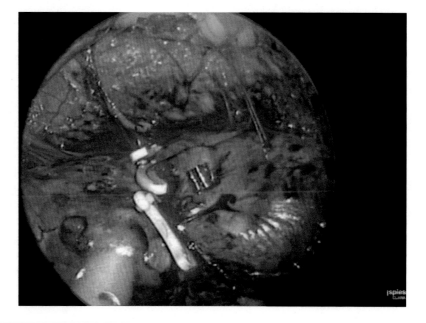

Mini Hybrid LESS Nephrectomy

LESS has been proposed as an evolutionary step beyond standard laparoscopy and has been increasingly adopted by surgeons worldwide since its introduction [8, 9, 24]. The main drawbacks of this technique are represented by crossing or collision of instruments, lack of triangulation and in-line vision that represent additional challenges for the surgeon compared with standard laparoscopy and may lead to increased operative times and complication rate. To overcome these limits, adjunctive ports are often required during LESS procedures [24]. In a recent multi-institutional analysis on 1,076 cases, Kaouk et al. reported that a planned, additional port was used in 23 % of cases of LESS and that overall conversion rate was 20.8 %, with 15.8 % of cases converting to reduced-port laparoscopy and 4 % to conventional laparoscopy (more than one unplanned extra port) [9].

When an adjunctive port is planned or needed to complete the procedure, a so-called hybrid LESS is performed. In our opinion, during these procedures, the use of mini-ports seems to be the best compromise between mini invasiveness and handiness and safety of the procedure. Mini-port wounds are almost invisible and do not add postoperative pain but make easier the intervention allowing surgeon to maintain correct triangulation of the instruments which is paramount for laparoscopy.

Herein, we present our technique of hybrid LESS nephrectomy by using adjunctive mini-ports [mini hybrid LESS nephrectomy].

- Indications: same of LESS nephrectomy.
- Limits/contraindications: severe obesity and previous significant abdominal surgery with extensive surgical scar in the upper abdomen.
- Preoperative preparation is the same of standard procedure.

Instruments

(At least) two mini-ports and two grasping forceps. Complete standard laparoscopic set.

Surgical Technique: Right Side

Patient Position

A Foley catheter is placed. The patient is placed on the flank at a 45° angle, on the table towards the edge of the table facing the surgeons. The legs are separated and protected with either pillow or foam mat. The head and neck are maintained in

neutral position whilst both arms are supported appropriately with armrests. The patient's thoracic and lumbar areas are supported in lateral position, and all pressure points are protected by foam mat. The table is broken at the level of the umbilicus by approximately 10–15°. Finally, light cohesive retention bandage is used to fix the patient to the table.

The surgeons stand in front of the patients, being the assistant seated down to allow the surgeon a complete range of movement without instruments clashing.

Port Placement

In slim patients, we prefer periumbilical access. A 4-cm incision is performed at the level of the umbilicus. After the suspension of fascial layers, GelPoint® Advanced Access Platform (Applied Medical, California, USA) is placed. Three 10-mm trocars are placed though this device: the first one for the scope and the other ones for the first surgeon. In our opinion, by using this system, the extra-long optic and pre-bent instruments are not mandatory; indeed, we use standard 10-mm 30° optic and standard laparoscopic instruments. After the induction of pneumoperitoneum and the inspection of the peritoneal cavity with the camera placed through one of the 10-mm ports of GelPoint, two adjunctive mini-ports for 3-mm instruments are placed under direct vision.

The first mini-port is placed just below the xyphoid; through this trocar, a 3-mm forceps is used by the assistant to lift up the liver. The second mini-port is placed at the level of the anterior axillary line, 4–6 cm cranially to the iliac crest (Fig. 18.38). The surgeon uses a 3-mm forceps inserted through this port with the left hand, to retract the tissues and all other instruments (scissors, suction device, Hem-o-lok clips or tissue-sealing devices) through one of the 10-mm ports of the GelPoint device with the right hand (Fig. 18.39). By using this configuration, the triangulation of the instruments is correct, and the clashing of instruments is dramatically reduced; thus, the main limitations of pure LESS are overcome (Figs. 18.40 and 18.41).

Fig. 18.38 Ports'
disposition in case of
right mini hybrid LESS
nephrectomy. We
routinely use GelPoint
Advanced Access
Platform which is
placed at the level of
the umbilicus

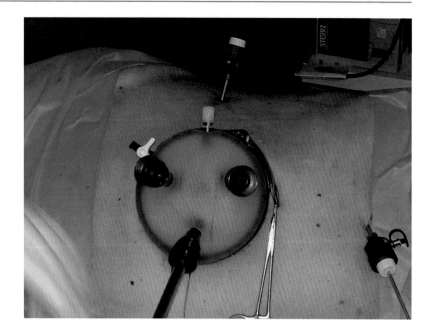

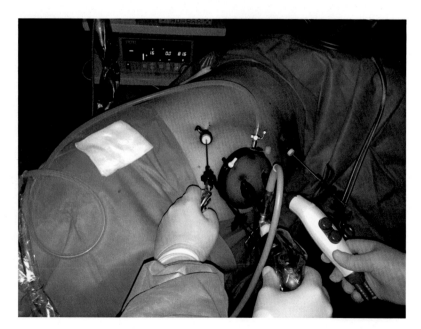

Fig. 18.39 Right mini hybrid LESS nephrectomy. The surgeon uses a 3-mm forceps inserted through the left (caudal) mini-port with the left hand, to retract the tissues and all other instruments (suction device in the picture) through one of the 10-mm ports of the GelPoint device with the right hand. The assistant holds the camera that is inserted through the GelPoint. The right (cranial) mini-port is used by the assistant to lift the liver. In this case, the forceps grasped superficially the inner part of the thoracic wall and "become" autostatic. Note that no dedicated (pre-bent or extra-long) instruments are used

Fig. 18.40 Initial step of nephrectomy for large renal tumour. Note two 3-mm grasping forceps: the first one is used through the right (cranial) mini-port to retract the liver and the second one is used by the surgeon to retract the peritoneum. A tissue sealer is introduced through GelPoint device. Note the wide triangulation of the instruments fully comparable to that of standard laparoscopy

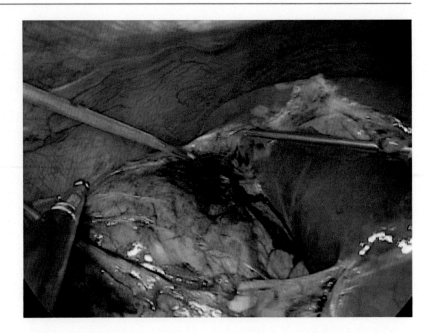

Fig. 18.41 Operative field after mini hybrid LESS right nephrectomy

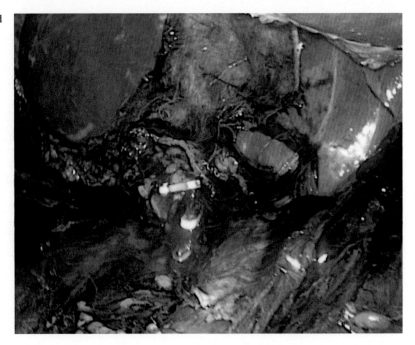

Thanks to these adjunctive ports, mini hybrid LESS nephrectomy follows exactly the same steps of a standard laparoscopic nephrectomy with transperitoneal approach.

Note that scars of mini incisions are almost invisible (Fig. 18.42).

Surgical Technique: Left Side

Patient position and GelPoint device placement are as for the right procedure.

Even in this case, two adjunctive mini-ports are suggested. The first one is placed at the level of the hemiclavear line, 2 cm below the costal arch; the second one is placed at the level of the anterior axillary line midline 4–6 cm cranially to the iliac crest (Fig. 18.43).

The surgeon uses a 3-mm forceps inserted through the subcostal mini-port with the left hand to retract the tissues and all other instru-

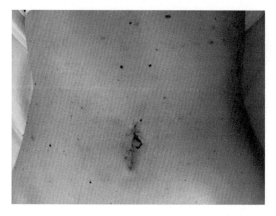

Fig. 18.42 Cosmetic results 3 months after surgery. Note that the scars of mini incisions are most invisible (same case as Fig. 18.33)

ments (scissors, suction device, Hem-o-lok clips or tissue-sealing devices) through one of the 10-mm ports of the GelPoint device with the right hand (Fig. 18.44). By using this configuration, the triangulation of the instruments is similar to the one of a standard laparoscopic procedure. Moreover, the other mini-port is used by the assistant to retract the colon (when it limits the laparoscopic vision) (Fig. 18.45) or to lift up the kidney during pedicle identification and management.

Thanks to these adjunctive ports, mini hybrid LESS nephrectomy follows exactly the same steps of a standard laparoscopic nephrectomy with transperitoneal approach.

Postoperative Management

- Start diet on postoperative day (POD) 1 and early mobilisation on POD 1.
- Remove catheter and drain on POD 1 (when minimal output).

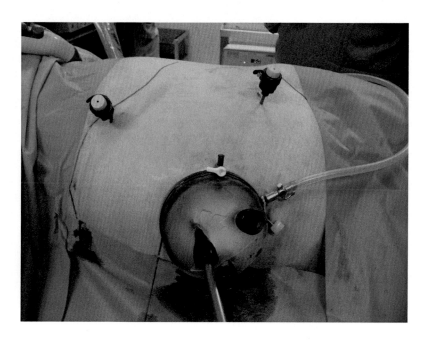

Fig. 18.43 Ports' disposition in case of left mini hybrid LESS nephrectomy. We routinely use GelPoint Advanced Access Platform, which is placed at the level of the umbilicus

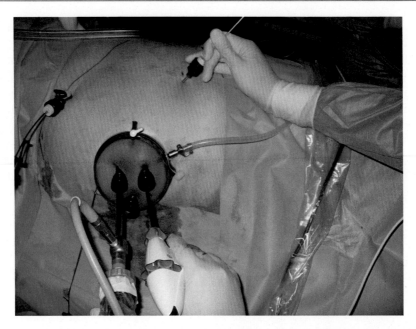

Fig. 18.44 Left mini hybrid LESS nephrectomy. The surgeon uses a 3-mm forceps inserted through the left (cranial) mini-port with the left hand and all other instruments (tissue sealer in the picture) through one of the 10-mm ports of the GelPoint device with the right hand. The assistant holds the camera that is inserted through the GelPoint. The right (caudal) mini-port is used by the assistant to displace the bowel

Fig. 18.45 Pedicle control during left mini hybrid LESS nephrectomy for large renal tumour. Note two 3-mm grasping forceps: the first one is used through the right (caudal) to displace the bowel by the assistant and the second one is used by the surgeon to lift up the kidney. A Hem-o-lok applier is introduced through GelPoint device. Even in this case, this port disposition allows a wide triangulation of the instruments, fully comparable to that of standard laparoscopy

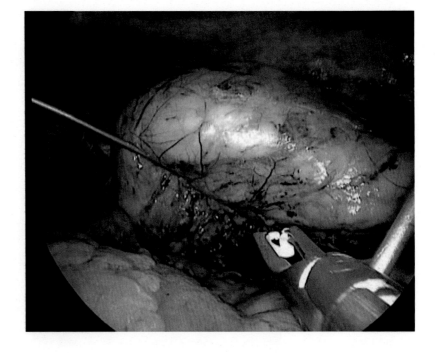

References

1. Mamazza J, Schlachta CM, Seshadri PA, et al. Needlescopic surgery: a logical evolution from conventional laparoscopic surgery. Surg Endosc. 2001;15:1208–12.
2. Pini G, Porpiglia F, Micali S, Rassweiler J. Minilaparoscopy, needlescopy and microlaparoscopy: decreasing invasiveness, maintaining the standard laparoscopic approach. Arch Esp Urol. 2012;65(3):366–83.
3. Kalloo AN, Singh VK, Jagannath SB, et al. Flexible transgastric peritoneoscopy: a novel approach to diagnostic and therapeutic interventions in the peritoneal cavity. Gastrointest Endosc. 2004;60:114–7.
4. Raman JD, Bensalah K, Bagrodia A, Stern JM, Cadeddu JA. Laboratory and clinical development of single keyhole umbilical nephrectomy. Urology. 2007;70:1039–44.
5. Autorino R, Yakoubi R, White WM, Gettman M, De Sio M, Quattrone C, Di Palma C, Izzo A, Correia-Pinto J, Kaouk JH, Lima E. Natural orifice transluminal endoscopic surgery (NOTES): where are we going? A bibliometric assessment. BJU Int. 2013;111(1):11–6.
6. Alcaraz A, Peri L, Molina A, Goicoechea I, García E, Izquierdo L, Ribal MJ. Feasibility of transvaginal NOTES-assisted laparoscopic nephrectomy. Eur Urol. 2010;57(2):233–7.
7. Humphrey JE, Canes D. Transumbilical laparoendoscopic single-site surgery in urology. Int J Urol. 2012;19(5):416–28.
8. Symes A, Rane A. Urological applications of single-site laparoscopic surgery. J Minim Access Surg. 2011;7(1):90–5.
9. Kaouk JH, Autorino A, Kim FJ, et al. Laparoendoscopic single-site surgery in urology: worldwide multi-institutional analysis of 1076 cases. Eur Urol. 2011;60:998–1005.
10. Tsai YC, Wu CC, Yang SSD. Minilaparoscopic nerve-sparing extravesical ureteral reimplantation for primary vesicoureteral reflux: a preliminary report. J Laparoendosc Adv Surg Tech. 2008;18(5):767–70.
11. Soble JJ, Gill IS. Needlescopic urology: incorporating 2-mm instruments in laparoscopic surgery. Urology. 1998;52:187–94.
12. Tan HL. Laparoscopic anderson-hynes dismembered pyeloplasty in children using needlescopic instrumentation. Urol Clin North Am. 2001;28(1):43–51.
13. Pini G, Goezen AS, Shulze M, Hruza M, Klein J, Rassweiler JJ. Small incision access retroperitoneoscopic technique (SMART) pyeloplasty in adult patients: comparison of cosmetic and post operative pain outcomes in a matched pair analysis with standard retroperitoneoscopy: preliminary report. World J Urol. 2012;30(5):605–11.
14. Gill IS, Soble JJ, Sung GT, Winfield HN, Bravo EL, Novick AC. Needlescopic adrenalectomy—the initial series: comparison with conventional laparoscopic adrenalectomy. Urology. 1998;52:180–6.
15. Chueh SC, Chen J, Chen SC, Liao CH, Lai MK. Clipless laparoscopic adrenalectomy with needlescopic instruments. J Urol. 2002;167:39–43.
16. Liao C-H, Lai M-K, Li H-Y, Chen S-C, Chueh S-C. Laparoscopic adrenalectomy using needlescopic instruments for adrenal tumors less than 5 cm in 112 cases. Eur Urol. 2008;54:640–6.
17. Porpiglia F, Morra I, Bertolo R, Manfredi M, Mele F, Fiori C. Pure mini-laparoscopic transperitoneal pyeloplasty in an adult population: feasibility, safety, and functional results after one year of follow-up. Urology. 2012;79(3):728–32.
18. Fiori C, Morra I, Bertolo R, Mele F, Chiarissi ML, Porpiglia F. Standard vs mini-laparoscopic pyeloplasty: perioperative outcomes and cosmetic results. BJU Int. 2013;111(3):E121–6. Epub 2012 Jul 12.
19. Fiori C, Morra I, Di Stasio A, Grande S, Scarpa RM, Porpiglia F. Flexible pneumocystoscopy for double J stenting during laparoscopic and robot assisted pyeloplasty: our experience. Int J Urol. 2010;17(2):192–4.
20. Porpiglia F, Billia M, Volpe A, Morra I, Scarpa RM. Transperitoneal left laparoscopic pyeloplasty with transmesocolic access to the pelvi-ureteric junction: technique description and results with a minimum follow-up of 1 year. BJU Int. 2007;101:1024–8.
21. Porpiglia F, Fiori C, Bertolo R, Cattaneo G, Amparore D, Morra I, Didio M, De Luca S, Scarpa RM. Mini-retroperitoneoscopic adrenalectomy: our experience after 50 procedures. Urology. 2014;84(3):596–601.
22. Ljungberg B, Cowan NC, Hanbury DC, Hora M, Kuczyk MA, Merseburger AS, Patard JJ, Mulders PF, Sinescu IC, European Association of Urology Guideline Group. EAU guidelines on renal cell carcinoma: the 2010 update. Eur Urol. 2010;58(3):398–406.
23. Khalifeh A, Autorino R, Hillyer SP, Laydner H, Eyraud R, Panumatrassamee K, Long JA, Kaouk JH. Comparative outcomes and assessment of trifecta in 500 robotic and laparoscopic partial nephrectomy cases: a single surgeon experience. J Urol. 2013;189(4):1236–42.
24. Autorino R, Cadeddu JA, Desai MM, et al. Laparoendoscopic single site and natural orifice transluminal endoscopic surgery in urology: a critical analysis of the literature. Eur Urol. 2011;59:26–45.

19 LESS in the Pediatric Population

Selcuk Sahin and Volkan Tugcu

Introduction

In the field of minimally invasive surgery, there has been a trend toward minimizing the number of incisions and ports required, and this has led to the development of laparoendoscopic single-site (LESS) surgery. There are theoretical advantages to this approach including less postoperative pain, a faster convalescence period, and improved cosmetic outcome [1].

Since the initial reporting of single-port nephrectomy in 2007 by Rane et al. [2], there are now several studies in the published literature demonstrating the feasibility and efficacy of LESS in both children and adults.

There is evidence to suggest that visible scarring in children can result in reduced self-esteem, impaired socialization skills, and lower self-ratings of problem solving ability [3]. LESS is performed via a single incision through the umbilicus; therefore, there is no psychosocial impact of visible abdominal scarring. LESS clearly resulted in excellent cosmesis [1]. Although improved cosmesis is the most apparent benefit of LESS, there may be benefits regarding postoperative pain and the recovery period [3].

The advantages of LESS in the pediatric age group are well-defined tissue planes, absence of fat, and thin abdominal walls. These characteristics of the pediatric age group help in easier dissection of surgical planes. The challenges in development of LESS revolve around technique and anesthesia-related issues. From a technical standpoint, the challenges include a need for specialized instrumentation and loss of triangulation. Although a few workers have used articulating and bent instruments. The technical challenges one encounters are in-line camera and instrument angles and a need for coordination with an experienced camera driver. The smaller working space in infants and toddlers also increases the level of difficulty [4].

Positioning

Laparoendoscopic single-site surgery performed with the patient in a position similar to that used for standard laparoscopy. The patient was placed at the edge of the table with the arms padded and secured. The eyes were padded and taped. The patients were secured with the help of tape; however, the use of a bean bag would also be suitable. The surgeon stood while the assistant (camera driver) sat to make space in the operating area. This made the procedure ergonomically less challenging [4].

S. Sahin, MD • V. Tugcu, MD (✉)
Urology Department, Bakırkoy Research and Training Hospital, Bakırkoy Dr. Sadi Konuk Training and Research Hospital, Istanbul, Turkey
e-mail: sahinsel78@gmail.com; Volkantugco@yahoo.com

© Springer Science+Business Media New York 2017
J.H. Kaouk et al. (eds.), *Atlas of Laparoscopic and Robotic Single Site Surgery*, Current Clinical Urology, DOI 10.1007/978-1-4939-3575-8_19

Anesthesia

The pneumoperitoneum pressures should be kept at 8–10 mmHg and all efforts made to prevent hypothermia. It is the responsibility of the anesthetist and the surgeon to ensure that the child is positioned properly on the table. It should be ensured that the access port fits snugly, thus preventing subcutaneous emphysema [4].

Instruments

LESS can be performed only by standard laparoscopic instruments. However, novel instruments are useful to reduce the size of the incision and facilitate the procedures. One more important point is to avoid instrument crowding. Small or articulating instruments may solve this problem.

Access Port

There are many alternatives depending on the surgeon's preference. Some of these are the TriPort or R-Port (Olympus, New York, USA, and Advance Surgical Concept, Wicklow, Ireland), SILS Port (Covidien, Chicopee, Massachusetts, USA), the Uni-X system (Pnavel Systems Inc., Morganville, New Jersey, USA), GelPort device (Applied Medical, Rancho Santa Margarita, CA), GelPOINT access port (Applied Medical, Rancho Santa Margarita, CA, USA), Octoport (DalimSurgNet, Seoul, Korea), and homemade access port device.

The ports were inserted by using the open technique. An umbilical skin crease incision was made and the fascia incised. The skin incision was hidden in the umbilical skin crease. The key to proper insertion is an optimal size of the facial opening. The opening should not be too large, because the port tends to slip out; neither should it be too small, because this may cause difficulty in introduction of both the port and the instruments. A larger facial incision causes gas leaks during surgery. Once the port was inserted, the plastic sleeve was pulled down so that the plastic rings (abdominal and peritoneal) approximated and the port fit snugly on the abdominal wall [4].

As an additional port, a 2–3-mm needlescopic port is used in some institutes. The common reasons for introduction of accessory ports included difficulty in upper pole dissection, inadequate exposure of the renal hilum, and difficulty in suturing in reconstructive procedures. The needlescopic port achieves a good cosmetic result.

Endoscope

A 5-mm 30° rigid laparoscope is the most popular scope in the previous studies, whereas a 5-mm flexible scope was used in some studies.

Other Instruments

The choice of instruments is a matter of surgeon's preference; the surgeon should choose instruments he or she is familiar with. Nonarticulating straight laparoscopic instruments were used in all procedures. Articulating and prebent instruments are commercially available. Some authors use articulating forceps in the operator's nondominant hand and standard instruments in the dominant hand. While some authors, use articulating forceps in the operator's nondominant hand and standard instruments in the dominant hand, the others choose vice-versa. In this combination, the instruments in each of the operator's hands usually cross in the access port and go to the opposite sides in the operative field.

Nephrectomy

The LESS simple nephrectomy (SN) procedure was carried out with the patient positioned in a 45° flank position for transperitoneal surgery (Fig. 19.1); a 2-cm semilunar-shaped skin incision was concealed completely within the umbilicus (Fig. 19.2) and deepened to the anterior rectus fascia, where a 2.5-cm fascial incision was made (Fig. 19.3); the peritoneum was incised; and the multichannel port was deployed (Fig. 19.4). A pneumoperitoneum was created by carbon dioxide insufflation. For LESS-SN

Fig. 19.1 A and B Patient's position of simple LESS nephrectomy

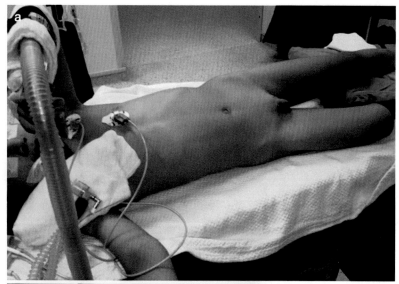

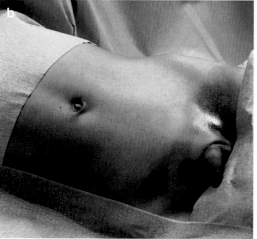

procedures, a 5 mm, 30° high-definition rigid laparoscope with integrated different cameras (Karl Storz, Tuttlingen, Germany and Gimmi, Tuttlingen, Germany) were used along with two working instruments (Fig. 19.5). During operations a combination of flexible forceps and scissors and a conventional laparoscopic (straight) instruments (e.g., scissors, ultrasonography scissors, bipolar forceps) were used to perform the procedures as necessary. During operations the straight instrument in the left hand was used to dissect the tissue, while roticulating laparoscopic graspers hold in the right hand were used to retract the tissues. In this procedure, an additional Prolene mesh was designed as a hammock

and attached to the abdominal wall with the help of sutures. Hem-o-lok clips were used for liver retraction during right nephrectomies. Sutures for liver retraction were passed transabdominally by 60-mm straight needle (Caprosyn, Covidien, Norwalk, USA) [5]. During operations the straight instrument in the left hand was used to dissect the tissue, while the peritoneal incision along the line of Toldt was performed with a roticulating laparoscopic scissors hold in the right hand (Fig. 19.6). The ureter was dissected free and transected between hemostatic clips (Fig. 19.7). Once the renal vessels were dissected free, the renal vessels were occluded separately with hemostatic clips (Hem-o-lock

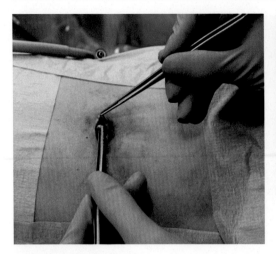

Fig. 19.2 Semilunar-shaped skin incision, concealed within the umbilicus

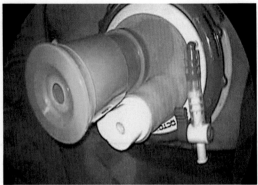

Fig. 19.4 The extracorporeal view of the Octoport

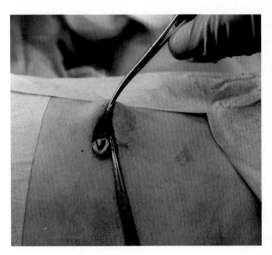

Fig. 19.3 Fascial and rectus muscle incision

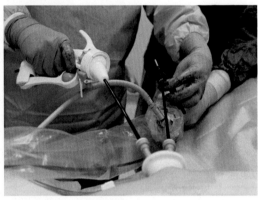

Fig. 19.5 The straight instrument was used in the left hand and roticulating laparoscopic scissors in the right hand

XL or L size clips, Teleflex Medical, Research Triangle Park, NC, USA) and then divided individually (Figs. 19.8 and 19.9). The kidney was then dissected free from all remaining attachments superiorly and laterally (Fig. 19.10). The morcellated specimens were removed through the umbilical incision or/and the specimen was removed intact using the single-port trocar site without extension of the skin incision (Figs. 19.11 and 19.12). The drain was removed in the next day morning after the procedure.

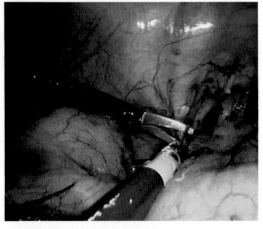

Fig. 19.6 Ureteral dissection

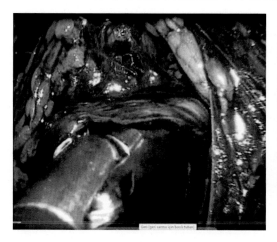

Fig. 19.7 Prolene mesh for liver retraction during right nephrectomies

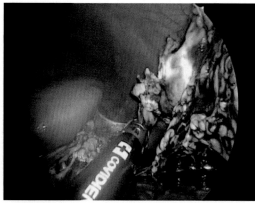

Fig. 19.10 Dissection of the upper renal pole

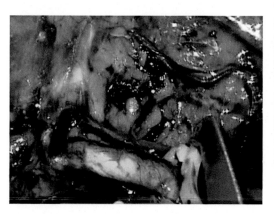

Fig. 19.8 Clipping of renal artery

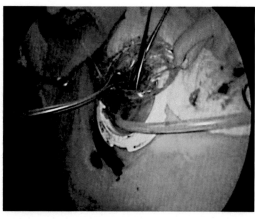

Fig. 19.11 Remove of the morcellated renal specimen

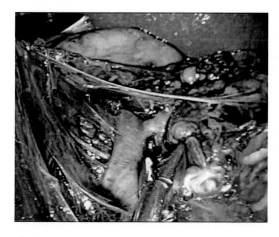

Fig. 19.9 Dissection of the renal vein

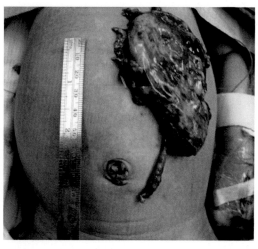

Fig. 19.12 Large left kidney specimen removed using umbilical incision after LESS nephrectomy (Courtesy of Chester Koh, MD)

Pyeloplasty

All procedure underwent cystoscopy with retrograde ureteral catheterization to define the stricture length and location more precisely and to rule out obstruction distal to the UPJ at the beginning of the procedure. After performing retrograde open-end stent placement cystoscopically, this stent was attached to a Foley catheter inserted into the bladder.

Some authors think that the previous insertion of a double J catheter by means of cystoscopy increases the surgical time, but may avoid failure of antegrade placement of a double J catheter intraoperatively. Others do not advocate insertion of a ureteral catheter before surgery because they think that antegrade placement involves no great technical difficulty, and having a distended pelvis at the time of surgery facilitates dissection of the UPJ. We think that antegrade placement of the ureteral catheter during LESS-P is technically demanding and time-consuming; therefore, retrograde placement of a double J catheter during the LESS-P procedure was performed in all cases.

The patient was placed in a 45° flank position for transperitoneal surgery after induction with general endotracheal anesthesia. A 2-cm semilunar-shaped skin incision was concealed completely within the umbilicus and deepened to the

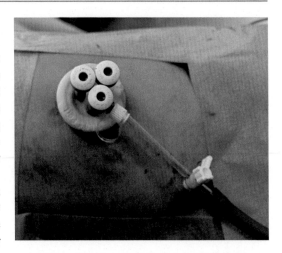

Fig. 19.14 The extracorporeal view of the SILS Port

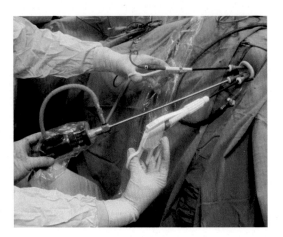

Fig. 19.15 The straight instrument was used in the left hand and roticulating laparoscopic scissors in the right hand

anterior rectus fascia, where a 2.5-cm median fascial incision was made, the peritoneum was incised, and the single-access multichannel laparoscopic port was deployed. Then pneumoperitoneum was established (Figs. 19.13 and 19.14). The instruments were inserted through channel of the port. A 5-mm 30° high-definition rigid laparoscope integrating different cameras (Karl Storz, Tuttlingen, Germany, and Gimmi, Tuttlingen, Germany) was used along with two working instruments. During the procedure a combination of flexible forceps and scissors and conventional laparoscopic (straight) instruments (e.g., scissors, ultrasound scissors, bipolar

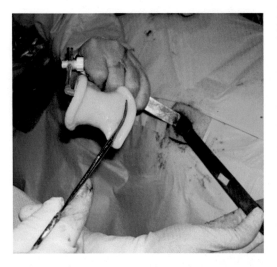

Fig. 19.13 SILS Port placed intraperitoneally with the help of a clamp

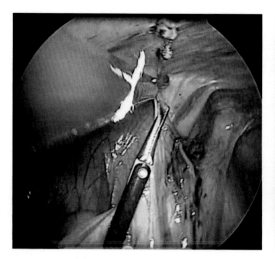

Fig. 19.16 Mobilization of the colon

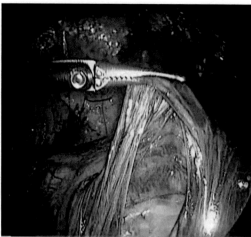

Fig. 19.17 Open of Gerota's fascia and dissection of the ureter

forceps) were used to perform the procedures as necessary (Fig. 19.15).

The dissection was begun with mobilization of the colon on the affected side medially by incising along the avascular line of Toldt (Fig. 19.16). The straight instrument in the left hand was used to dissect the tissue, while the peritoneal incision along the line of Toldt was performed with roticulating laparoscopic scissors held in the right hand. After Gerota's fascia was opened, dissection was carried down to the level of the kidney (Fig. 19.17). The adventitia around the proximal ureter and UPJ was cleared (Fig. 19.18). After complete laparoscopic mobilization of the UPJ, the renal pelvis and the proximal ureter were brought out to the abdominal wall by hitching the redundant pelvis.

A standard Anderson-Hynes dismembered pyeloplasty was performed (Fig. 19.19). The strictured region was excised sharply. The ureter was spatulated on its lateral aspect, and if necessary, the redundant renal pelvis was excised. The excision of the strictured region and the ureteral spatulation were performed using the reticulating scissors (Fig. 19.20). When UPJ obstruction was caused by a crossing vein or small artery, the vessel was dissected free. However, if the crossing vessel was a large arterial branch, the renal pelvis and ureter were transposed to the anterior of the vessel. The anastomosis between the ureter and

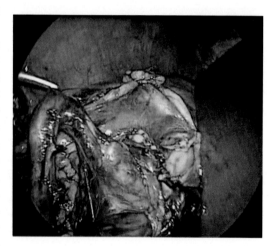

Fig. 19.18 Dissection of the renal pelvis

the renal pelvis was performed with a 4–0 Vicryl suture with an atraumatic needle in a running fashion (Fig. 19.21). After completion of the posterior wall anastomosis and before completion of the anterior wall anastomosis, a retrograde double J stent was advanced over the previously placed 0.035-in. guidewire, and the proximal end of the double J stent was passed into the renal pelvis (Fig. 19.22). After the anastomosis was completed (Fig. 19.23), a closed suction drain was placed through the SILS Port site (Figs. 19.24 and 19.25). The pneumoperitoneum was reduced and the port site was closed. A Foley catheter

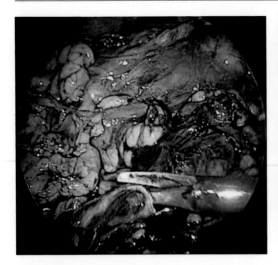

Fig. 19.19 Spatulation of the ureter

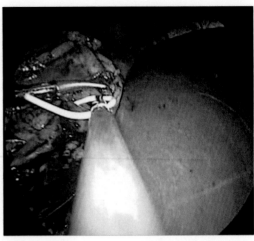

Fig. 19.22 Double J catheter placement

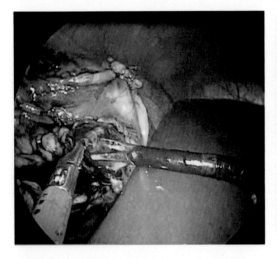

Fig. 19.20 The strictured region was excised sharply

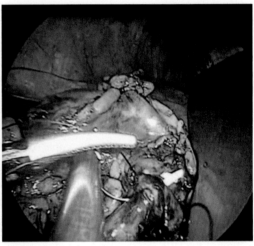

Fig. 19.23 Completing of anastomosis

remained in situ in all patients for 24 h after surgery (Fig. 19.26).

Complications in Pediatric LESS Reports

Vricella et al. reported three cases of LESS nephrectomy. The postoperative complication of hematoma was observed in one of the bilateral cases. In that case, blood transfusion and percutaneous drainage were needed [6].

Koh et al. reported 11 patients undergoing LESS nephrectomies for poorly functioning, hydronephrotic kidneys. Postoperatively, two

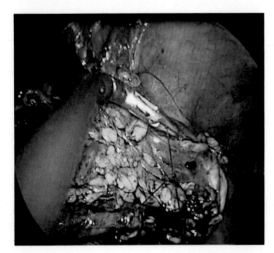

Fig. 19.21 Anastomosis

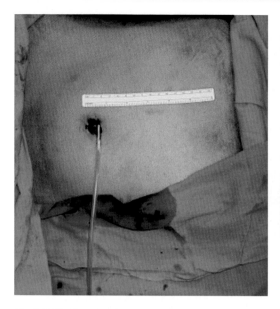

Fig. 19.24 Postoperative appearance

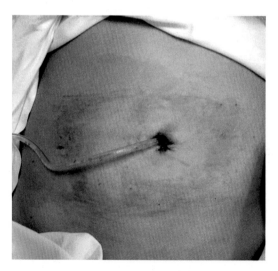

Fig. 19.25 Postoperative appearance (day 1)

male patients developed unilateral ipsilateral hydroceles on postoperative days 3 and 8, respectively. The hydrocele in the 39-day-old boy spontaneously resolved within 4 weeks after surgery. A surgical repair of the hydrocele was performed in the 3.9-year-old boy. The cause of the hydroceles was presumed to be secondary to a subclinical pattern processus vaginalis in both cases [7].

Tugcu et al. reported early experience with LESS pyeloplasty in children. There was no

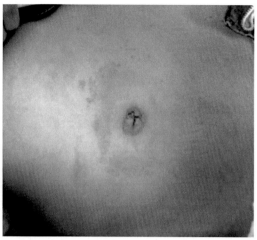

Fig. 19.26 Postoperative appearance (after 2 weeks)

major complication. The two minor complications, of wound infection at port site and urinary infection, were managed with conservative care [1].

References

1. Tugcu V, Ilbey YO, Polat H, Tasci AI. Early experience with laparoendoscopic single-site pyeloplasty in children. J Pediatr Urol. 2011;7(2):187–91.
2. Rane A, Rao P, Bonadio F, Rao P. Single port laparoscopic nephrectomy using a novel laparoscopic port (R-port) and evolution of single laparoscopic port procedure (SLIPP). J Endourol. 2007;21:A287.
3. Broder HL, Smith FB, Strauss RP. Effects of visible and invisible orofacial defects on self-perception and adjustment across developmental eras and gender. Cleft Palate Craniofac J. 1994;31(6):429–43.
4. Ganpule A, Sheladiya C, Mishra S, Sabnis R, Desai M. Laparoendoscopic single-site urologic surgery in children less than 5 years of age. Korean J Urol. 2013;54(8):541–6.
5. Tugcu V, Ilbey YO, Mutlu B, Tasci AI. Laparoendoscopic single-site surgery versus standard laparoscopic simple nephrectomy: a prospective randomized study. J Endourol. 2010;24(8):1315–20.
6. Vricella GJ, Ross JH, Vourganti S, Cherullo EE. Laparoendoscopic single-site nephrectomy: initial clinical experience in children. J Endourol. 2010;24(12):1957–61.
7. Koh CJ, De Filippo RE, Chang AY, Hardy BE, Berger A, Eisenberg M, Patil M, Aron M, Gill IS, Desai MM. Laparoendoscopic single-site nephrectomy in pediatric patients: initial clinical series of infants to adolescents. Urology. 2010;76(6):1457–61.

Part IV

Robotic LESS Surgery

Robotic Laparoendoscopic Single-Site Radical Nephrectomy

Dinesh Samarasekera and Jihad H. Kaouk

Introduction

It has been established that robotic-assisted laparoscopic surgery has several advantages when compared to standard laparoscopic surgery. Optics, ergonomics, dexterity, and precision are all enhanced with the use of the robotic platform for a number of urologic procedures. For these reasons, it was postulated that the application of robotics to laparoendoscopic single-site surgery (LESS) could overcome some of the constraints seen with the conventional laparoscopic approach. Issues such as instrument clashing, inability to achieve effective triangulation for dissection, and difficulties with intracorporeal suturing have limited the widespread adoption of conventional LESS in urology.

Kaouk et al. [1] reported the first experience with R-LESS in 2008 (radical prostatectomy and nephrectomy, pyeloplasty). It was noted that intracorporeal suturing and dissection were

easier, as compared with standard LESS. Since then there have been numerous reports and refinements in technique from the same group, for a number of different urologic procedures [2–4]. Furthermore there have been a number of series that have compared R-LESS to either standard laparoscopy, conventional LESS, or standard robotic surgery [2, 5, 6]. While these studies have been small and retrospective in nature, they have shown that R-LESS is not inferior with regard to perioperative outcomes and may offer better cosmesis. Additionally, the surgeons found the EndoWrist technology and three-dimensional high-definition camera beneficial. However, despite the advantages of the robotic platform, R-LESS is not free of challenges which are similar to conventional LESS. Instrument clashing remains an issue, due to the bulky external profile of the current robotic system. Other issues include lack of space for the assistant at the bedside, inability to incorporate the fourth robotic arm for retraction, and difficulties with triangulation. Although solutions for some of these issues are currently under development [7, 8], R-LESS is still very much in its infancy.

Standard robotic surgery and R-LESS share numerous similarities. The setup of the operating room is identical, as well as all the instruments, drapes, sutures, etc. Docking of the robot is also identical, although the arms may be angled differently to minimize instrument clashing. With regard to radical nephrectomy, almost all of the

D. Samarasekera, BSc, MD, FRCSC (✉)
Urology, Surrey Memorial Hospital,
207-13710 94a Ave., Surrey, BC V3V 1N1, Canada
e-mail: samarad@ccf.org; samarasekera@gmail.com

J.H. Kaouk, MD, FACS
Professor of Surgery, Cleveland Clinic Lerner College of Medicine, Zagarek Pollock Chair in Robotic Surgery, Center for Robotic and Image guided Surgery, Glickman Urologic Institute, Cleveland, OH, USA
e-mail: kaoukj@ccf.org

© Springer Science+Business Media New York 2017
J.H. Kaouk et al. (eds.), *Atlas of Laparoscopic and Robotic Single Site Surgery*,
Current Clinical Urology, DOI 10.1007/978-1-4939-3575-8_20

steps of standard robotic surgery are carried out in R-LESS. That being said, there are improvisations that are made because of the limited space with R-LESS. For example, because there is no space for the fourth arm, which is often used to retract tissue, various other techniques have been employed (i.e., stay and marionette sutures). Also other strategies are employed to minimize instrument clashing, such as moving the two arms and camera together in unison. For this reason, this chapter will focus on the equipment and procedural aspects that are specific to R-LESS radical nephrectomy and differ from standard robotic surgery.

Port Selection and Instrumentation

Multichannel Port Selection

A number of different multichannel ports have been used for R-LESS (radical nephrectomy and other procedures) (Table 20.1); however, there have been no direct head-to-head comparisons. In Kaouk et al.'s initial R-LESS series, the R-port (Advanced Surgical Concepts, Dublin, Ireland) was used. This port consists of one 12-mm channel, two 5-mm channels, and an insufflation cannula. The port is placed using the Hasson technique through a 2-cm umbilical incision. The authors made no specific comments with regard to

the performance of the port, and there were no reported issues with pneumoperitoneum leakage or instrument crowding. White et al. [3] reported their experience with 50 patients, which included 24 renal procedures and 26 pelvic procedures. They used three different commercially available ports, including the SILS port, the R-port, and the GelPort/GelPOINT. The authors mentioned of the three multichannel ports used, they preferred the SILS port because of its durability, the free exchange of cannulas of varying size, and the ease of passage of staplers, clip appliers, sutures, and entrapment bags through the port. However, they noted that gas leakage was experienced with three multichannel ports, which was usually caused by a fascial incision that was too large. To combat this, they placed a fascial suture or petroleum-impregnated gauze along the tract of the port. Stein et al. [2] used the GelPort laparoscopic access system to perform four R-LESS upper-tract procedures (pyeloplasty $n=2$, partial nephrectomy $n=1$, radical nephrectomy $n=1$). They concluded that the GelPort was beneficial for R-LESS, because it allowed for greater spacing and flexibility of port placement and easier access to the surgical field for the bedside assistant. Although the fascial incision they used was larger to place the port (2–2.5 cm), they found that this facilitated specimen extraction, especially during the radical nephrectomy. Finally, there have been a number of centers that have had

Table 20.1 Currently available multichannel ports

Instrument	Study	Features	Advantages	Disadvantages
SILS port (Covidien)	White et al. [4]	Flexible Expands after insertion to prevent air leak	Accommodates 3 variable-sized ports and instruments	Difficult insertion with large abdominal wall
GelPort/ GelPOINT (Applied Medical)	White et al. [3] Olweny et al. [6] Stein et al. [2] Fareed et al. [11]	GelSeal cap creates pseudoabdomen Insufflation port on side	Larger working platform for spacing of trocars Easier specimen extraction	Requires larger fascial incision Gas leakage during longer procedures
Homemade	Lee et al. [10] Arkoncel et al. [5]	Surgical glove placed over a wound retractor	Low cost Widely available Flexible port placement	Fragile; tears with inserting/reinserting robotic instruments Ballooning of port with high insufflation pressures

Table adapted from White et al. [4] and Autorino et al. [13]

experience using a homemade port, both for conventional LESS and R-LESS. Lee et al. [10] reported the largest series of R-LESS procedures using a homemade port, which consisted of an Alexis wound retractor (Applied Medical, Rancho Santa Margarita, CA) and a standard size 7 surgical glove stretched over the top. They utilized a 5–6 cm fascial incision to place the wound retractor. Four trocars were placed through the fingers of the glove, including two 8-mm robotic trocars and two 12-mm optical trocars. They performed 68 upper-tract procedures, including 51 partial nephrectomies, 12 nephroureterectomies, 2 adrenalectomies, 2 radical nephrectomies, and 1 simple nephrectomy. The authors felt that the homemade port offered greater flexibility of port placement than any of the commercially available multichannel devices, as well as being extremely cost-effective. Limitations included the susceptibility of the glove to tearing with insertion of the robotic instruments, the larger fascial incision required to place the wound retractor, and ballooning of the glove under higher pneumoperitoneum pressures (>20 mmHg). However, the authors concluded that their homemade port was a

safe, effective, low-cost alternative to commercially available multichannel ports.

Instrumentation

The vast majority of the R-LESS procedures to date have been performed with standard instruments (Table 20.2), as task-specific tools are currently under development and testing. Two of the larger clinical series both report the use of standard 8-mm and 5-mm instruments for a wide range of R-LESS procedures [9, 10]. White et al. [4] described using an 8-mm instrument in the right hand and a 5-mm pediatric instrument in the left hand for their R-LESS prostatectomy series of 20 patients. The authors felt this configuration maximized the benefit of each instrument. The 5-mm instruments do not articulate but instead deflect, which greatly increased their range of motion. Conversely the authors found that the EndoWrist action of the standard 8-mm instruments greatly facilitated complex tasks, such as suturing. Furthermore, they reported that the 8-mm robotic Hem-o-lok clip applier was

Table 20.2 Instrumentation currently available for robotic LESS procedures

Instrument	Features	Advantages	Disadvantages
8-mm EndoWrist monopolar shears	7° of freedom 90° of articulation Intuitive motion and fingertip control Motion scaling and tremor reduction	Instrument articulation allows access to difficult operative angles	Larger profile; increased instrument clashing because of lack of deflection
8-mm EndoWrist monopolar hook			
8-mm EndoWrist Prograsp grasper			
8-mm/5-mm needle drivers		Clips can be applied by operating surgeon	Time consuming; extra large clip size is not available
8-mm Hem-o-lok applier			
5-mm Schertel grasper	Robust snake-wrist architecture Intuitive motion and fingertip control Motion scaling and tremor reduction	Lower profile; triangulation is increased secondary to instrument deflection; functional in a tight working space	Lack of distal instrument tip articulation decreases overall range of motion; decreased grip strength
5-mm Harmonic scalpel	Nonwristed instrument based on Ethicon Endosurgery Harmonic technology Simultaneously cuts and coagulates Motion scaling and tremor reduction	Can be applied by the operating surgeon; time efficient	Does not articulate; increased amount of instrument clashing

Table adapted from White et al. [4] and Autorino [13]

beneficial during nerve sparing, as clip placement was in the surgeon's console control and clashing with the bedside assistant's instruments was minimized.

Surgical Technique

Patient Positioning and Port Placement

The patient is positioned in the modified flank position at approximately 60°, and the arms are supported with a double arm board (Fig. 20.1). The table is flexed, positioned in slight Trendelenburg, and the patient is secured. The umbilicus is identified and an incision is made, intraumbilically, 2 cm above and 1 cm below the umbilicus (Fig. 20.2). The abdomen is entered in the midline using an open technique. When the SILS port is to be used, the fascial incision is enlarged enough to accommodate two fingers. The robotic trocars are placed inside the skin incision at the apices of the incision. The trocars are tunneled into the abdomen atop two fingers and directed lateral to the midline. The SILS port is inserted with the premade trocars, and the abdomen is insufflated (Fig. 20.3). When the

GelPort or GelPOINT port is used, the fascial incision is enlarged, and the device is deployed in the standard fashion (Fig. 20.4). The robotic trocars are inserted at the most cephalad and caudal aspects of the device, while the camera trocar is placed at the most medial and central portion (Fig. 20.5). Either the da Vinci S or da Vinci Si system (in a three-arm approach) is then positioned over the patient's shoulder, with the camera oriented in line with the kidney, and docked (Fig. 20.6). No modifications to the robotic system are done, and the system is docked in the same fashion as traditional robotic renal procedures. The 12-mm robotic scope with a 30° lens directed downward is introduced, and either a 5-mm channel in the SILS port or an additional 12-mm port added through the GelPort or GelPOINT port remains free for assistance.

Colon Mobilization

Colon mobilization is performed using the 8-mm EndoWrist (Intuitive Surgical) monopolar shears in the right hand and an 8-mm EndoWrist Prograsp grasper in the left (Fig. 20.7). Instruments are not intentionally crossed throughout the procedure. The bowel is mobilized medially, and

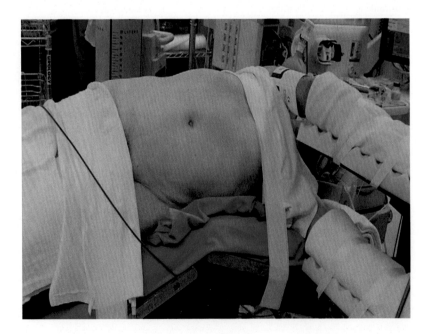

Fig. 20.1 Patient positioning

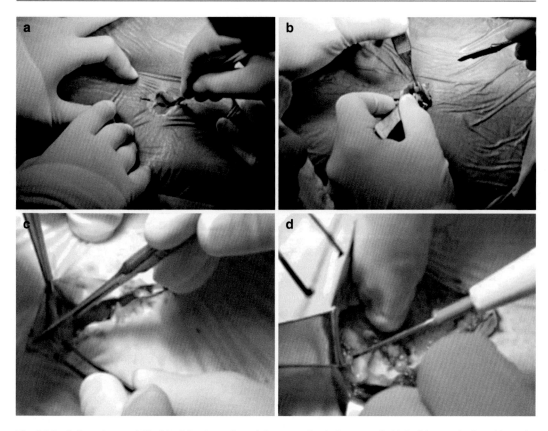

Fig. 20.2 A 3-cm intraumbilical incision is made and the rectus fascia is exposed. (**a**) Incision made thru skin at the umbilicus. (**b**) Umbilicus is carefurlly everted. (**c**) Incision taken deeper into the facia. (**d**) Meticulous hemostasis is carefully achieved to avoid later seromas

dissection continues cephalad to mobilize the spleen or liver. Colon mobilization proceeds similarly to conventional laparoscopic nephrectomy, except that the assistant's suction retraction is more vital to the dissection.

Ureteral Identification

The ureter and gonadal vein are identified, and dissection proceeds cephalad along the psoas muscle, with slight anterior elevation of the ureter to identify the renal hilum. The assistant provides counter retraction with the suction device (Fig. 20.8).

Hilar Dissection and Control

After the hilum is identified, it is dissected using either the 8-mm EndoWrist monopolar curved

shears or the 8-mm EndoWrist permanent cautery hook (Fig. 20.9). The 8-mm EndoWrist Hem-o-lok clip applier (Teleflex Medical, Research Triangle Park, NC, USA) is used to control the artery and then the vein (Fig. 20.10). If difficulty of immobilization of the renal hilum is encountered, an endovascular stapler is introduced through a vacant SILS port trocar site after the 5-mm trocar has been removed or directly through the GelPort/GelPOINT faceplate, and the artery and vein are controlled separately.

Kidney Mobilization

The remaining attachments to the kidney are freed by a combination of blunt and sharp dissection (Fig. 20.11). If the spleen or liver cannot be retracted adequately, an additional 5-mm trocar can be placed outside the initial incision, in a reduced port fashion, to allow for assistant

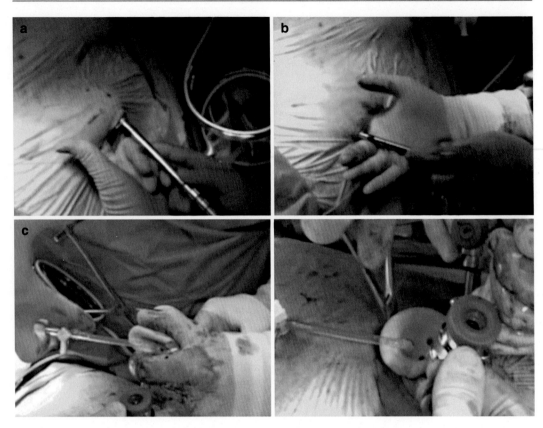

Fig. 20.3 (**a**, **b**) 8-mm robotic trocars are tunneled under the skin into the abdomen through separate fascial stab incisions. (**c**, **d**) The SILS port is placed cranial to the robotic trocars through a separate fascial incision

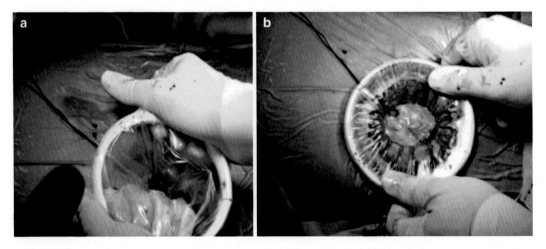

Fig. 20.4 The wound protector is placed through a single fascial incision when the GelPOINT device is used. (**a**) Using both hands the gelport ring is rolled on itself to tighten. (**b**) Adequate positioning of the gelport as shown

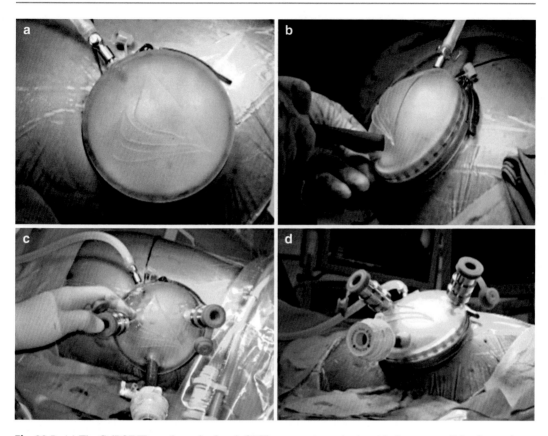

Fig. 20.5 (**a**) The GelPOINT membrane is placed. (**b**) The camera trocar is placed in the most medial and central portion. (**c**, **d**) The robotic trocars are placed in the most cephalad and caudal aspects

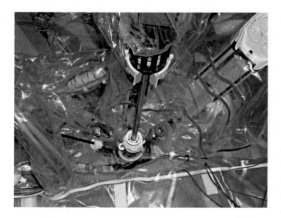

Fig. 20.6 The robot is docked using a three-arm approach over the patient's shoulder with the camera in line with the kidney

retraction and completion of upper-pole mobility. Finally, the ureter and gonadal vein are clipped and divided in a standard fashion (Fig. 20.12).

Kidney Extraction and Closure

A 15-mm entrapment sac is inserted through one of the premade trocar sites of the SILS port after the 5-mm trocars have been removed or directly through the faceplate of the GelPort or GelPOINT port (Fig. 20.13). The specimen is removed and, if needed, the skin incision is enlarged. The fascia is closed with a large absorbable suture, and the

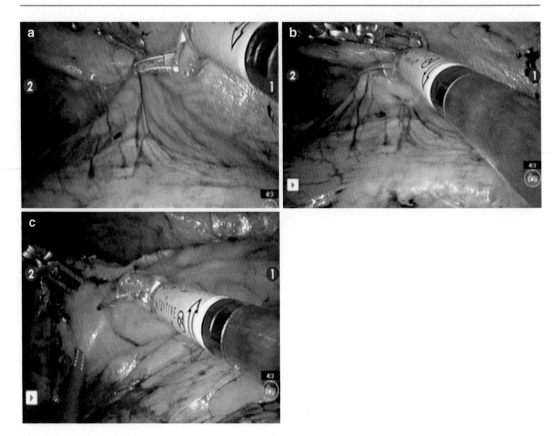

Fig. 20.7 (**a, b**) Colon mobilization proceeds similarly to conventional laparoscopic nephrectomy. (**c**) The assistant provides retraction with the suction-irrigator which aids dissection

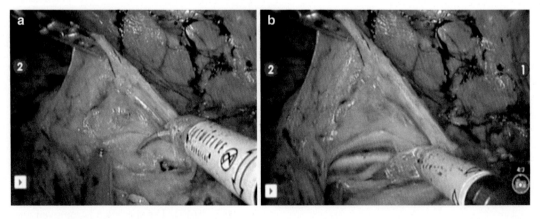

Fig. 20.8 (**a, b**) The ureter and gonadal vein are identified in the retroperitoneum. (**b, c**) A plane is created out to the psoas muscle and the ureter and gonadal vein are lifted (*left side dissection*)

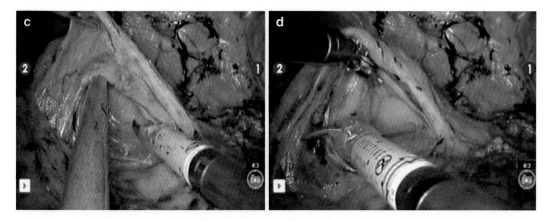

Fig. 20.8 (continued)

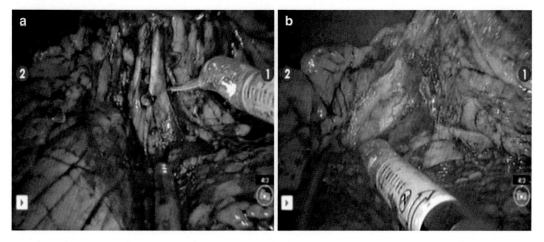

Fig. 20.9 (**a**, **b**) The renal hilum is dissected in a standard fashion

umbilicus is reapproximated to the fascia with the same suture. The subcutaneous adipose tissue is closed with a 3-0 absorbable suture to reduce seroma formation, and the skin is sutured in a subcuticular fashion (Fig. 20.14). No drain is placed.

Outcomes

Unfortunately, there is a paucity of data with regard to R-LESS radical nephrectomy, and no prospective comparative analyses exist. Conventional LESS radical nephrectomy was compared to standard laparoscopic radical nephrectomy in a recent meta-analysis, which included 1,094 cases [12]. A longer operative time and a higher conversion rate were found for the LESS group, as compared with conventional laparoscopic nephrectomy. However, LESS nephrectomy was associated with less postoperative pain, lower analgesic requirement, shorter hospital stay, shorter recovery time, and a better cosmetic outcome. No significant differences were found in perioperative complications or estimated blood loss. Theoretically these benefits would apply to R-LESS as well; however, only one comparative study exists. White et al. [3] performed a retrospective comparative analysis of ten patients who underwent R-LESS radical

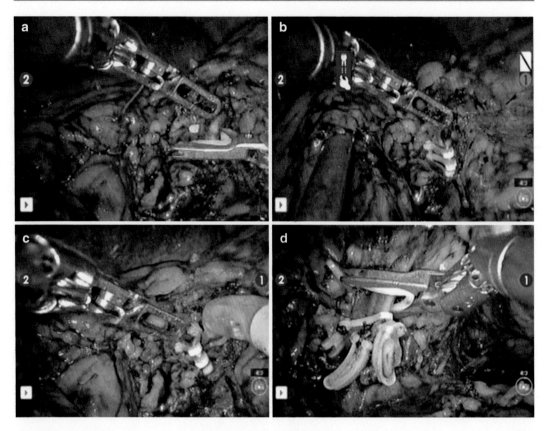

Fig. 20.10 The artery and vein can be controlled with Hem-o-lok clips or an endovascular stapler. (**a**) Artery clipped. (**b**) Artery clipped and cut. (**c**) Renal vein dissected. (**d**) Renal vein double clipped

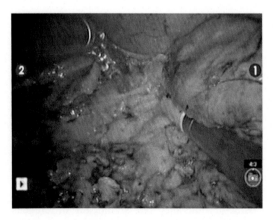

Fig. 20.11 The kidney is then mobilized completely in preparation for extraction

nephrectomy. They were matched to a similar cohort of ten patients who underwent conventional laparoscopic radical nephrectomy. Patients were similar at baseline, with no significant difference in ASA score, BMI, or tumor size. The SILS port and the GelPort were both used, and the robot was docked in a three-arm approach. There was no difference between R-LESS and conventional laparoscopy nephrectomy with regard to median operative time, estimated blood loss, visual analogue scale, or complication rate. The R-LESS group had a lower median narcotic requirement during hospital admission (25.3 morphine equivalents vs 37.5 morphine equivalents; $p = 0.049$) and a shorter length of stay (2.5 days vs 3.0 day; $p = 0.03$).

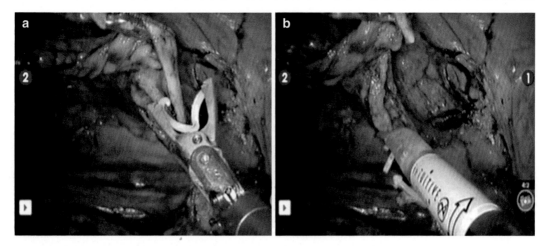

Fig. 20.12 (**a, b**) The ureter and gonadal vein are clipped and divided

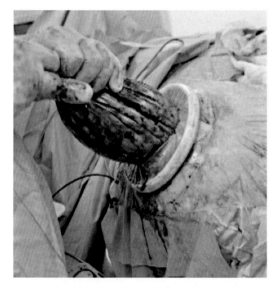

Fig. 20.13   The ports are removed and the specimen is extracted

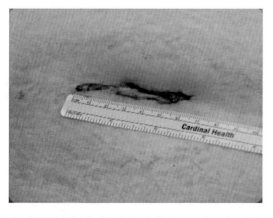

Fig. 20.14   The final incision is 5–6 cm in length and is hidden in the umbilicus

Conclusions

Robotic laparoendoscopic single-site surgery radical nephrectomy is technically feasible. The surgical technique is similar to a standard laparoscopic nephrectomy, with a few modifications. The assistant plays an even larger role, as the fourth robotic arm is not available for retraction. There are a number of different access ports which all seem to perform similarly, and the choice should be at the discretion of the surgeon. Currently, standard robotic instruments can be used; however, single-site-specific tools are currently under design. External clashing can be minimized by moving the robotic instruments in concert with the camera. Furthermore, the use of the GelPort facilitates spacing of the instruments, by providing a larger surface area for port placement. Other strategies like crossing the instruments at the abdominal wall have also been attempted. Unfortunately there are only a few studies comparing R-LESS radical nephrectomy to the standard technique. However, there does seem to be a trend toward improved cosmesis and lower postoperative analgesic requirements. Finally, task-specific, cost-effective robotic platforms that are specifically designed for single-site use are likely required if this technique is to gain widespread adoption.

References

1. Kaouk JH, Goel RK, Haber GP, Crouzet S, Stein RJ. Robotic single-port transumbilical surgery in humans: initial report. BJU Int. 2008;103:366–9.
2. Stein RJ, White WM, Goel RK, Irwin BH, Haber GP, Kaouk JH. Robotic laparoendoscopic single-site surgery using GelPort as the access platform. Eur Urol. 2010;57:132–7.
3. White MA, Autorino R, Spana G, et al. Robotic laparoendoscopic single-site radical nephrectomy: surgical technique and comparative outcomes. Eur Urol. 2011;59:815–22.
4. White MA, Haber G-P, Autorino R, et al. Robotic laparoendoscopic single-site radical prostatectomy: technique and early outcomes. Eur Urol. 2010;58:544–50.
5. Arkoncel FR, Lee JW, Rha KH, Han WK, Jeoung HB, Oh CK. Two-port robot-assisted vs standard robot-assisted laparoscopic partial nephrectomy: a matched-pair comparison. Urology. 2011;78:581–5.
6. Olweny EO, Park SK, Tan YK, Gurbuz C, Cadeddu JA, Best SL. Perioperative comparison of robotic assisted laparoendoscopic single-site (LESS) pyeloplasty versus conventional LESS pyeloplasty. Eur Urol. 2012;61:410–4.
7. Joseph RA, Goh AC, Cuevas SP, et al. Chopstick surgery: a novel technique improves surgeon performance and eliminates arm collision in robotic single-incision laparoscopic surgery. Surg Endosc. 2010;24:1331–5.
8. Haber GP, White MA, Autorino R, et al. Novel robotic da Vinci instruments for laparoendoscopic single-site surgery. Urology. 2010;76:1279–82.
9. White MA, Autorino R, Spana G, Hillyer S, Stein RJ, Kaouk JH. Robotic laparoendoscopic single site urological surgery: analysis of 50 consecutive cases. J Urol. 2012;187:1696–701.
10. Lee JW, Arkoncel FRP, Rha KH, et al. Urologic robot-assisted laparoendoscopic single-site surgery using a homemade single-port device:a single-center experience of 68 cases. J Endourol. 2011;25:1481–5.
11. Fareed K, Zaytoun OM, Autorino R, et al. Robotic single port suprapubic transvesical enucleation of the prostate (R-STEP): initial experience. BJU Int. 2012;110(5):732–7.
12. Fan X, Lin T, Xu K, et al. Laparoendoscopic single-site nephrectomy compared with conventional laparoscopic nephrectomy: a systematic review and meta-analysis of comparative studies. Eur Urol. 2012;62:601–12.
13. Autorino R, Kaouk JH, Stolzenburg J, et al. Current status and future directions of robotic single-site surgery: a systematic review. Eur Urol. 2013;63:266–80.

Robotic LESS Partial Nephrectomy

21

Christos Komninos, Tae Young Shin,
and Koon Ho Rha

Introduction

Partial nephrectomy (PN) has become the standard of care for the management of small renal
masses [1]. For appropriately selected patient,
nephron-sparing surgery has equivalent oncologic outcomes to radical nephrectomy with the
added benefits of parenchymal preservation and
evidence of improved overall survival [2].

PN is well suited for robotic assistance
because of the requirement for instrument dexterity during the excision of the tumor and reconstruction of the collecting system and renal

C. Komninos, MD, MSc, PhD
Urology Department, Severance Hospital, Yonsei
University College of Medicine, Seoul, South Korea,
Korea
e-mail: CHRKOM@yuhs.ac

T.Y. Shin, MD
Department of Urology, ChunCheon Sacred Heart
Hospital, Hallym University, Chuncheon, Kangwon,
South Korea
e-mail: shinergy@hallym.or.kr

K.H. Rha, MD, PhD (✉)
Urology Department, Severance Hospital, Yonsei
University College of Medicine, Seoul, South Korea

Department of Urology and Urological Science
Institute, Yonsei University College of Medicine,
Seoul, South Korea
e-mail: khrha@yuhs.ac

cortex. The first robotic partial nephrectomy
study was published in 2004, by Gettman et al.
[3]. Since then, robot-assisted multi-port laparoscopic partial nephrectomy (RPN) gained
momentum worldwide in the treatment of small-
and medium-size renal masses.

With widespread acceptance of minimal
access operations among patients and surgeons in
the urologic community, surgical evolution has
gone one step further by reducing access to a
single port. Although the da Vinci Surgical
System (Intuitive Surgical, Sunnyvale, CA, USA)
has been designed for multi-port procedures,
robotic single-port surgery (R-LESS) has been
developed in an attempt to perform major surgery
with minimal incisions and nearly scar-free outcome. Kaouk and colleagues were the first to
report their experience in R-LESS PN operations
in humans, in an effort to merge the beneficial
attributes of the da Vinci Surgical System to the
minimally invasive approach of R-LESS PN [4].
The advantages of the da Vinci Surgical System
for LESS include; easier articulation using
EndoWrist instruments, three-dimensional visualization, motion scaling, and tremor filtration.
Thenceforth, nephron-sparing surgery is increasingly performed by R-LESS approach. The
worldwide experience with R-LESS PN procedures is summarized in Table 21.1.

However, R-LESS PN is remains challenging
and more complicated for surgeons compared
with conventional RPN. Therefore, when start-

© Springer Science+Business Media New York 2017
J.H. Kaouk et al. (eds.), *Atlas of Laparoscopic and Robotic Single Site Surgery*,
Current Clinical Urology, DOI 10.1007/978-1-4939-3575-8_21

Table 21.1 Worldwide published studies in R-LESS PN procedures

Author	Y	Ports	N	TS	OT	WIT	EBL	PM	Conv
Kaouk et al. [4]	2009	Triport	2	2	170	nm	100	0	0
Stein et al. [33]	2010	GelPort	1	11	180	nm	600	0	0
Jeon et al. [33]	2010	Glove technique	11	3.7	227	30.7	667	0	1
[a]Haber et al. [15]	2010	da Vinci platform	4	–	37.5	14.8	30	–	0
Lee et al. [35]	2011	Glove technique	51	3.0	217	27	322	nm	2
Han et al. [36]	2011	Glove technique	14	3.2	233	30	464	0	2
Choi et al. [37]	2011	Glove technique	56	2.8	198	26	273	2	2
[b]Seo et al. [38]	2011	Glove technique	1	2.8	350	29	522	0	0
Khanna et al. [39]	2011	Triport/GelPort/SILS	5	4	172	NM	242	0	1
[a]Kaouk et al. [40]	2012	da Vinci platform	1	–	nm	21	nm	–	nm
Tiu et al. [41]	2013	Glove technique	39	3	185	25	150	1	0

Y year, *N* number of subjects, *TS* tumor size (cm), *OT* operative time (minutes), *WIT* warm ischemia time (minutes), *EBL* estimated blood loss (ml), *PM* positive surgical margins, *Conv* conversion to conventional PN, *nm* not mentioned in the study
[a]Studies in animals
[b]Bilateral R-LESS PN

ing R-LESS PN surgery, proper patient selection and adequate robotic experience are recommended to minimize complications and conversions [5].

Indications-Contraindications

Although indications and contraindications for R-LESS have not been recommended, studies have shown that all patients who are candidates for open PN are also eligible for RPN [6]. Traditional indications for PN have included patients with renal insufficiency, hereditary kidney cancer, bilateral renal masses, or renal mass in an anatomical or functional solitary kidney. Nowadays, PN is also indicated in patients with T1a and T1b tumors, with a normally functioning contralateral kidney [7].

Patient selection for R-LESS PN is essential. Strict patient selection criteria should be applied by surgeons to minimize the likelihood of complications [8]. In a recent analysis, Autorino and colleagues found that PN represents by far the procedure most likely to be converted during LESS [9]. Thus, only highly selected masses should be approached with LESS to maintain acceptable outcomes.

From a technical standpoint, mainly masses with low complexity (PADUA and RENAL score) are the one suitable for R-LESS PN [10–12]. However, R-LESS PN has been also reported as a safe and effective procedure in high complexity tumors in experienced surgeons [13].

Relative contraindications of R-LESS PN include over-obese patients, patients with extensive previous abdominal surgery, and patients with chronic renal failure who cannot tolerate warm ischemia [7].

Access Platforms in R-LESS PN

According to current endorsed nomenclature, R-LESS access can be obtained either by performing a single skin and fascial incision, through which a single multichannel access platform is placed (single-port), or by placing several low-profile ports through separate fascial incisions (single site) [5]. Although several commercially available single-port access devices have been reported in published studies, it is inevitable that more research is required for the development and design of an ideal robotic platform [14]. Loss of triangulation and clashing of instruments are usual limitations occurring independently of the device used.

The following single-port devices have been used in R-LESS PN studies:

- *Glove technique and Alexis retractor (Applied Medical, Rancho Santa Margarita, CA,USA)*
A surgical glove is folded around the outer ring of an Alexis retractor, and two robotic ports, the camera port, and the assistant port are inserted through the fingers of the glove.
- *Triport (Advanced Surgical Concepts, Bray, Co. Wicklow, Ireland)*
This platform is a multichannel port with three soft valves, in which one robotic port, the camera, and the assistant port are inserted. The robotic port for the second instrument is placed directly in the wound, in tandem with the Triport.
- *GelPort (Applied Medical, Rancho Santa Margarita, CA, USA)*
The GelPort is an Alexis wound retractor adapted with a gel seal cap. The robotic ports are directly inserted in the gel.
- *SILS port (Covidien, Dublin, Ireland)*
This device is made of elastic polymer. The top of the port has small perforations for insertion of rigid ports.
- *da Vinci single-site platform (Intuitive Surgical, Sunnyvale, CA, USA)*
Intuitive Surgical International has recently developed a new set of instruments and accessories for robotic single incision laparoscopy, to be used with the da Vinci Si Surgical System: the da Vinci Single-Site Instrumentation (VeSPA surgical instruments) [15]. The access device is a soft silicon reel-shaped port with four channels. Two channels accommodate curved cannulae for the flexible robotic instruments, while the third and fourth channels remain for the laparoscope and the assistant's instrument. The left robotic instrument is directed downward to the right, whereas the right one is directed downward to the left. Although the robotic instruments are crossed at the entrance site, the instruments are automatically reassigned by the system software, such as the left hand of the surgeon's control would control the left instrument and vice versa. With this "chopstick" surgery technique,

collision of the external robotic arms can be prevented as was reported by Joseph et al. [16].

The benefits and disadvantages of several access devices which have been used in R-LESS PN procedures are summarized in Table 21.2.

Patient Evaluation

A staging evaluation with an abdominal CT or MRI and a chest X-ray should be undertaken in all patients. CT angiography is of major importance since it can provide us information about the renal vessels' anatomy. Additional imaging such as chest CT, head CT, and bone scan is ordered based on clinical signs and symptoms of metastasis. Regular blood testing with electrolytes, creatinine, blood urea nitrogen, liver function tests, and coagulation tests is also necessary.

Patient Preparation

Anticoagulants and antiplatelets should be stopped at least 5 days before the operation. Mechanical bowel preparation is not necessary. Our current practice is to just allow clear liquids the day before. On the night before surgery, patients are instructed not to drink or eat anything after midnight. Prevention of thrombosis (low molecular weight heparin) is mandatory, and single-shot i.v. antibiotics using a cephalosporin should be administered 30 min before incision, unless there is a history of allergy to penicillin. We also advocate calf stimulators to reduce the potential risk of deep vein thrombosis.

Instruments and Equipment

We generally use three robotic instruments during R-LESS PN (Intuitive Surgical, Sunnyvale, CA):

- EndoWrist Hot Shears monopolar curved scissors in the dominant hand
- Fenestrated bipolar grasper or Maryland bipolar forceps in the nondominant hand
- Robotic needle drivers for renorrhaphy

Table 21.2 Advantages and disadvantages of several ports used in R-LESS PN operations

Port	Additional incisions	Advantages	Disadvantages
Triport	1 additional trocar through separate facial incision	Small device	Less flexibility Rigid outer ring inducing interference with the ports Conflicts
GelPort	No	Large working platform Flexibility of port placement Easy specimen extraction Minimal collisions	Large incision (>2.5 cm) Bulging of the GelCap with insufflation
SILS port	2 additional trocars through separate facial incisions	Durable Free exchange of varying cannula sizes Easy passage of equipments	
Glove technique	5 mm subxiphoid port for right kidney tumors	Large working platform Broad range of motion Low cost Flexibility Effective in keeping pneumoperitoneum	Fragility Ballooning of glove
da Vinci single-site platform	No	Triangulation Minimal collisions Adequate ergonomics Wide range of movements 30° downward camera	Loss of distal tip articulation Restricted space for the bedside assistant Unavailable 4th robotic arm

Single-port device, long suction tip and irrigator, laparoscopic needle drivers, grasper and scissors, laparoscopic ultrasound, laparoscopic bulldog clamp applier, polyglactin sutures, 5 mm Hem-o-lok clip applier, haemostatic agents, and drain are also indispensable equipment. Moreover, equipment for conversion to either robot-assisted laparoscopic radical nephrectomy or open procedure must be always prepared in the table.

Surgical Technique

Regardless of tumor location, complete exposure and mobilization of the kidney are preferred to allow optimal visualization and positioning of the tumor in the middle of the surgeon's field of view. In case of severe adhesions and difficulty in progression, a conversion to LESS port laparoscopy, standard laparoscopy, or open approach is recommended.

Patient Positioning and Single-Port Device Placement: Glove Technique

After induction of general endotracheal anesthesia, a Foley catheter and a nasogastric tube are placed to decompress the urinary bladder and stomach. The patient is placed in a 45-degree flank position with the ipsilateral side elevated and secured to the operating table, after padding the pressure points. The lower leg is flexed, the upper leg is straightened, and a pillow is placed between them. When the patient is positioned securely, the table is rolled to a classic flank position to verify the stability of the system (Fig. 21.1).

The table is tilted to position the patient supine, and a 4 cm midline periumbilical incision is made and dissected deep to the rectus fascia, down through the peritoneum (Figs. 21.2 and 21.3). The fascial incision is slightly larger at 5 cm. Access to the peritoneum is then obtained, and an Alexis wound retractor is inserted through the incision in the peritoneal cavity and rolled up. Thereafter, a common size 7 surgical glove is applied over the external side of the wound retractor, the retractor is rolled down till the abdominal wall and the fingers of the glove are secured by sutures (Fig. 21.4). Four trocars (two 12 mm and two 8 mm) are inserted through incisions on the fingertips of the surgical glove and fixed by using rubber bands (Fig. 21.5). A 12 mm trocar for the camera is placed in the most medial position (finger 3), and 8 mm robotic trocars are placed laterally (fingers 1 and 4). An assistant

Fig. 21.1 Patient's
position in Left
R-LESS PN

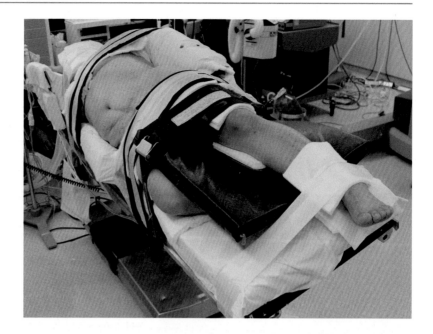

Fig. 21.2 The patient is
positioned supine in order
to insert the single-port
device

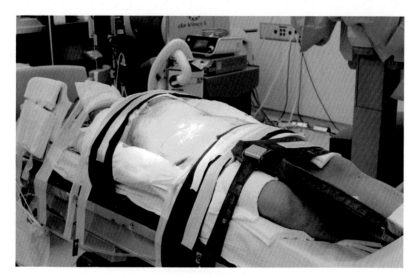

12 mm port is positioned near the edge of the cap
(finger 5).

Pneumoperitoneum is achieved through the
12 mm camera port and set at 15 mmHg. A 30°
robotic scope is used viewing upward. For right-
sided cases, an additionally 5 mm port may be
inserted in the subxiphoid area for liver retraction. Afterward, the table is rolled at 60°.

The robot is then introduced to the surgical
field toward the back side of the patient and
docked, with the camera oriented in line with the
kidney (Fig. 21.6).

Bowel Mobilization

The kidney is exposed by incising along the
white line of Toldt at the lateral border of the
colon (Fig. 21.7). After colon is mobilized
medially, sharp and blunt dissection is used to
develop the avascular plane between Gerota's
fascia and the posterior mesocolon (Fig. 21.8).
This dissection is continued along the upper
pole of the kidney to mobilize the spleen or the
liver. Care must be taken to avoid thermal injury
to the bowel.

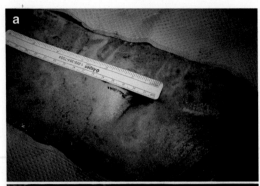

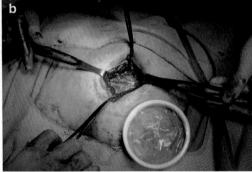

Fig. 21.3 (a) 4 cm umbilical incision is made; (b) the incision is dissected down through the peritoneum, with the fascial incision slightly larger

Spleen/Liver Mobilization-Duodenum Dissection

Attachments to the spleen (splenocolic, splenore-nal, lienophrenic ligaments) are released allowing the spleen and the tail of the pancreas to be separated from the upper pole of the kidney, and the adrenal is spared (Fig. 21.9).

For right-sided renal tumors, we primarily incise along the posterior hepatic ligament to free the posterior liver edge from the specimen, and then we incise the peritoneum parallel to ascending colon and above the hepatic flexure. The duodenum, which is medial to the vena cava, is identified and dissected free from Gerota's fascia and retracted medially (Fig. 21.10). The inferior vena cava and the right renal vein can usually be exposed posterior to the duodenum.

Ureteral Identification, Hilar Dissection, and Tumor Exposure

Once the colon has been mobilized caudally, till the common iliac vessels, to expose the lower pole of the kidney, the retroperitoneum can be dissected layer by layer until the ureter and gonadal vessels are identified. The ureter with surrounding fibro-fatty tissue is lifted, and the psoas muscle is widely exposed. Ureter is then retracted upward alongside the lower pole to facilitate hilar dissection (Fig. 21.11).

The hilum is identified by tracing the gonadal vein in cranial direction. On the left side, the gonadal vein is traced to its insertion in the renal vein, while on the right side the gonadal is traced to the inferior vena cava (Fig. 21.12). The renal vein at first and the renal artery afterward are identified. The renal artery is located posteriorly to the renal vein, and visualization of arterial pulsations can aid in identifying its location. Ligation of the left gonadal vein may be performed in order to increase mobility of the left renal vein for better exposure of the renal artery.

The preparation of the renal vessels is mandatory, in order to proceed to clamping of the artery in the presence of serious bleeding during the resection of the tumor (Fig. 21.13). Hilar lymphatic vessels and small accessory veins can usually be divided using the monopolar or bipolar cautery. Attention should be paid to avoid inadvertent injury to adrenal vein and posterior lumbar vein on the left side.

Thence, the posterior-lateral attachments to the abdominal wall are released, and after incising Gerota's fascia, the kidney is defatted to expose the tumor. Laparoscopic ultrasound with TilePro projection (Intuitive Surgical, Sunnyvale, CA, USA) onto the console screen is introduced through the 12 mm assistant port to confirm the tumor margin and depth (Fig. 21.14). The mass is identified and circumferentially marked by electrocautery to provide a line by which excision of the tumor can follow.

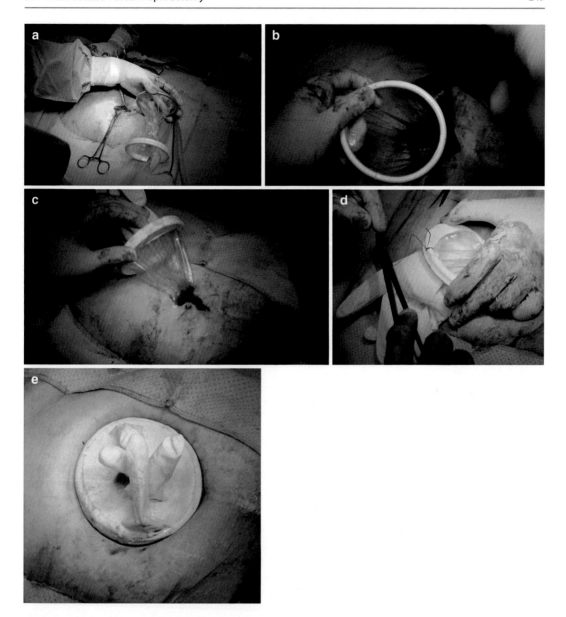

Fig. 21.4 Development of glove technique: (**a**) an Alexis wound retractor is inserted in the peritoneal cavity; (**b**) the retractor is rolled up; (**c**) a surgical glove is attached into the wound retractor; (**d**) the glove is secured by sutures; (**e**) the retractor is rolled down

Clamping of the Renal Vessels

Based on the location of the tumor, hilar control is important to safely resect the tumor and achieve adequate hemostasis. In an attempt to minimize warm ischemia time (WIT), all necessary material including sutures and hemostatic agents are inserted before hilar clamping. We usually ask the anesthesiologists to prescribe intravenous 12.5 g mannitol and 20 mg

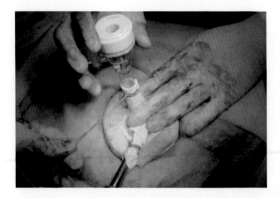

Fig. 21.5 Four trocars are inserted into the fingers of the glove and fixed using rubber bands

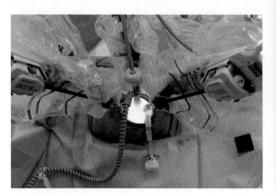

Fig. 21.6 The robot is docked at the back side of the patient. A camera trocar is placed in the most medial position, the robotic trocars are placed laterally, and the assistant 12 mm port is positioned near the edge of the cap

furosemide 30 min and 1 min before occlusion, respectively.

Temporary occlusion of the renal artery and vein is performed by placement of laparoscopic bulldog clamps through the assistant port, by the assistant. The renal artery is clamped first, followed by the renal vein (Fig. 21.15). Care must be taken to avoid movement of the clamp or collision with any of the robotic instruments, which might result to renal vessel injury.

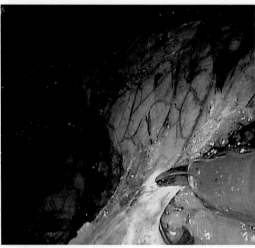

Fig. 21.8 Development of the plane between Gerota's fascia and the posterior mesocolon, in the anterior surface of the kidney, up to the spleen

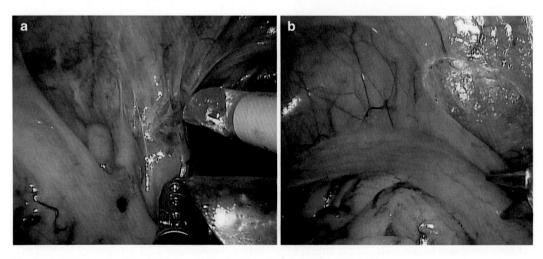

Fig. 21.7 (**a**) The colon is mobilized medially, (**b**) along the white line of Toldt

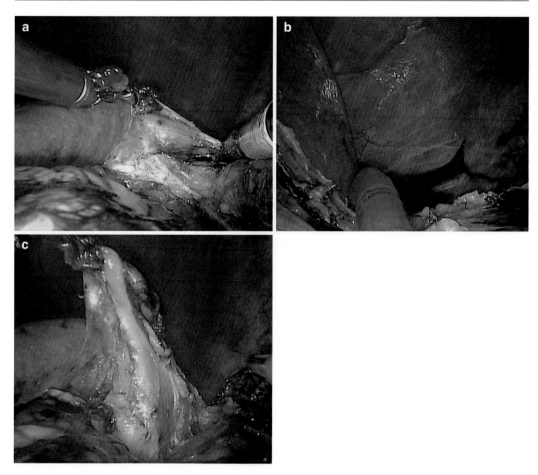

Fig. 21.9 Spleen mobilization and adrenal detachment: (**a**) release of the spleen attachments, allowing the spleen and the tail of the pancreas to be separated from the upper pole of the kidney; (**b**) spleen is mobilized; (**c**) the adrenal is detached medially

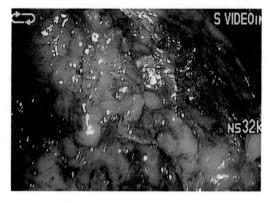

Fig. 21.10 On the *right side*, the duodenum is retracted medially. The inferior vena cava and right renal vein usually can be exposed posterior to the duodenum

In an effort to shorten WIT, early unclamping technique can be performed after placement of the first layer of parenchymal sutures [17].

Occasionally, exophytic small renal masses can be approached without ischemia in selected patients with cT1a disease and low PADUA score (off-clamping technique). Although a higher blood loss is encountered, operative time is shorter and estimated glomerular filtration rate (eGFR) is better preserved than complete hilar control, while potential ischemic and vascular injury to the kidney is avoided [18–20]. Additionally, sometimes we perform the "zero ischemia" technique, in which only the

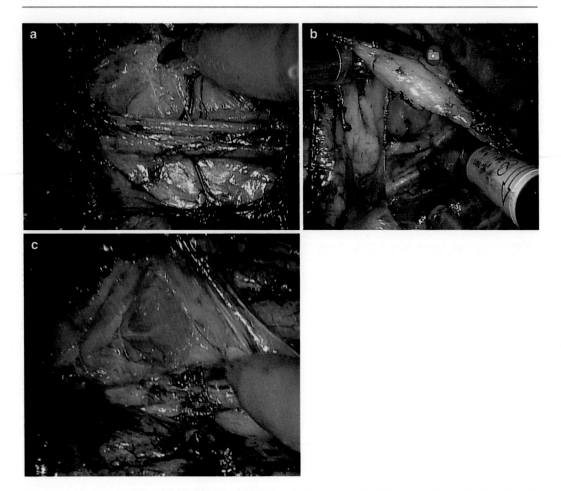

Fig. 21.11 Ureteral identification: (**a**) the ureter is identi-fied. Gonadal vein and artery are above the ureter, crossing to it; (**b**) the ureter with surrounding fat tissue is lifted up on the lower pole of the kidney to facilitate hilar dissection; (**c**) only the ureter is pulled *upward*, allowing the identification of renal hilum by tracing the gonadal vein cranially

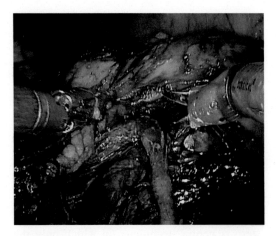

Fig. 21.12 The renal vein is recognized by tracing the gonadal vein in cranial dissection. On the *left side*, the gonadal vein is inserted into the renal vein, while on the *right*, it is inserted into the inferior vena cava

segmental artery supplying the tumor is clamped, minimizing the bleeding and allowing tumor excision and renorrhaphy to proceed without the constraint of main arterial clamping [21]. In the above cases, the intra-abdominal pressure of the pneumoperitoneum is increased to 20 mmHg, to avoid possible bleeding from small vessels, allowing a precise resection of the tumor even with unclamped renal vessels. If excessive intraoperative bleeding is encoun-tered, the renal hilum must be clamped.

Tumor Excision-Frozen Biopsies

We usually leave in place a small amount of perire-nal fat on the top of the tumor, allowing us to pull

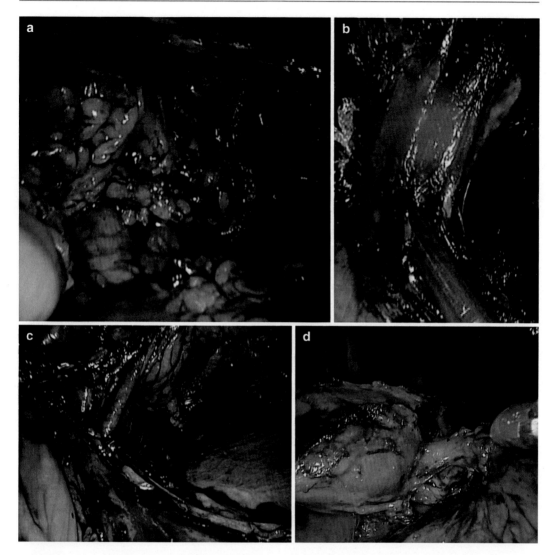

Fig. 21.13 The renal hilum: (**a**) the renal vein is identified firstly, just in anterior position to the renal artery; (**b**) preparation of renal vessels is mandatory for appropriate renal clamping; (**c**) after pulling the ureter upward, we can identify the left gonadal vein inserting into the renal vein, which is anterior to the renal artery; (**d**) the right renal hilum and the inferior vena cava medially to it

the mass during resection and achieving better visualization without the danger of tumor fragmentation (Fig. 21.16a). The tumor is excised using the EndoWrist monopolar curved scissors initially directed away from the tumor (Fig. 21.16b). Retraction is provided by the fenestrated bipolar forceps, and the assistant uses the suction tip to clear any blood from surgical field and to apply traction on the renal parenchyma to ensure adequate visualization during tumor resection (Fig. 21.16c).

Frozen section biopsy specimens of renal parenchyma from the base of the operative bed are always obtained. The excised specimen is then placed aside within the operative field.

Renorrhaphy

The monopolar scissors are exchanged with a robotic needle driver for suturing and renal reconstruction. To shorten the time taken for renorrhaphy, we use the sliding-clip technique for renorrhaphy which has been already described [22]. Running suturing with 25 cm polyglactin

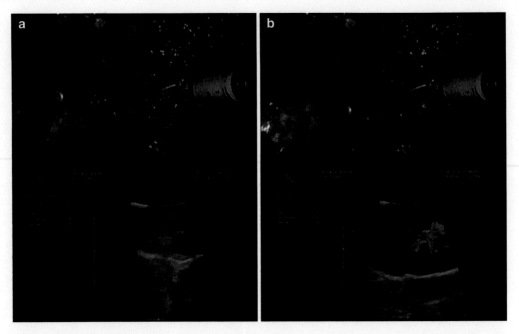

Fig. 21.14 Laparoscopic ultrasound is introduced to identify tumor margin and depth: (**a**) identification of the tumor and (**b**) identification of tumor margin

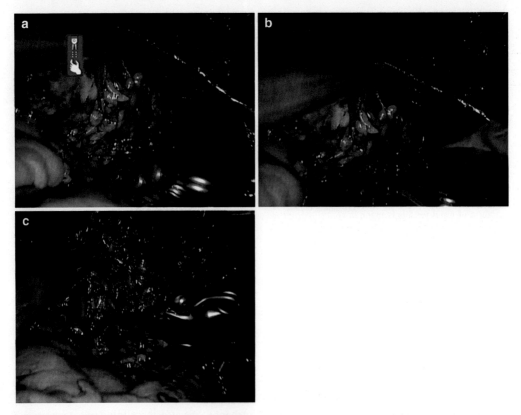

Fig. 21.15 Hilar clamping with bulldog clamps: (**a**) the renal artery is clamped first; (**b**) clamping of the renal vein; (**c**) reverse order is followed during unclamping of the hilum, i.e., renal vein is unclamped primarily

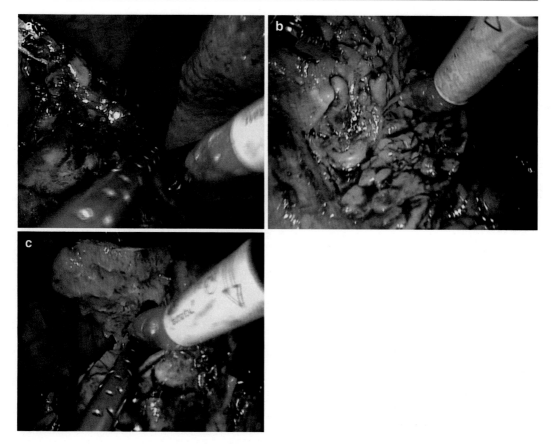

Fig. 21.16 Tumor resection: (**a**) small amount of perirenal fat on the *top* of the tumor has been left in order to pull the tumor during resection; (**b**) resection is performed by using the monopolar scissors directed away from the tumor; (**c**) the assistant applies traction with the suction irrigator to ensure adequate visualization during tumor resection

sutures 3-0 and 2-0 is performed in two layers, a deep layer closure of the resection bed (3-0) and an outer layer closure of the renal capsule (2-0). Sutures are anchored with a knot and a 5 mm Weck Hem-o-lok clip (Teleflex, Research triangle Park, NC).

Suturing in the deep layer (deep cortex, collecting system, blood vessels) is always directed toward the shorter axis of the renal bed and secured by using absorbable clips (Lapra-Ty, Ethicon Endosurgery, Ohio) (Fig. 21.17). After running the entire resection bed, the suture is passed out through the cortex and anchored with a Hem-o-lok clip placed by the assistant. Deep bites within this layer are avoided, as this could injure deeper blood vessels, predisposing to formation of arteriovenous fistulas or pseudoaneurysms.

Sutures in the outer layer are secured with Hem-o-lok clips, placed by the assistant, after each pass through the cortex, and additional clips are placed at the edges of the sutures to prevent them from sliding back. Large bites of capsule are taken to ensure that the suture does not cut through.

Renorrhaphy can also be performed by using barbed sutures (V-loc, Covidien, MA, USA) which facilitate tight renorrhaphy without sliding of sutures [23].

Hilar Unclamping-Hemostatic Agents

After the completion of renal reconstruction, the hilar clamps are removed by the assistant. The venous clamp is unclamped first. If bleeding is

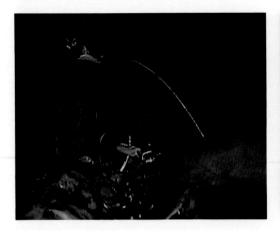

Fig. 21.17 Renorrhaphy is performed in two layers using the sliding-clip technique. Suturing in the inner layer is directed toward the *shorter axis* of the renal bed

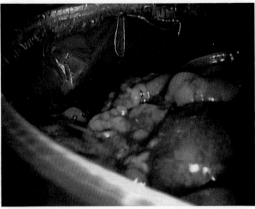

Fig. 21.18 Tumor is entrapped in an endocatch bag

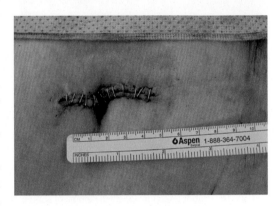

Fig. 21.19 Skin is closed by using metallic clips

present, Hem-o-lok clips may be cinched down a little further and additional sutures may be required.

The pneumoperitoneum is then decreased to 12 mmHg to check for adequate hemostasis.

The sutures are cut and the needles are removed. Additionally, we always apply gelatin matrix thrombin sealant (FloSeal, Baxter, Deerfield, IL, USA) as well as fibrin sealants to the parenchymal defect in order to reduce hemorrhagic complications [24, 25]. However, hemostatic agents and tissue sealants should not be considered as a surgical alternative technique but rather as an adjunct to facilitate and achieve the optimal surgical outcome.

Tumor Extraction-Drain Placement

Afterwards, the specimen is placed in an endocatch bag, and extracted through the same umbilical incision (Fig. 21.18). A closed suction drain is then placed, and the trocars are removed following robot's undocking. The overlying fascia and the skin are closed with absorbable sutures and metallic clips, respectively (Fig. 21.19).

Postoperative Care

The nasogastric tube is removed immediately postoperatively. Intravenous fluids, antibiotics, analgesics, and prophylaxis for deep venous thrombosis are given. Hemoglobin levels, hematocrit, and renal function are monitored in the postoperative period. The drain output is recorded and fluid is sent for measurement of creatinine levels. If there is no creatinine elevation and no postoperative bleeding, the drain can be removed. The morning after surgery, the Foley catheter is removed, patients are encouraged to ambulate, and liquid diet is started. Usually, the patients are discharged from the hospital after 2 days.

Complications and Intraoperative Troubleshooting

In R-LESS PN approach, surgical complications can occur due to the surgical procedure, as also because of the single-port device usage.

Many authors recognize that there are difficulties in performing R-LESS PN operations, since the current da Vinci system is not designed to be used in this fashion. The most common problems are; instrument collision (internal or external), significant gas leak, and insufficient retraction due to the absence of the fourth robotic arm [26]. One additional disadvantage of the improvised single-port device is its fragility because of the use of a standard glove. We have experienced accidental tears when inserting the robot instruments and ballooning at high insufflation pressures when the inner edge of the robotic trocar is partially or totally occluded by the glove. To prevent this from occurring, during construction of the improvised device, the robotic trocars should be fixed in such a way that its inner edge is well beyond the base of the finger of the glove. If during the procedure leakage of carbon dioxide occurs through the single-port device, the trocar sites are packed with petroleum gauze to maintain pneumoperitoneum. Ballooning can be prevented by avoiding use of high insufflation pressures. Moreover, if we want to retract a tissue, we use internal retraction sutures in a marionette fashion.

Common surgical complications during R-LESS PN are hemorrhage, urine leakage, and bowel injury. The perioperative venous bleeding can usually be controlled by direct pressure and increased pneumoperitoneum. Clips and cautery are usually sufficient for minor bleeders, but sutured vascular repair with polyglactin suture 4-0 and a Lapra-Ty clip at its end may be required for larger vessels. In case of injury to the inferior vena cava, direct control of bleeding can be achieved by applying direct pressure with the suction irrigator below the injury during suturing. Bleeding from the parenchyma is usually controlled by applying direct pressure, while the renorrhaphy clips are retightened and cinched down. In case of uncontrolled bleeding, radical nephrectomy or open conversion may be indicated. The postoperative hemorrhage can be usually managed by blood transfusions. Delayed postoperative bleeding may result from an arteriovenous fistula or a pseudoaneurysm, and consideration should be given for angiography and embolization.

If urine leak is suspected, a CT urography may be ordered, and a retrograde placement of a ureteral stent is an option in case of ureteral obstruction or continuous leak. Percutaneous drain may be necessary if there is a urinoma and the drain has been removed.

In case of bowel injury, immediate surgical repair is required. Postoperative symptoms and signs such as abdominal pain, tenderness, vomiting, fever, and leukocytosis may indicate bowel injury.

Surgical Tips

- Use a 30° robotic scope viewing upward in the most medial position of the glove to minimize clashing between the robotic scope and instruments externally.
- Use 5 mm suction tube for suction, irrigation, and retraction.
- The lateral attachments of the kidney to the abdominal wall should be dissected last to avoid the kidney from falling medially into the operative field.
- During hilar dissection, it is important to place the kidney on upward traction, to improve identification of the vessels, and to facilitate dissection of the hilar vessels.
- Maintain a small amount of fat on the tip of the tumor for traction.
- Suturing must be directed toward the shorter axis of the renal bed.
- Absorbable clips (Lapra-Ty) must be used during renal bed reconstruction. Nonabsorbable clips must not be adjacent to

the collecting system, to prevent migration within the system.

- Apply hemostatic agents and tissue sealants as an adjunct to reduce postoperative bleeding.

Studies

When compared to conventional laparoscopy, no clear benefits on postoperative course and patient convalescence have been definitively proven in R-LESS. Potential benefits of LESS might be improvement in cosmetic outcomes and decrease in postoperative pain [5, 27]. Park and associates elegantly demonstrated that scar satisfaction is higher than that for alternative surgical approaches and 86 % of patients who underwent LESS would undergo future LESS at equivalent risk [28]. However, Golkar et al. reported that patients' utmost concern is safety reminding that in the application of any procedure, patient's safety is always of paramount importance [29].

As LESS surgery still remains an evolving field, there is a limited amount of literature comparing R-LESS PN with multi-port approaches. In the largest, worldwide, multi-institutional study of 1076 LESS urological procedures, a total of 127 laparoscopic single-site PNs and R-LESS PNs were included in the analysis. The conclusions from that analysis were that LESS techniques can be effectively and safely performed in PN cases [30].

Moreover, in a recently published multi-institutional study, Springer and colleagues demonstrated that LESS PN is also effective in renal function preservation and oncologic control at a short and intermediate follow-up interval [31]. The authors analyzed the data from 190 patients who underwent R-LESS PN and laparoscopic single-site PN and concluded that LESS PN can be effectively performed in experienced hands. The same group, in another study, reported that patients presenting with low PADUA score tumors represent the best candidates for LESS PN and that the application of robotic platform is likely to reduce the overall risk of postoperative complications [12].

In contrast, Tiu and associates analyzed the outcomes of patients with renal tumors >4 cm who underwent R-LESS PN and found that patients with tumors >4 cm had a statistically significant longer warm ischemia time, but there was no increased risk of conversion rates in comparison to subjects with masses ≤4 cm [13].

However, patients who usually undergo R-LESS PN are highly selected individuals, and therefore, results must be interpreted with caution. Recently, in a review of the literature focused on this kind of surgery, it was noted that R-LESS PN is usually performed in small masses (<3 cm) [32].

Reviewing our data, we found that Trifecta (defined as the combination of WIT <20 min, negative margins, and no surgical complications) in robotic partial nephrectomies is better accomplished by multi-port procedure (unpublished data). We compared the data of 89 and 78 patients with renal tumor who underwent multi-port and single-port robotic partial nephrectomy and distinguished that patients in single-port group had longer operative and warm ischemia time and increased eGFR percentage change in comparison to multi-port patients. Our analysis suggests that R-LESS PN technique can achieve similar results with conventional approach only in elective patients with small tumor size, low PADUA and RENAL score, and without renal sinus or collecting system involvement. In conclusion, we believe that the previous single-port devices used in R-LESS PN procedures could be applicable in patients with small sized tumor and complexity and should not be routinely applied in all cases at current robotic platform.

In summary, current studies demonstrate that R-LESS PN is a feasible procedure performed in an acceptable length of operative and warm ischemia time and resulting in an excellent cosmetic outcome. Since R-LESS PN is still in its clinical infancy, there is a lack of comparative studies between R-LESS PN and multi-port RPN technique in the existing literature. For the time being, R-LESS PN is indicated as a useful alternative approach in elective patients with small sized tumor and complexity.

The results of worldwide studies in R-LESS PN surgery are summarized in Table 21.1, while Table 21.3 includes the published comparative and multi-institutional studies regarding this procedure.

Table 21.3 Comparative and multi-institutional laparoendoscopic single-site partial nephrectomy studies

Author	Y	Instit	Comp	N	TS	OT	WIT	GFR	EBL	PM	Conv
Tiu et al. [13]	2013	One	>4 cm	20	5.4	197	31	78.9	408	5 %	5 %
			≤4 cm	47	2.4	178	24	75.4	271	4 %	0 %
						p=ns	p=s	p=ns	p=ns	p=ns	p=ns
[a]Jeon et al. [34]	2010	One	R-LESS	11	3.7	227	30.7	nm	667	0	9 %
			LESS	2	3.3	220	37	nm	60	0	0 %
[b]Springer et al. [31]	2013	Multi	No	190	2.6	170	16.5	84.7 p=ns	150	4.2 %	5.8 %
[b]Kaouk et al. [30]	2011	Multi	No	127	nm	208	18.4	nm	276	nm	5 %

Y year, *Instit* one institution or multi-institutional study, *Comp* comparative study, *N* number of subjects, *TS* tumor size (cm), *OT* operative time (minutes), *WIT* warm ischemia time (minutes), *GFR* estimated glomerular filtration rate (ml/min/1.73 m²), *EBL* estimated blood loss (ml), *PM* positive surgical margins, *Conv* conversion to conventional PN, *nm* not mentioned in the study, *p* p value, *ns* not significant, *s* significant
[a]p value is not mentioned in the study
[b]These studies include both R-LESS and Laparoscopic single-site PN

Conclusions

Despite the increasing interest in LESS worldwide, the actual role of this novel approach in the field of R-LESS PN remains to be determined and its claimed advantages to be demonstrated. Randomized evaluation and long-term assessment and follow-up are requisite. Moreover, actual instrumentation for R-LESS surgery is still not adequate to allow proper diffusion of this technique. Significant improvements in robotic and access platform designs are needed.

For the time being, R-LESS PN can be an alternative approach to conventional RPN in elective patients with low complexity tumors. With increasing surgical experience and improved instrumentation, we can extend the indications to select patients with more complex tumors.

References

1. Fergany AF, Hafez KS, Novick AC. Long term results of nephron sparing surgery for localized renal cell carcinoma: 10-year follow up. J Urol. 2000;163:442–5.
2. Thompson RH, Boorjian SA, Lohse CM, et al. Radical nephrectomy for T1a renal masses may be associated with decreased overall survival compared with partial nephrectomy. J Urol. 2008;179:468–73.
3. Gettman M, Blute M, Chow G, Neururer R, Bartsch G, Peschel R. Robotic-assisted laparoscopic partial nephrectomy: technique and initial clinical experience with Da Vinci robotic system. Urology. 2004;64:914–8.
4. Kaouk JH, Goel RK. Single-port laparoscopic and robotic partial nephrectomy. Eur Urol. 2009;55:1163–9.
5. Gill IS, Advincula AP, Aron M, et al. Consensus statement of the consortium for laparoendoscopic single-site surgery. Surg Endosc. 2010;24:762–8.
6. Rogers CG, Patard JJ. Open to debate. The motion: robotic partial nephrectomy is better than open partial nephrectomy. Eur Urol. 2009;56:568–70.
7. Ljungberg B, Hanbury DC, Kuczyk MA, et al. Renal cell carcinoma guideline. Eur Urol. 2007;51:1502–10.
8. Greco F, Cindolo L, Autorino R, et al. Laparoendoscopic single-site upper urinary tract surgery: assessment of postoperative complications and analysis of risk factors. Eur Urol. 2012;61:510–6.
9. Autorino R, Kaouk JH, Yakoubi R, et al. Urological laparoendoscopic single site surgery: multi-institutional analysis of risk factors for conversion and postoperative complications. J Urol. 2012;187:1989–94.
10. Ficarra V, Novara G, Secco S, et al. Perioperative aspects and dimensions used for an anatomical (PADUA) classification of renal tumours in patients who are candidates for nephron-sparing surgery. Eur Urol. 2009;56:786–93.
11. Kutikov A, Uzzo RG. The R.E.N.A.L. Nephrometry score: a comprehensive standardized system for quantitating renal tumor size, location and depth. J Urol. 2009;182:844–53.
12. Greco F, Cindolo L, Autorino R, et al. Laparoendoscopic single-site partial nephrectomy: a multi-institutional outcome analysis. Eur Urol. 2013;64:314–22.
13. Tiu A, Kwang KH, Shin TY, Woong HK, Han SW, Rha KH. Feasibility of robotic laparoendoscopic single-site partial nephrectomy for renal tumors >4 cm. Eur Urol. 2013;63:941–6.
14. Khanna R, White MA, Autorino R, et al. Selection of a port for use in laparoendoscopic single-site surgery. Curr Urol Rep. 2011;12:94–9.

15. Haber GP, White M, Autorino R, et al. Novel robotic Da Vinci instruments for laparoendoscopic single-site surgery. Urology. 2010;76:1279–82.

16. Joseph RA, Goh AC, Cuevas SP, et al. Chopstick surgery: a novel technique improves surgeon performance and eliminates arm collision in robotic single incision laparoscopic surgery. Surg Endosc. 2010;24:1331–5.

17. San Francisco IF, Sweeney MC, Wagner AA. Robot-assisted partial nephrectomy: early unclamping technique. J Endourol. 2011;25:305–8.

18. White WM, Goel RK, Haber GP, Kaouk J. Robotic partial nephrectomy without renal hilar occlusion. BJU Int. 2010;105:1580–4.

19. George A, Herati A, Srinivasan A, Rais-Bahrami S, et al. Perioperative outcomes of off-clamp vs complete hilar control laparoscopic partial nephrectomy. BJU Int. 2012;111:235–41.

20. Springer C, Veneziano D, Wimpissinger F, Inferrera A, Fornara P, Greco F. Clampless laparoendoscopic single-site partial nephrectomy for renal cancer with low PADUA score: technique and surgical outcomes. BJU Int. 2013;111:1091–8.

21. Gill IS, Eisenberg M, Aron M, et al. 'Zero ischemia' partial nephrectomy: novel laparoscopic and robotic technique. Eur Urol. 2011;59:128–34.

22. Benway BM, Wang AJ, Cabello JM, Bhayani SB. Robotic partial nephrectomy with sliding-clip renorrhaphy: technique and outcomes. Eur Urol. 2009;55:592–9.

23. Sammon J, Petros F, Sukumar S, et al. Barbed suture for renorrhaphy during robot-assisted partial nephrectomy. J Endourol. 2011;25:529–33.

24. Gill IS, Ramani AP, Spaliviero M, et al. Improved hemostasis during laparoscopic partial nephrectomy using gelatin matrix thrombin sealant. Urology. 2005;65:463–6.

25. Galanakis I, Vasdev N, Soomro N. A review of current hemostatic agents and tissue sealants in laparoscopic partial nephrectomy. Rev Urol. 2011;13:131–8.

26. White MA, Autorino R, Spana G, Hillyer S, Stein RJ, Kaouk JH. Robotic laparoendoscopic single-site urological surgery: analysis of 50 consecutive cases. J Urol. 2012;187(5):1696–701.

27. Fan X, Lin T, Xu K, et al. Laparoendoscopic single-site nephrectomy compared with conventional laparoscopic nephrectomy: a systematic review and meta-analysis of comparative studies. Eur Urol. 2012;62:601–12.

28. Park SK, Olweny EO, Best SL, et al. Patient-reported body image and cosmesis outcomes following kidney surgery: comparison of laparoendoscopic single-site, laparoscopic, and open surgery. Eur Urol. 2011;60:1097–104.

29. Golkar FC, Ross SB, Sperry S, et al. Patients' perceptions of laparoendoscopic single-site surgery: the cosmetic effect. Am J Surg. 2012;204:751–61.

30. Kaouk JH, Autorino R, Kim FJ, et al. Laparoendoscopic single-site surgery in urology: worldwide multi-institutional analysis of 1076 cases. Eur Urol. 2011;60:998–1005.

31. Springer C, Greco F, Autorino R, Rha KH, et al. Analysis of oncologic outcomes and renal function after laparoendoscopic single site partial nephrectomy: a multi-institutional outcome analysis. BJU Int. 2013. doi:10.1111/bju.12376 [Epub ahead of print].

32. Cindolo L, Greco F, Fornara P, Mirone V, Schips L. Nephron sparing less: technique and review of the literature. Arch Esp Urol. 2012;65:303–10.

33. Stein RJ, White WM, Goel RK, Irwin BH, Haber GP, Kaouk JH. Robotic laparoendoscopic single-site surgery using GelPort as the access platform. Eur Urol. 2010;57:132–7.

34. Jeon HG, Jeong W, Oh CK, et al. Initial experience with 50 laparoendoscopic single site surgeries using a homemade, single port device at a single center. J Urol. 2010;183:1866–71.

35. Lee JW, Arconcel FR, Rha KH, et al. Urologic robot-assisted laparoendosopic single-site surgery using a homemade single-port device: a single-center experience of 68 cases. J Endourol. 2011;25:1481–5.

36. Han WK, Kim DS, Jeon HG, et al. Robot-assisted laparoendoscopic single-site surgery: partial nephrectomy for renal malignancy. Urology. 2011;77:612–6.

37. Choi KH, Ham WS, Rha KH, et al. Laparoendoscopic single-site surgeries: a single center experience of 171 consecutive cases. Korean J Urol. 2011;52:31–8.

38. Seo IY, Rim JS. Bilateral robotic single-site partial nephrectomy. J Laparoendosc Adv Surg Tech. 2011;21:435–8.

39. Khanna R, Stein RJ, White MA, et al. Single institution experience with robotic laparoendoscopic single site renal procedures. J Endourol. 2011;26:230–4.

40. Kaouk JH, Autorino R, Laydner H, et al. Robotic single-site kidney surgery: evaluation of second-generation instruments in a cadaver model. Urology. 2012;79:975–9.

41. Tiu A, Shin TY, Kwang KH, Lim SK, Han WK, Rha KH. Robotic laparoendoscopic single-site transumbilical partial nephrectomy: functional and oncologic outcomes at 2 years. Urology. 2013;82:595–9.

Robotic-Assisted Laparoendoscopic Single-Site (RLESS) Pyeloplasty

Jeffrey C. Gahan and Jeffrey A. Cadeddu

Introduction

The performance of the first laparoscopic nephrectomy in 1991 marked a new surgical era in urology [1]. Since that time, urologists have continued to embrace the advantages of laparoscopic surgery, while continuing to push its boundaries through the use of fewer and smaller trocars. The report of the first laparoscopic nephrectomy through a single fascia incision ushered in yet another era of urologic surgery. This approach, dubbed laparoendoscopic single-site surgery or LESS, was promoted to offer better cosmetic results as well as quicker convalescence compared to conventional laparoscopy [2]. However, since its inception, LESS has proven to be technically demanding due to a loss of triangulation, instrument clashes, and limited instrument articulation.

With the introduction of the da Vinci robot, laparoscopic surgery was again revolutionized. The robot recreated the wristed action of the human hand, while at the same time maintaining the minimally invasive nature of laparoscopic surgery. These advantages naturally led to its application in LESS surgery, with the first robotic LESS (RLESS) pyeloplasty reported in 2008 [3]. Since then, RLESS strategies have continued to improve both through advances in single-site platforms and newly designed robotic arms.

For a number of reasons, pyeloplasty has been identified as a rational application of LESS. As a non-extirpative surgery, it does not require specimen extraction and thus the incision can remain small. LESS pyeloplasty can also be performed through the umbilicus, allowing the incision to stay hidden and maximizing cosmetic results. In addition, many of the patients presenting with ureteropelvic junction obstruction (UPJO) are young and have a greater concern for favorable cosmesis. Lastly, the majority of these individuals have not had previous abdominal surgeries, making them ideal candidates for LESS. However, the extent of intracorporeal suturing needed during LESS pyeloplasty tended to make these surgeries prohibitive to most surgeons. With the inception of the robot, LESS pyeloplasty has become a more ergonomic and technically feasible operation. The strategies involved in setting

J.C. Gahan, MD
Department of Urology, UT Southwestern Medical Center, VA North Texas Health System, Dallas, TX, USA
e-mail: Jeffrey.gahan@utsouthwestern.edu

J.A. Cadeddu, MD (✉)
Department of Urology, J8.106, UT Southwestern Medical Center, 5323 Harry Hines Blvd., Dallas, TX 75202, USA

Urology and Radiology, University of Texas Southwestern Medical Center, Dallas, TX, USA
e-mail: jeffrey.cadeddu@utsouthwestern.edu

© Springer Science+Business Media New York 2017
J.H. Kaouk et al. (eds.), *Atlas of Laparoscopic and Robotic Single Site Surgery*, Current Clinical Urology, DOI 10.1007/978-1-4939-3575-8_22

up and performing RLESS pyeloplasty will be discussed in this chapter, along with the key points for patient selection and a brief discussion of the reported outcomes.

Diagnosis and Planning

The most common presenting symptom of UPJO is flank pain, which can be associated with nausea and vomiting, although other symptoms may include hematuria, recurrent episodes of pyelonephritis, recurrent stone formation, or vague abdominal pain. In some instances, UPJO may not present with pain, but may be identified surreptitiously on abdominal imaging, although this presentation is rare.

The work-up for UPJO is generally no different for RLESS pyeloplasty than for standard pyeloplasty and should be performed with the goal of identifying the anatomic site and functional significance of the obstruction. A CT scan is often performed when the adult patient presents with flank or abdominal pain and usually shows a dilated pelvicalyceal system with a normal caliber ureter. If the diagnosis is already suspected, a CT angiography can help to identify a crossing vessel etiology. A CT further can delineate the extent of perinephric fat, a large amount of which may significantly hinder the ability to perform RLESS pyeloplasty. The diagnosis can be confirmed with a diuretic renal scan, with a $T \frac{1}{2} > 20$ min considered conclusive for the presence of obstruction [4–6]. In addition, the renal scan can give an estimation of the differential function of the kidney. While there is no well-defined cutoff, a kidney with less than 15–20 % function should be considered for nephrectomy. If there is concern for stricture length, a retrograde pyelogram may be helpful in planning a more extensive repair.

Additional considerations must be made when considering RLESS pyeloplasty compared to conventional pyeloplasty. In the author's opinion, BMI plays the primary role in patient selection. All series in the RLESS literature report an average BMI between 22 and 25, with many using a BMI >30 as exclusionary criterion for surgery [7–9]. Further, because RLESS pyeloplasty is often performed through the umbilicus, greater abdominal girth can increase the working distance from the fascial incision which may create difficulties with reach and visualization. Also of concern is previous abdominal surgery. Not only may port placement be compromised, but lysis of medial adhesions may not be possible in RLESS given the difficult working angles. Previous operations to the kidney, including endoscopic procedures, may cause significant fibrosis, which can cause difficulties when using single-site approach. Lastly, we advise ureteral stents to be removed at least 4 weeks prior to pyeloplasty to allow for a reduction in inflammation at the UPJ.

Other considerations for RLESS include the administration of a partial bowel preparation to reduce bowel volume due to the limited camera mobility. This can be performed with a bottle of magnesium citrate given the night prior to surgery. Sterile urine is also mandatory prior to any pyeloplasty.

Surgical Procedure

In most cases of RLESS, a ureteral stent is placed prior to the patient being placed in the flank position as LESS does not afford favorable angles when placing a stent in an antegrade manner. Stent placement may be performed under fluoroscopic guidance to give an idea of the location and extent of the UPJO and will ensure proper stent positioning. Conversely, other authors have reported using a flexible scope at the time of surgery to place a stent in a retrograde fashion in an effort to save time and avoid repositioning [8]. We have also positioned a stent antegrade over a guidewire introduced through a 14-gauge angiographic catheter inserted into the abdomen in the midclavicular line below the costal margin. Of note, it is encouraged to upsize the stent length by approximately 2 cm to ensure that it is not displaced from the bladder during manipulation of the anastomosis.

Patient Positioning

The patient is positioned in a manner similar to conventional pyeloplasty. The patient is placed in a modified or full flank position. It is the author's preference to use a modified flank position which eliminates the need for an axillary role. The arm can be secured safely at the side as shown with the table in slight flexion (Fig. 22.1). Alternatively, the arm can be draped over the face and supported with a pillow or Krause arm support. A Foley catheter should be placed prior to the start of surgery and remain accessible to the circulating nurse throughout the case as clamping and unclamping may be necessary. The bed is then maximally rotated away from the side on which the robot docks.

Abdominal Access and Port Placement

A curvilinear 2–3 cm incision is made at the umbilicus, and dissection is carried down to the rectus fascia. Once exposed, the fascia is cleaned of fat and two 0-Vicryl stay sutures on a UR-6 needle are placed on each side of the fascia. These are then used to lift the fascia as it is divided. Once the muscle layer is separated, atraumatic forceps are used to lift the peritoneum and scissors are used to divide this sharply. Once peritoneal access has been achieved, the fascial incision is extended to accommodate the single-site platform of choice.

Our preference is to use the GelPoint access platform (Applied Medical, Rancho Santa Margarita, CA, USA). This is placed in the standard manner through the fascial incision. Care must be taken when the device is secured, ensuring no bowl loops become pinned between the device and abdominal wall. This can be verified with a finger sweep outside the device and confirmed with a 30° lens in the upward position. The gel portion of the device is then attached and insufflation is started. The ports are positioned as shown in Fig. 22.2. A 12 mm camera port is placed at the top or on the most lateral portion of the gel, and the gel ports are positioned in a triangular pattern as shown.

The robotic 5 mm cannulas are placed through the gel ports, and the camera is placed through

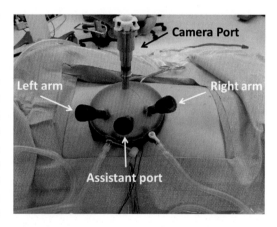

Fig. 22.2 Trocar placement using the GelPoint for RLESS pyeloplasty

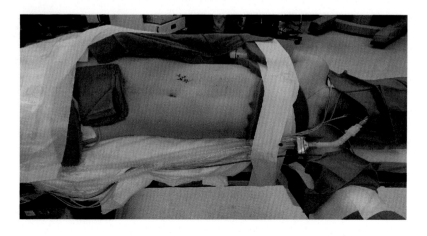

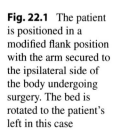

Fig. 22.1 The patient is positioned in a modified flank position with the arm secured to the ipsilateral side of the body undergoing surgery. The bed is rotated to the patient's left in this case

Fig. 22.3 Robot docked for RLESS pyeloplasty with robotic instruments and cannulas placed through the GelPoint trocars. The camera trocar is placed directly through the GelPoint

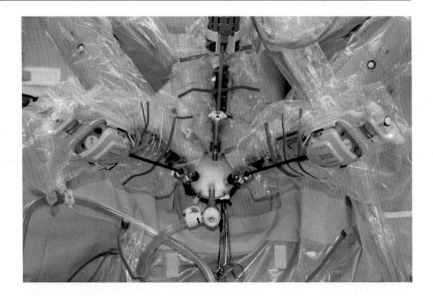

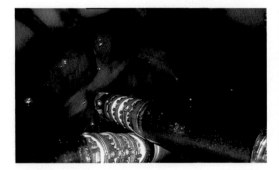

Fig. 22.4 Ports are positioned with their remote center at the level of the fascia, and the robotic arms are crossed inside the abdomen

the most lateral port in the 30° upward position. The upward angle keeps the extracorporeal portion of the camera arm away from the other robotic arms. The robot is then docked and the 5 mm arms are brought through the trocars (Fig. 22.3).

The remote center of the robot ports is positioned just above the fascial level, and the arms are crossed inside the patient (Fig. 22.4). The master control is then reprogrammed so that the right hand controls the left instrument and the left controls the right. This is done so intuitive control is gained by the surgeon once the arms are crossed. Once inside the body, the point at which the arms cross cannot be seen unless the camera is pulled back. The advantage of this method is that articu-

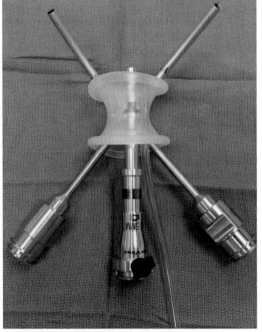

Fig. 22.5 Da Vinci single-site surgical platform

lating instruments can still be used; however, the arms must be continually crossed and uncrossed depending on the retraction needed.

An alternative to the GelPoint used by other centers is the da Vinci single-site platform (Intuitive Surgical, Sunnyvale, CA, USA) (Fig. 22.5) [10]. This surgical platform is specifically designed for

RLESS. It is a multichannel, single-site port that accommodates two curved robotic cannulas which allow for semirigid instruments to cross inside the patient. Similar to the setup described previously, the master control is reprogrammed so that the left and right are reversed. One disadvantage to this system is that the semirigid instruments do not have articulating abilities. The camera is placed in the 30° downward position. Currently, this platform is FDA approved only for single-site cholecystectomy and hysterectomy.

Initial Steps

The operation is started by reflecting the colon medially. This is performed by grasping the mesenteric fat just lateral to the colon and lifting this off from the kidney (Fig. 22.6). A plane of loose areolar tissue between the colon/mesentery and Gerota's is encountered. This can be dissected through using the hook cautery with blunt or hot dissection. It is the author's preference to perform the majority of the dissection with the Maryland graspers and hook cautery, as the 5 mm scissors do not have cautery capability.

Once the colon is mobilized medially, the ureter is then identified. This is accomplished by grasping Gerota's fascia just inferior to the lower pole of the

kidney and lifting this upward. The gonadal vein is identified and an incision is made in the fascia just above it, dropping it medially (Fig. 22.7). The ureter is located in nearly all cases just lateral and posterior to the gonadal vein. The ureter can be easily identified if a stent has been preplaced.

Alternatively, other centers have described a transmesenteric approach to locate the ureter, although this approach is not widely used [9]. This approach may offer the advantage of decreased bowel manipulation and quicker identification of the ureter. However, this approach does lend itself to consequences if a mesenteric vessel is inadvertently divided.

Once isolated, a grasper is then placed under the ureter and is lifted up toward the abdominal wall (Fig. 22.8). Circumferential access to the

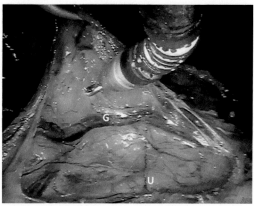

Fig. 22.7 The Gerota's fascia just caudal to the lower pole is lifted and incised, dropping the gonadal vessels (*G*) to expose the ureter (*U*)

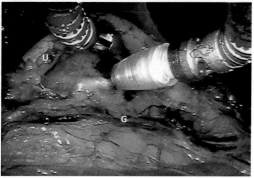

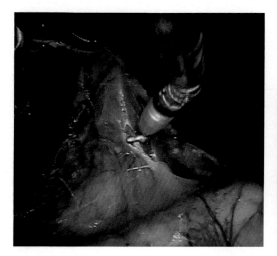

Fig. 22.6 The tissue lateral to the colon is elevated to reveal the loose, areolar tissue which is dissected off of Gerota's fascia

Fig. 22.8 The ureter (*U*) is dissected free and elevated to provide tension for subsequent dissection. *G* gonadal vessels

ureter is gained so that it can be placed on traction. The dissection of the ureter is then carried out cranially, with care taken to conserve as much periureteral tissue as possible so as to not devascularize the ureter. Care must also be taken to avoid crossing vessels as the dissection progresses toward the renal pelvis, as these may be encountered even in situations where they are not the etiology of UPJO.

If a crossing vessel is identified, the ureter below the crossing vessel and the renal pelvis

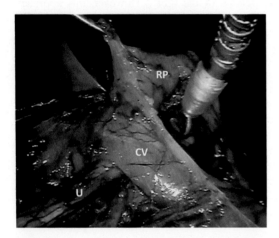

Fig. 22.9 The dissection of the ureter (*U*) is carried up to the crossing vessels (*CV*) at which point the renal pelvis (*RP*) is further dissected. The pelvis can be manipulated safely with a grasper, so long as the portion undergoing the anastomosis is not damaged

above should be dissected free, rather than trying to dissect out the vessels themselves (Fig. 22.9). In addition, it is always prudent to dissect the renal pelvis to a greater degree than what is thought needed, as this will aid in sewing the anastomosis. Once clearly dissected and the cause of the UPJO determined, the method of reconstruction must be chosen.

Anderson-Hynes Dismembered Pyeloplasty

The dismembered pyeloplasty is the surgery of choice in most instances of UPJO. It is an effective repair given a number of etiologies including crossing vessels, strictured segments, or high insertions. Further, it allows for a reduction pyeloplasty to be performed. It also allows for anterior or posterior transposition of the UPJ and, unlike the flap techniques, allows for the removal of strictured segments.

Once the renal pelvis and ureter have been completely mobilized and dissected, the point of division must be decided. In the case of a crossing vessel, it is recommended that the dismemberment occur at the renal pelvis above the UPJ, as this etiology is rarely associated with internal stricture (Fig. 22.10). This allows for a more wide open anastomosis.

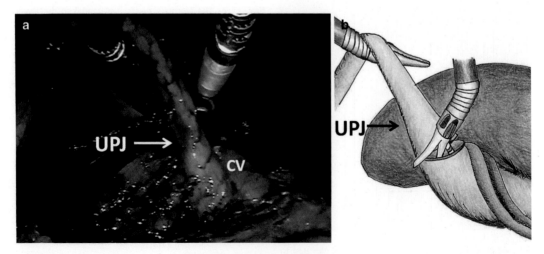

Fig. 22.10 (**a**) The UPJ can be brought below the crossing vessels with sufficient mobilization (**b**) and the renal pelvis divided proximal to the UPJ to facilitate a wide anastomosis. *UPJ* ureteral pelvic junction, *CV* crossing vessel

Care must be taken to avoid cutting the pre-placed stent. Once divided, the ureteral portion should spatulated along the lateral aspect and then cannulated with an instrument to ensure its patency (Figs. 22.11 and 22.12).

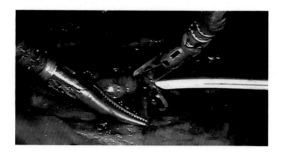

Fig. 22.11 The ureter is rolled using the periureteral tissue to facilitate spatulation along its lateral edge

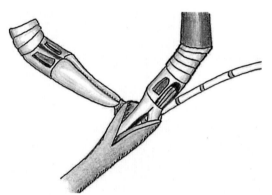

Fig. 22.12 The ureter is calibrated with the robotic scissors to ensure the lumen is widely patent

The ureter and renal pelvis are then transposed over the crossing vessel and the anastomosis is performed. We prefer to us a 4-0 Vicryl suture. The ureteral stitch is always thrown "in-to-out" to ensure the mucosa is obtained and the back wall is not inadvertently incorporated into the anastomosis (Fig. 22.13). Once the posterior aspect is completed, the ureteral stent is placed in the renal pelvis and the anterior anastomosis is completed.

A drain is placed either through a lateral stab incision or through the umbilicus and Gerota's fascia reapproximated over the anastomosis using Hem-o-lok clips. The LESS platform is removed and the fascia and skin are closed. The end result is shown in Fig. 22.14.

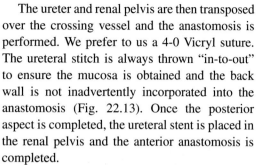

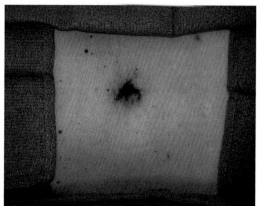

Fig. 22.14 The resulting skin incision of an RLESS pyeloplasty

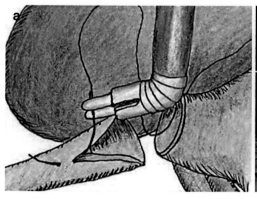

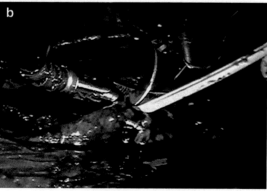

Fig. 22.13 (**a**) The renal pelvis is transposed over the crossing vessels and the first stitch is placed out-to-in through the renal pelvis, followed by (**b**) a stitch placed in-to-out through the ureter. A needle driver and Maryland grasper are used

In situations where a strictured UPJ is encountered, a dismembered pyeloplasty can be performed with excision of the strictured segment. Unlike a crossing vessel etiology, this requires division both above and below the strictured segment. Spatulation and anastomosis are then performed as previously described. For cases where a large, redundant renal pelvis is associated with a UPJO, a reduction pyeloplasty is sometimes warranted. This is performed by simply removing a greater portion of the renal pelvis and sewing this portion to itself.

Foley Y-V Pyeloplasty

The Foley Y-V plasty was originally implemented to treat UPJO resulting from a ureter inserting high in the renal pelvis. This technique currently has a somewhat limited role as it is not efficacious when treating UPJO due to crossing vessels or when there is a redundant renal pelvis requiring reduction. It further is not useful when treating a strictured UPJ.

To perform a Y-V plasty, a wide inverted "V" incision is made to the point of high insertion on the medial aspect of the renal pelvis. The incision is then carried down the lateral aspect of the proximal ureter incorporating several millimeters of normal caliber ureter creating a "Y" (Fig. 22.15a). The apex of the generated flap is then sutured to the apex of the spatulated ureter (Fig. 22.15b). The posterior aspect of the anastomosis is completed in a run-

ning fashion followed by a running closure of the anterior component (Fig. 22.15c).

Fenger Non-dismembered Pyeloplasty

Focal stenosis of the ureter at the UPJ may be treated with a non-dismembered Fengerplasty. This assumes no crossing vessels or high insertion of the ureter. This is performed by making a 2 cm incision through the stenotic area extending approximately 1 cm on either side of the strictured segment. The incision is then closed transversely over a ureteral stent effectively increasing the luminal diameter at the strictured point. The advantage to this procedure is its relative ease and shorter operative time due to less reconstruction and intracorporeal suturing.

Vertical and Spiral Flap Pyeloplasty

In cases where the strictured segment is long, a vertical or spiral flap may be used. For this to be performed, the ureter must be inserted at the dependent portion of the renal pelvis. One disadvantage to this approach is that the strictured segment is not removed. Additional length may be gained from spiraling the flap around the renal pelvis. This is performed by making a ureterotomy into normal ureter approximately 1 cm distal to the ureteral stricture and caring this incision to the renal pelvis as shown in Fig. 22.16.

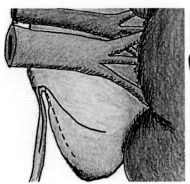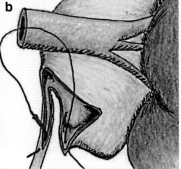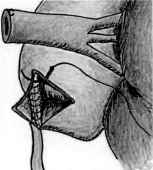

Fig. 22.15 (a) An outline depicting of the incision to be used in a high-insertion Y-V plasty. (b) An out-to-in stitch is placed in the renal pelvis, followed by in-to-out stitch at the apex of the ureteral incision. (c) The anterior wall is closed after the back wall of the Y-V plasty has been completed

Fig. 22.16 (**a**) The creation of a vertical flap is shown, (**b**) followed by the running repair of the back wall once the flap has been created (Note: the stricture is not excised)

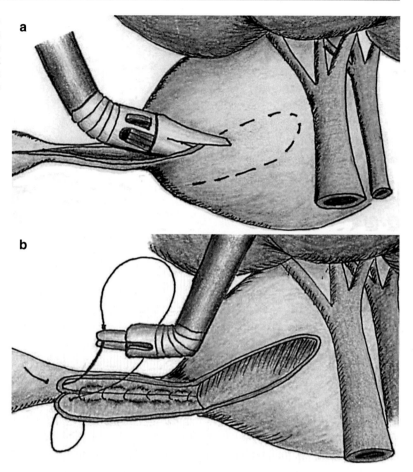

The flap is then taken medially with the amount of renal pelvis incised directly related to the length of the ureter stricture to be repaired. The back wall is then closed with a running 4-0 Vicryl suture, followed by a repair of the front wall. Although this is a more complex reconstruction technique, this repair is possible because of the wristed action of the robotic instruments.

Postoperative Management

The care for patients undergoing RLESS pyeloplasty is no different than patient undergoing other forms of pyeloplasty. Typically, a Foley catheter and drain are left in place. The Foley catheter is typically removed the night after surgery and the drain output monitored until the next morning. If the drain output dramatically increases, the Foley catheter is replaced and the patient is discharged with the drain and catheter in place. If there is no significant increase in output, and the 24 h drain volume is minimal, the drain is removed prior to discharge. If there is a concern for leak due to equivocal drain output, or there are concerns with the integrity of the anastomosis, the drain fluid can be sent for creatinine level. The stent is left in place for 4 weeks and removed in the clinic with cystoscopy. A diuretic renal scan is obtained 6 weeks after stent removal to evaluate kidney drainage.

Outcomes

LESS pyeloplasty is a highly technical surgery and therefore is often associated with an increased learning curve when compared to traditional laparoscopic pyeloplasty or even extirpative LESS surgeries. Indeed, this has been shown in a multi-institutional study focusing on LESS procedures, whereby the majority of complications were identified in the LESS reconstruction cohort compared to the extirpative cohort (27.1 vs. 7.8 %) [11]. Demonstrating this steep learning curve, Best et al. reported that 71 % of their complications occurred in the first ten cases of their 28 case series of conventional LESS (CLESS) pyeloplasty. However, it is hypothesized that RLESS pyeloplasty can shorten the learning curve and minimize complications compared to CLESS. One study comparing these two approaches concluded there was in fact a shortened learning curve for RLESS based on common surrogates such as conversion rates and complications [7]. This study also reported a reduction in the number of accessory ports used [7]. It is the author's opinion that RLESS does in fact offer significant advantages compared to CLESS for the following reasons: (1) there is enhanced visualization using a 3-D high-definition camera; (2) the endowrist affords greater maneuverability and facilitates sewing; (3) intuitive control is gained by reprogramming the robot; and (4) removal of the surgeon from the crowded extracorporeal working space yields improved ergonomics (Table 22.1).

Despite these advantages, RLESS pyeloplasty remains a relatively new and infrequently performed operation, and as such, the literature concerning outcomes is limited. Currently, most RLESS pyeloplasty series demonstrate clinical success (defined as resolution of pain) in greater than 90 % of patients. This rivals the success of conventional robotic and laparoscopic series [12–14]; however, the RLESS series are small with limited follow-up (Table 22.1). There are also no series directly comparing RLESS to conventional laparoscopic or robotic pyeloplasty, making conclusions regarding its true efficacy difficult. Another limitation to the RLESS data is the relatively short follow-up. Published series report follow-up ranging from 3 to 12 months, although longer-term failures are known to occur with pyeloplasty. Despite these inadequacies, as RLESS technology continues to evolve both with the improvement of current equipment and the development of new devices such as the Titan robot (Titan Medical Inc., Toronto, Canada), RLESS pyeloplasty will undoubtedly have an increasing role in the management of UPJO.

> **Key Points**
> - Patient selection is critical for RLESS pyeloplasty: ideal patients are those with BMI <30 and with no previous abdominal surgeries.
> - Success rates for RLESS do not appear to differ from conventional laparoscopic pyeloplasty, although complication rates may be higher initially as learning curve develops.
> - RLESS may shorten the learning curve for LESS pyeloplasty in terms of complication and conversion rate, although the data is limited.

Table 22.1 Outcomes of selected RLESS pyeloplasty series

	N	BMI (kg/m²)	OR time (min)	Conversions	Complications (Clavien grade)	Success[a]
Harrow et al. [4]	22	22.0	208	0/22	2–3a	22/22
Olweny et al. [7]	10	21.8	226	0/10	1–3a	8/8
Tobis et al. [9]	8	24.0	181	0/8	1–3a	8/8
Cestari et al. [8]	9	22.5	169	0/8	1–2	5/5
Khanna et al. [15]	7	26.4	247	2/7	2	6/7

[a]Success defined as resolution of clinical symptoms

References

1. Clayman RV, et al. Laparoscopic nephrectomy. 1991. J Urol. 2002;167(2 Pt 2):862; discussion 863.
2. Park SK, et al. Patient-reported body image and cosmesis outcomes following kidney surgery: comparison of laparoendoscopic single-site, laparoscopic, and open surgery. Eur Urol. 2011;60(5):1097–104.
3. Desai MM, et al. Scarless single port transumbilical nephrectomy and pyeloplasty: first clinical report. BJU Int. 2008;101(1):83–8.
4. Harrow BR, et al. Renal function after laparoendoscopic single site pyeloplasty. J Urol. 2013;190(2):565–9.
5. Stein RJ, et al. Laparoendoscopic single-site pyeloplasty: a comparison with the standard laparoscopic technique. BJU Int. 2011;107(5):811–5.
6. Ost MC, et al. Laparoscopic pyeloplasty versus antegrade endopyelotomy: comparison in 100 patients and a new algorithm for the minimally invasive treatment of ureteropelvic junction obstruction. Urology. 2005;66(5 Suppl):47–51.
7. Olweny EO, et al. Perioperative comparison of robotic assisted laparoendoscopic single-site (LESS) pyeloplasty versus conventional LESS pyeloplasty. Eur Urol. 2012;61(2):410–4.
8. Cestari A, et al. Feasibility and preliminary clinical outcomes of robotic laparoendoscopic single-site (R-LESS) pyeloplasty using a new single-port platform. Eur Urol. 2012;62(1):175–9.
9. Tobis S, et al. Robot-assisted transumbilical laparoendoscopic single-site pyeloplasty: technique and perioperative outcomes from a single institution. J Laparoendosc Adv Surg Tech A. 2013;23(8):702–6.
10. Kaouk JH, et al. Robotic single-site kidney surgery: evaluation of second-generation instruments in a cadaver model. Urology. 2012;79(5):975–9.
11. Irwin BH, et al. Complications and conversions of upper tract urological laparoendoscopic single-site surgery (LESS): multicentre experience: results from the NOTES Working Group. BJU Int. 2011;107(8):1284–9.
12. Gettman MT, et al. A comparison of laparoscopic pyeloplasty performed with the daVinci robotic system versus standard laparoscopic techniques: initial clinical results. Eur Urol. 2002;42(5):453–7; discussion 457-8.
13. Link RE, Bhayani SB, Kavoussi LR. A prospective comparison of robotic and laparoscopic pyeloplasty. Ann Surg. 2006;243(4):486–91.
14. Tracy CR, et al. Perioperative outcomes in patients undergoing conventional laparoscopic versus laparoendoscopic single-site pyeloplasty. Urology. 2009;74(5):1029–34.
15. Khanna R, Stein RJ, White MA, Isac W, Laydner H, Autorino R, Hillyer S, Spana G, Shah G, Haber GP, Kaouk J. Single institution experience with robot-assisted laparoendoscopic single-site renal procedures. J Endourol. 2012;26(3):230–4. doi:10.1089/end.2011.0187. Epub 2012 Feb 21. PubMed PMID: 22192077.

Single-Site Robotic Pyeloplasty Employing the Novel-Dedicated da Vinci Platform

23

Andrea Cestari, Matteo Ferrari, Matteo Zanoni, Mattia Sangalli, Massimo Ghezzi, Fabio Fabbri, Francesco Sozzi, and Patrizio Rigatti

Introduction

In the last two decades, after the pioneering and fundamental codification of the laparoscopic nephrectomy procedure by Clayman and colleagues [1], minimally invasive surgery in urology (i.e. laparoscopic and robotic surgery) experienced a dramatic development and worldwide diffusion.

More recently, laparoendoscopic single-site surgery (LESS) was proposed with the aims to further reduce the limited invasiveness of conventional laparoscopy in order to offer not only an increased better cosmetic result (incision hidden by the umbilical scar) but also to potentially reduce the postoperative pain and offer a quicker convalescence [2]. Nevertheless, LESS remains a challenging surgical technique mainly due to the lack of triangulation among the surgical instruments. Proper laparoscopic suturing techniques and great surgical skills are required for procedures requiring a reconstructive phase such as pyeloplasty, as proper suturing is mandatory to provide adequate repair of the stenotic upper urinary tract junction (UPJ). In order to overcome this hurdles, some authors tried to adapt the traditional da Vinci robotic system to the LESS concept, trying to solve the lack of triangulation and limited instrument movement with the aid of the endowristed instruments of the robotic system [3, 4].

Recently, the da Vinci Single-Site® Surgery technique has been introduced into clinical practice to properly perform cholecystectomy procedures robotically in a LESS surgery scenario, with encouraging preliminary results [5, 6].

Moreover, to our knowledge, we were the first to describe the feasibility in urology of robotic laparoendoscopic single-site (R-LESS) pyeloplasty procedures, using the new Single-Site® da Vinci platform, reporting encouraging preliminary clinical outcomes [7].

We herein describe in details the surgical technique of single-site pyeloplasty employing the novel da Vinci Single-Site® platform. The clinical outcomes of the first series of patients submitted to this pyeloplasty technique will be also reported.

A. Cestari, MD (✉) • M. Ferrari, MD • M. Zanoni, MD
M. Sangalli, MD • M. Ghezzi, MD • F. Fabbri, MD
F. Sozzi, MD • P. Rigatti, MD
Urology Department, Scientific Institute
"Istituto Auxologico Italiano", via Mercalli 30,
Milan 20122, Italy
e-mail: a.cestari@auxologico.it;
ma.ferrari@auxologico.it; m.sangalli@auxologico.it;
m.ghezzi@auxologico.it; f.fabbri@auxologico.it;
f.sozzi@auxologico.it; p.rigatti@auxologico.it

© Springer Science+Business Media New York 2017
J.H. Kaouk et al. (eds.), *Atlas of Laparoscopic and Robotic Single Site Surgery*,
Current Clinical Urology, DOI 10.1007/978-1-4939-3575-8_23

Surgical Technique

Characteristics of the da Vinci Single-Site® Platform

The new da Vinci Single-Site robotic surgery platform is a robotic operative system designed to work with the Intuitive da Vinci Si Operative System (Intuitive Surgical – Sunnyvale, Ca, USA). The system incorporates a multichannel siliconic single port that has the peculiarity to be able to accommodate two curved robotic cannulas. This allows for the passage of interchangeable 5 mm diameter, semi-rigid instruments that cross each other within the trocar so that the right entering instrument becomes the left-sided operative instrument in the abdominal cavity and vice versa. There are two different kinds of cannulas of different lengths: the short ones are better suitable for procedures on the kidney.

The master-slave software of the da Vinci platform automatically exchanges the master-slave controls allowing the surgeon at the console to control the tip of the instrument with his right hand at the right side of the surgical field and the opposite for the left. Unfortunately, the surgical instruments do not have the wrist at the tip as conventional robotic da Vinci instruments do. Altough very recently wristed needle holders become available into clinical practice. In addition to the robotic-controlled instruments and a 7.5 mm diameter optic (a 30° scope down oriented), the specifically designed port allows for the access of additional one or two conventional laparoscopic entrances for the assistant (Fig. 23.1).

Patient Preparation

Patients were invited to have a non-gas-producing diet 1 week prior to hospital admission and receive a bowel preparation the day before surgery in order to decompress the intestine and reduce the risk of auxiliary port placement in order to better expose the surgical area. Whenever possible, if a DJ stent was already in place to

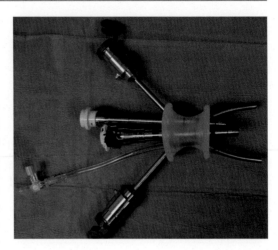

Fig. 23.1 Scheme of da Vinci Single-Site platform (From Cestari et al. [7]. Reprinted with permission from Elsevier Limited)

temporarily solve the patient's symptoms, it was removed at least 3 weeks prior to surgery.

A broad-spectrum third-generation cephalosporin antibiotic prophylaxis was administered at anaesthesia induction, as well as a nasogastric tube in order to decompress the stomach on the left side and duodenum on the right side.

Patients were positioned in a 75° flank position with the bed flexed (30°) in order to elevate and better expose the surgical area (Fig. 23.2). The surgical field was prepared in order to have full access to the target abdominal area and the penis in males and vagina in females, providing access to the external urinary meatus to perform the flexible cystoscopy for DJ stent positioning during the surgical procedure.

Surgical Technique

A 2–2.5 cm totally intra-umbilical skin incision was performed with dissection of musculo-fascial planes to reach the peritoneal cavity. In patients with particular abundant subcutaneous fatty tissue, two stay sutures are appositioned on the fascia at the two edges of the surgical incision in order to reduce the thickness of the planes and easy the port placement.

The da Vinci Single-Site port was then inserted shaping the siliconic port as shown in Fig. 23.2

Fig. 23.2 Patient positioning (**a**) and single-site port inserted in the umbilical scar (**b**) (From Cestari et al. [7]. Reprinted with permission from Elsevier Limited)

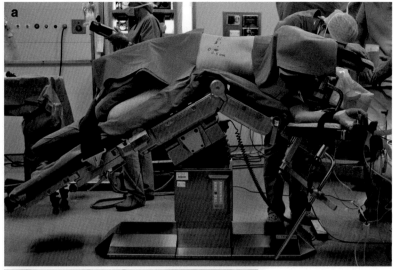

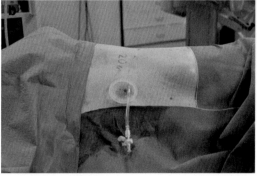

with a Satinsky clamp and pneumoperitoneum induced.

Once the abdominal cavity was inspected and the surgical area identified, a proper precise alignment of the robotic arms is required. Docking of the Single-Site® system to the patient is as follows: first the optical port is connected to the optical robotic arm; then, under direct vision, the curved trocar n° 2 is docked to arm n° 2 of the robotic system; and as the third step the curved trocar n° 1 is docked to arm n°1. Finally, one or two 5 mm assistant trocars are inserted in the remaining dedicated holes in the multichannel port (Fig. 23.3).

The transperitoneal pyeloplasty surgical technique was carried out similarly as previously described for standard robotic pyeloplasty at our institution [8] with slight differences between the right and left side. On the right side, the posterior peritoneum overlying the Gerota's fascia is incised with identification of the dilated renal pelvis and proximal ureter that were dissected free. If crossing vessels were encountered, it was judged case-by-case whether a decrossing was necessary or not in order to solve the UPJ obstruction.

On the left side, if the dilated renal pelvis and proximal ureter were identifiable in transparency, a transmesocolic approach was routinely employed; otherwise, the left colon is medialised, incising the line of Toldt and the Gerota's fascia exposed. The pelvis and proximal ureter are similarly dissected as for the right side (Fig. 23.4). In all patients, a dismembered pyeloplasty was carried out. The stenotic UPJ obstruction was dissected and removed; the proximal ureter was spatulated; and, if required, the redundant renal pelvis reduced.

For the plasty reconfiguration, 5-0 Vicryl sutures with RB2 needle were routinely

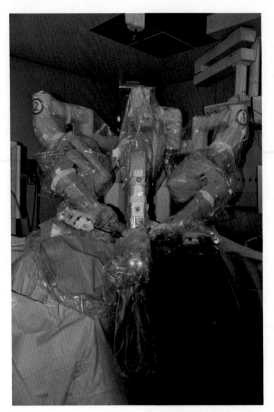

employed. The needles are inserted and removed under direct vision through the assistant port employing a laparoscopic needle driver. Once the posterior plate of the anastomosis was completed, a DJ stent was inserted retrogradely employing a flexible cystoscope in order not to modify patient positioning and the undocking-redocking of the robotic arm system in order to easy the procedure and avoid time consuming. The technique includes retrograde guide wire insertion through the flexible cystoscope into the renal pelvis and subsequently the DJ positioning. Once the DJ stent was correctly placed, a Foley catheter was inserted in the urinary bladder, and the anterior aspect of the anastomosis was completed and the remaining open pelvis closed in a similar fashion when necessary. A drain is left in place in all cases.

Postoperative Patient Care

Patients were mobilised and were allowed to resume an oral diet from the evening of the operative day. Postoperative management included catheter removal from post-operative day 2, based on clinical evaluation. The drain was

Fig. 23.3 Single-Site da Vinci platform docked to the patient (From Cestari et al. [7]. Reprinted with permission from Elsevier Limited)

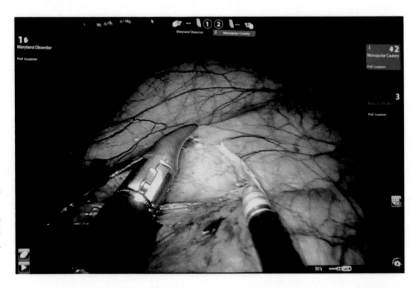

Fig. 23.4 Intra-operative dissection of the idrone-phrotic renal pelvis (From Cestari et al. [7]. Reprinted with permission from Elsevier Limited)

removed 12/24 h after surgery if the output was inferior to 50 cc and the patient was subsequently discharged from hospital. The DJ stent was removed by means of cystoscopy in an office-based setting 4 weeks after surgery, following negative urine culture and ultrasound evaluation. The follow-up protocol included a clinical and ultrasound evaluation 3 months after surgery and clinical, ultrasound and renal scan evaluation at 6-month follow-up.

Complications were reported according the Clavien-Dindo classification system [9].

Demographics and Results

Thirty-two patients were selected for robotic LESS pyeloplasty for symptomatic UPJ obstruction using the novel da Vinci Single-Site® between July 2011 and December 2013 by the same experienced robotic surgeon (A.C.).

Patients were selected according to the results of imaging techniques, MAG-3 diuretic renal scans showing evident obstruction not solved following furosemide injection ($t_{1/2}$ greater than 20 min) and the presence of symptoms, e.g. recurrent flank pain, fever and recurrent UTI episodes.

Exclusion criteria were BMI >33 kg/m^2, previous upper abdominal and renal surgery, concomitant multiple renal stones, extremely large renal pelvis (i.e. pelvis diameter greater than 6 cm), pelvic kidney and horseshoe kidney.

Demographics and preoperative characteristics of the patients are listed in Table 23.1.

Patients signed an informed consent before surgery and were made aware of the possibility that the surgery may be converted into traditional robotic pyeloplasty or open surgery.

Table 23.2 reports the perioperative outcomes of the series.

Each procedure was completed as programmed with the new robotic platform without converting into classic robotic surgery or open surgery and the DJ stent was positioned using a

Table 23.1 Demographics and pre-operative data of the series of R-LESS pyeloplasty employing the new single-port platform

N patients	32
Age (years) – median (range)	Mean 34 Median 32 Range 19–65
Side (right/left)	10 left 22 right
BMI (kg/m^2) – median (range)	Mean 22.5 Median 22.5 Range 18.7–29.7
Symptoms	Flank pain: 25 Urinary tract infections : 3 Asymptomatic: 5
Pre-operative renal scan t1/2 post-Lasix (min) – median (range)	28 (21–34)

Table 23.2 Perioperative outcomes of the series of patients submitted to R-LESS pyeloplasty employing the new single-port platform

Surgical time (min) – median (range)	Median 135, mean 140, range 90–210
Foley catheter removal (days) – median (range)	Median 2, mean 2.7, range 2–6
Drain removal (days) – median (range)	Median 3, mean 2.94, range 2–7
Hospital stay (days) – median (range)	Median 4, mean 4.67, range 3–13
Crossing vessels (n°)	24
Intra-operative complications	0

cystoscope during the procedure without any difficulties.

In one patient with congenital hepatomegaly, it was necessary to employ an auxiliary 3 mm trocar to properly retract the liver and expose the surgical field. Mean operative time was 140 min (range 90–210). No intraoperative complications were recorded and blood loss was minor. All patients were discharged the following day, after drain removal, while three patients on the same day of drain removal. Two patients experienced transient hyperpyrexia and were treated with antibiotics (Clavien-Dindo grade II), while one patient developed a dehiscence of the pyeloplasty the day of catheter removal requiring a standard robotic pyeloplasty the same night and one patient required a DJ substitution on post-operative day 2 for clot retention and flank pain (Clavien-Dindo grade III).

No other complications were observed. All patients had the DJ stent removed 4 weeks after surgery following negative urine culture and abdominal ultrasound evaluation. The 29 patients who reached a 3-month follow-up revealed resolution of pre-operative symptoms and resolution of hydronephrosis at the ultrasound evaluation. Moreover, the same results and absence of urinary obstruction at the renal scan ($t_{1/2}$ ≤20 min) were maintained in the 24 patients that reached the 6-month follow-up.

Discussion

Minimally invasive surgery is progressively expanding its role in the management of UPJ obstruction [10, 11], with LESS pyeloplasty reported for the first time as a feasible minimally invasive surgical option for UPJ repair by Desai et al. [12], hiding the surgical incision inside the umbilical scar while allowing to perform a dismembered technique.

Due to the lack of proper intra-abdominal instrument triangulation, LESS suturing appears to be extremely demanding, even for a skilled laparoscopist [13, 14], and it is unanimously considered the most challenging step of LESS pyeloplasty [15], often with the necessity to frequently employ an auxiliary 3 or 5 mm port to achieve proper instrument triangulation for correct suturing. Best et al. [16] reported a urinary anastomotic leak in 11 % of patients submitted to LESS pyeloplasty; the increased risk of urinary fistula formation led to subsequent increased risk of UPJ obstruction recurrence.

More recently, the advent of da Vinci platform eased the more complex and important step of the pyeloplasty: the suturing phase. Stein et al. [17] reported the feasibility of da Vinci single-port pyeloplasty on two patients employing 5 mm surgical instruments and a gel-port platform for the access. In their preliminary experience, they reported large skin incisions (up to 5 cm) and the problem of external conflict of the robotic arms during the procedures.

More recently, Olweny et al. [18] reported the feasibility of single-site robotic pyeloplasty employing 5 mm diameter robotic instrumentation: the skin incision in their series was 2.5–3 cm, and frequently a transposition of robotic instruments during dissection and sewing was required. Moreover, for all right-side procedures, an auxiliary 3 mm port was required to retract the liver.

The da Vinci Single-Site® technology was specifically developed to overcome some of the disadvantages and problems of LESS surgery [19, 20]. One of the greatest advantages of this system is restoration of intra-abdominal triangulations of the instruments by the use of semi-rigid tools passing through rigid curved cannulas. This creates instrument separation and sufficient triangulation at the working edges with adequate rigidity of the instruments themselves. Furthermore, the space between the robotic arms is sufficient for the assistant to do his job, although with some movement limitations. The employment of an HD-3D camera allows for an optimal visualisation of the surgical field with a stable image. The 30° laparoscope is also necessary to minimise the internal conflicts between the surgical instruments and the optical system.

In our experience, the skin incision required to properly insert the Single-Site® port was limited to 2–2.5 cm offering the opportunity for an optimal cosmetic result (Fig. 23.5). We never experienced external collisions between the robotic arms in any of the procedures, and only in one case it was necessary to add a 3 mm port to retract the liver in a patient with congenital hepatomegaly.

Already existing and potential limitations of R-LESS pyeloplasty employing the new single-port platform are mainly related to the limited availability of surgical instruments including the lack of monopolar curved scissors although very recently (July 2013) bipolar forceps become available on the market for clinical use. Most importantly, the lack of endowrist movement at the tip of the instruments requires the surgeon to

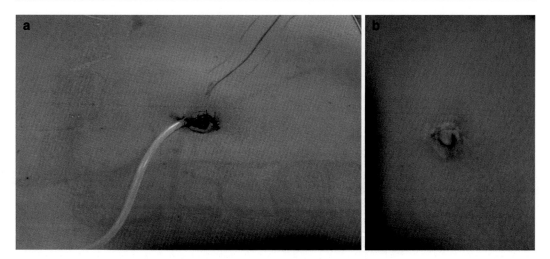

Fig. 23.5 Aesthetic results at the end of the procedure (**a**) and after 1 month (**b**) from surgery (From Cestari et al. [7].
Reprinted with permission from Elsevier Limited)

have excellent standard laparoscopic suturing skills. Due to these restrictions, we limit the indications for R-LESS pyeloplasty employing the new single-port platform to patients with BMI <33 kg/m^2, without previous major abdominal or renal surgery and/or previous renal inflammatory diseases or renal stones. The recent introduction of wristed needle holders allows for a further easing of suturing during the procedure.

Although the instrument triangulation offered by the da Vinci Single Site® has always been adequate for both the dissection and reconstructive phases, we prefer to insert the DJ stent retrogradely, via a flexible cystoscope, in order to simplify this step of the procedure.

We were the first to report the successful employment of da Vinci Single-Site® technology in urology. We successfully performed R-LESS pyeloplasty employing the new single-port platform on 32 patients including cases where aberrant crossing vessels were found and decrossed. We demonstrated the feasibility and reproducibility of the technique along with patient satisfaction as they experienced a short post-operative stay and convalescence and had an excellent aesthetical result. However, clinical benefits for the patient to standard laparoscopic or robotic pyeloplasty remain unproven, although the preliminary results appear promising.

References

1. Clayman RV, Kavoussi LR, Soper NJ, Dierks SM, Merety KS, Darcy MD, Long SR, Roemer FD, Pingleton ED, Thomson PG. Laparoscopic nephrectomy. N Engl J Med. 1991;324:1370–1.
2. Kaouk JH, Autorino R, Kim JF, et al. Laparoendoscopic single-site surgery in urology: worldwide multi-institutional analysis of 1076 cases. Eur Urol. 2011;60:998–1005.
3. White MA, Haber GP, Autorino R, Khanna R, Altunrende F, Yang B, Stein RJ, Kaouk JH. Robotic laparoendoscopic single-site surgery. BJU Int. 2010;106:923–7.
4. Haber GP, White MA, Autorino R, Escobar PF, Kroh MD, Chalikonda S, Khanna R, Forest S, Yang B, Altunrende F, Stein RJ, Kaouk JH. Novel robotic da Vinci instruments for laparoendoscopic single-site surgery. Urology. 2010;76:1279–82.
5. Kroh M, El-Hayek K, Rosenblatt S. First human surgery with a novel single-port robotic system: cholecystectomy using the da Vinci Single-Site platform. Surg Endosc. 2011;25:3566–73.
6. Wren SM, Curet MJ. Single-port robotic cholecystectomy results from a first human use clinical study of the new da Vinci single-site surgical platform. Arch Surg. 2011;146:1122–7.
7. Cestari A, Buffi NM, Lista G, Lughezzani G, Larcher A, Lazzeri M, Sangalli M, Rigatti P, Guazzoni G. Feasibility and preliminary clinical outcomes of robotic laparoendoscopic single-site (R-LESS) pyeloplasty using a new single-port platform. Eur Urol. 2012;62:175–9.
8. Cestari A, Buffi NM, Lista G, et al. Retroperitoneal and transperitoneal robot-assisted pyeloplasty in adults: techniques and results. Eur Urol. 2010;58:711–8.

9. Dindo D, Demartines N, Clavien PA. Classification of surgical complications: a new proposal with evaluation in a cohort of 6336 patients and results of a survey. Ann Surg. 2004;240:205–13.

10. Seideman CA, Bagrodia A, Gahan J, Cadeddu JA. Robotic-assisted pyeloplasty: recent developments in efficacy, outcomes, and new techniques. Curr Urol Rep. 2013;14:37–40.

11. Braga LHP, Pace K, DeMaria J, Lorenzo JA. Systematic review and meta-analysis of robotic-assisted versus conventional laparoscopic pyeloplasty for patients with ureteropelvic junction obstruction: effect on operative time, length of hospital stay, postoperative complications, and success rate. Eur Urol. 2009;56:848–58.

12. Desai MM, Rao PP, Aron M, Pascal-Haber G, Desai MR, Mishra S, Kaouk JH, Gill IS. Scarless single port transumbilical nephrectomy and pyeloplasty: first clinical report. BJU Int. 2008;101:83–8.

13. Islam A, Castellvi AO, Tesfay ST, Castellvi AD, Wright AS, Scott DJ. Early surgeon impressions and technical difficulty associated with laparoendoscopic single-site surgery: a Society of American Gastrointestinal and Endoscopic Surgeons learning center study. Surg Endosc. 2011;25:2597–603.

14. Sodergren M, McGregor C, Farne HA, Cao J, Lv Z, Purkayastha S, Athanasiou T, Darzi A, Paraskeva P. A randomised comparative study evaluating learning curves of novices in a basic single-incision laparoscopic surgery task. J Gastrointest Surg. 2013;17:569–75.

15. Kommu SS. Ex-vivo training model for laparoendoscopic single-site surgery. J Minim Access Surg. 2011;7:104–8.

16. Best SL, Donally C, Mir SA, Tracy CR, Raman JD, Cadeddu JA. Complications during the initial experience with laparoendoscopic single-site pyeloplasty. BJU Int. 2011;108:1326–9.

17. Stein RJ, White WM, Goel RK, Irwin BH, Haber GP, Kaouk JH. Robotic laparoendoscopic single-site surgery using GelPort as the access platform. Eur Urol. 2010;57:132–6.

18. Olweny EO, Park SK, Tan YK, Gurbuz C, Cadeddu JA, Best SL. Perioperative comparison of robotic assisted laparoendoscopic single-site (LESS) pyeloplasty versus conventional LESS pyeloplasty. Eur Urol. 2012;61:410–4.

19. Eisenberg D, Vidovszky TJ, Lau J, Guiroy B, Rivas H. Comparison of robotic and laparoendoscopic single-site surgery systems in a suturing and knot tying task. Surg Endosc. 2013;27:3182–6.

20. Seideman CA, Tan YK, Faddegon S, et al. Robotic-assisted laparoendoscopic single-site pyeloplasty: technique using the da Vinci® Si robotic platform. J Endourol. 2012;19:1–15.

Robotic Laparoendoscopic Single-Site Radical Prostatectomy

24

Michael A. White and Jihad H. Kaouk

Introduction

Laparoendoscopic single-site surgery (LESS) can be regarded as the latest progression in laparoscopic surgery and has garnered much enthusiasm. LESS is evolving, and robotic assistance and other technical developments may well lead to its further advancement. Early clinical experiences with LESS have pointed out several limitations related to technical constraints, including lack of triangulation, clashing of instruments, and limited operating space. To help overcome these limitations, the da Vinci surgical system has been applied to LESS and termed robotic LESS (R-LESS) [1–6].

Kaouk et al. first reported an initial feasibility study of LESS radical prostatectomy (RP) in humans [7]. At that time, the authors acknowledged the limitation of embarking on this procedure due to challenges related to ergonomics and intracorporeal suturing, and they claimed a potential application of robotics. This chapter will detail R-LESS RP in a comprehensive description. The aim is to demonstrate the procedure by describing the technique.

Since the introduction of laparoscopic nephrectomy by Clayman et al. [8] in 1991, laparoscopy has been applied to nearly every urological procedure and has improved postoperative pain, reduced hospital stays, and decreased convalescence. Yet, laparoscopy is not without drawbacks including port site complications, such as bleeding, hernia, internal organ damage, and scarring. Additionally, multiple incisions lead to visible scars and decreased cosmesis. To further decrease the invasiveness of minimally invasive therapy, newer techniques such as laparoendoscopic single-site surgery (LESS) are currently being investigated. LESS is attractive because it allows for traditional abdominal access, a familiar anatomical working environment, specimen extraction, and avoidance of hollow viscera and their inherent difficulties with closure. LESS is challenging and requires an experienced laparoscopic surgeon and assistant. To help overcome current limitations, we have introduced the da Vinci surgical system to LESS.

M.A. White, DO, FACOS (✉)
Urology San Antonio, Clinical Instructor University
of Texas Health Science Center San Antonio,
424 Normandy Ave, San Antonio, 78209 TX, USA
e-mail: michael.white@urologysa.com;
mikeawhite@sbcglobal.net; wwhite@utmck.edu

J.H. Kaouk, MD, FACS
Professor of Surgery, Cleveland Clinic Lerner College of
Medicine, Zagarek Pollock Chair in Robotic Surgery,
Center for Robotic and Image guided Surgery,
Glickman Urologic Institute, Cleveland, OH, USA
e-mail: kaoukj@ccf.org

Positioning

The patient is placed in the dorsal lithotomy position atop a gel pad and drawsheet. The arms are fully padded and tucked in the neutral position along the patient's torso. Foam crating is placed across the chest and the patient is secured to the table with 3-in. cloth tape for three revolutions

© Springer Science+Business Media New York 2017
J.H. Kaouk et al. (eds.), *Atlas of Laparoscopic and Robotic Single Site Surgery*,
Current Clinical Urology, DOI 10.1007/978-1-4939-3575-8_24

around the operating table. The legs are slightly bent and the knees are angled in line with the contralateral shoulder. Intermittent pneumatic devices are placed on the lower extremities bilaterally. The legs are then lowered toward the ground.

Port Placement

There is not a specific port that must be used for R-LESS RP, and access can be accomplished in a variety of means that are truly a variation on a theme. An incision is created intraumbilically (3–4.5 cm), and the umbilicus is released from the rectus fascia. A 2-cm incision is created through the linea alba. The initial robotic port (8 mm) is placed at the most caudal portion of the incision on the right side and directed as far laterally as possible by guiding the port into place atop a finger (Fig. 24.1). This is repeated on the opposite side with a 5-mm pediatric or standard 8-mm robotic port (Fig. 24.2). A SILS port (Covidien, Cupertino, CA, USA) is inserted through the fascial incision into the abdomen (Fig. 24.3). The 12-mm trocar provided with the SILS port is inserted, as are the two 5-mm trocars (Fig. 24.4). The patient is positioned in steep Trendelenburg, and either the da Vinci S or Si system (Intuitive Surgical, Sunnyvale, CA, USA)

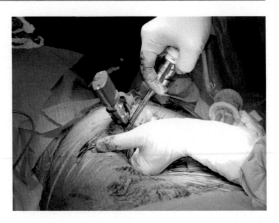

Fig. 24.2 The left robotic trocar is placed through the fascia atop two fingers and directed as lateral as possible

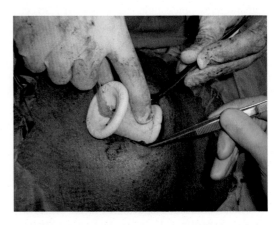

Fig. 24.3 The SILS port is inserted. This can be accomplished in an efficient manner by compressing the port with a clamp while directing through the fascia

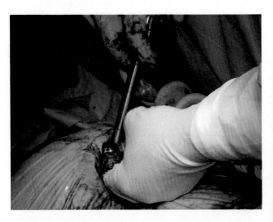

Fig. 24.1 A 3–4.5-cm incision has been made directly through the umbilicus and carried down through the skin, subcutaneous tissue, and fascia. The right-sided robotic trocar is placed through the fascia atop two fingers, for safety, and directed as lateral as possible

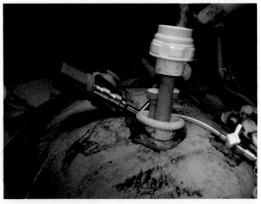

Fig. 24.4 The provided 12-mm trocar and 5-mm trocars are inserted through the SILS port

(in a three-arm approach) is docked (Fig. 24.5). The robotic 12-mm scope is introduced through the SILS port, and a 5-mm channel remains free in case the suction needs to be repositioned or sutures need to be passed (Fig. 24.6).

An alternative is to utilize standard trocars positioned through the same incision as described above but in a rhomboid fashion. This technique has been described [6]. The ports are placed in a rhomboid fashion with the endoscope in the upper corner (12 mm), a 5-mm trocar in the lower corner for suction and traction purposes, and

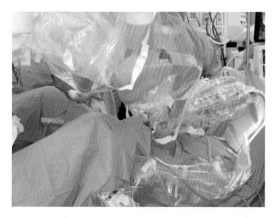

Fig. 24.5 The patient is placed in steep Trendelenburg and the robot is docked

8-mm working ports at either side, without need of any other instrument (Fig. 24.7).

Bladder Mobilization

Bladder mobilization is performed using the 8-mm EndoWrist (Intuitive Surgical) monopolar shears in the right hand and a 5-mm EndoWrist Schertel Grasper or 8-mm EndoWrist ProGrasp forcep in the left. Instruments are not intentionally crossed throughout the procedure. Using a 30° lens looking upward or a 0° lens, the peritoneum is widely incised high on the undersurface of the anterior abdominal wall, and dissection of the bladder is performed (Figs. 24.8 and 24.9). The camera is close to the desired operative target at this particular step, and withdrawing the cannula or the camera in to the cannula can assist with visual obstruction from smoke or condensation.

Defatting of the Prostate and Incision of the Endopelvic Fascia

Using the 8-mm EndoWrist monopolar shears in the right hand and a 5-mm EndoWrist Schertel Grasper or 8-mm EndoWrist ProGrasp forcep in

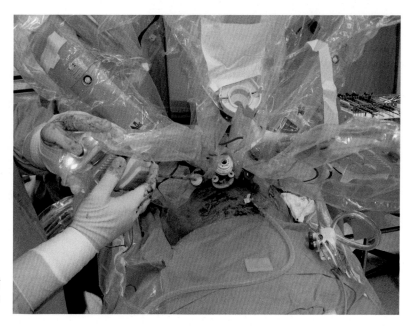

Fig. 24.6 Appearance of the robot and instruments docked

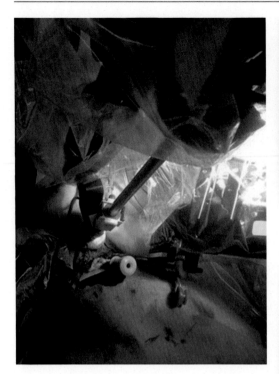

Fig. 24.7 Demonstration of alternate access configuration using standard trocars. Notice the 12-mm trocar is placed more caudal and the robotic trocars are placed more cranial and lateral (From Barret E. et al. [3])

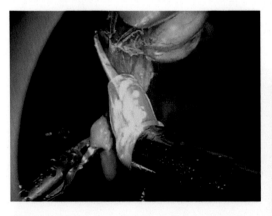

Fig. 24.8 The urachus is incised as high as possible and the space of Retzius is entered. The camera is close to the operative target at this step, and withdrawing the camera into the cannula reduces visual obstruction from smoke or condensation

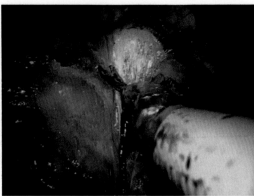

Fig. 24.9 Attachments to the pubic symphysis are taken down

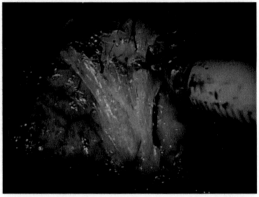

Fig. 24.10 Adipose tissue is incised just below the pubic symphysis

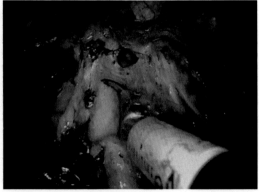

Fig. 24.11 The prostatic capsule is visualized

the left, fatty tissue is swept free from the pubic symphysis exposing the white surface of the prostatic capsule (Figs. 24.10 and 24.11). The superficial dorsal vein is cauterized and

transected. The adipose tissue is dissected from a caudal-to-cranial direction until an abrupt termination indicates the most distal aspect of the bladder. The tissue is amputated and grasped with a laparoscopic grasper introduced through the SILS port (5-mm trocar removed) or a 12-mm assistant port. The specimen is sent to pathology for permanent analysis.

The endopelvic fascia is identified and incised at the level of the most mobile portion of the prostate, the base (Fig. 24.12). The prostate is mobilized off the levator fibers from a cranial-to-caudal direction until the junction between the dorsal vein and urethra is identified (Fig. 24.13). It is important to note that at the periphery of the operative field, instrument clashing is more likely to occur and can be prevented by moving the camera and robotic instruments together in near unison.

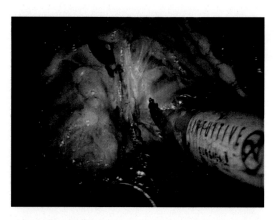

Fig. 24.12 The right-sided endopelvic fascia is identified and tensioned near the base of the prostate prior to incision

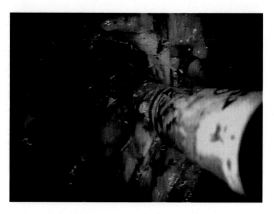

Fig. 24.13 The prostate is tractioned laterally and left-sided dissection proceeds toward the apex

Ligation of the Dorsal Venous Complex

Either two 8-mm EndoWrist robotic needle drivers or an 8-mm and a 5-mm EndoWrist robotic needle driver are used to ligate the dorsal venous complex with a 2.0 polyglactin suture (Vicryl) (Figs. 24.14, 24.15, and 24.16). The suture is introduced directly through the SILS port once the 5-mm trocar has been removed or through an assistant 12-mm trocar. Furthermore, to enhance the continence outcomes, the dorsal vein stitch is also secured to the pubic symphysis. A back-bleeding stitch is placed across the anterior surface of the prostate for hemostatic purposes and for a handle if additional traction is needed (Fig. 24.17).

Bladder Neck Dissection

Bladder neck dissection requires adjustments to the standard robotic technique. One way of compensating for the lack of a fourth robotic arm is to lift up on the back-bleeding suture with the left instrument and have the assistant apply downward pressure on the anterior bladder neck (Fig. 24.18). This can be a challenge for the assistant, and the introduction of a 15–30° of downward deflection to the suction can make this more manageable. An easier means to achieve retraction is to place a suture through the abdominal wall and through the distal bladder neck or prostatic base and then exit back out of the abdominal wall. This serves a self-retractor suspended in a "marionette" fashion. The anterior bladder neck is transected (Fig. 24.19). The urethral catheter is suspended from the abdominal wall with a 2-0 suture in the previously described marionette fashion (Fig. 24.20). The posterior bladder neck is then gradually dissected away from the prostate (Figs. 24.21 and 24.22).

Seminal Vesicle Dissection

The anterior layer of Denonvillier's fascia is incised, and the vas deferens and seminal vesicles are mobilized with the 5-mm harmonic scalpel in

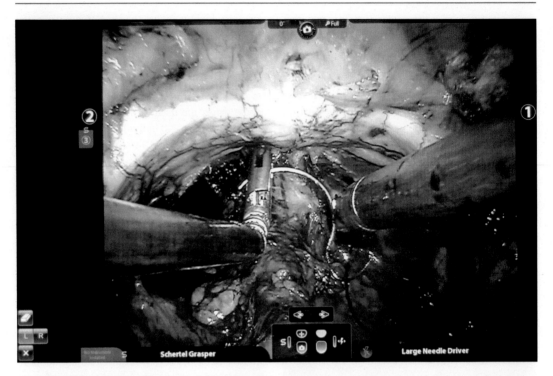

Fig. 24.14 The needle is grasped at the proximal portion

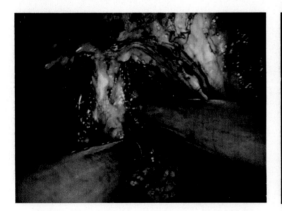

Fig. 24.15 The needle is passed around the dorsal vein

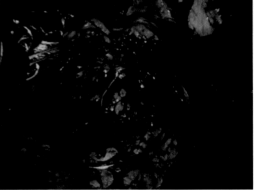

Fig. 24.16 The dorsal vein is ligated

a non-nerve-sparing approach and athermally with Hem-o-lok clips (Teleflex Medical, Research Triangle Park, NC, USA) in a nerve-sparing approach (Figs. 24.23 and 24.24). The robotic clip applier is very useful at this portion of the procedure as it can be difficult for the assistant to apply the clips via the assistant port. The vas deferens and seminal vesicles are retracted anteriorly with either the left or right robotic instrument or with marionette sutures if needed.

Prostatic Dissection

In a non-nerve-sparing procedure, a 5-mm harmonic scalpel is used in the right hand to cauterize the lateral pedicles bilaterally. Additionally, the harmonic scalpel is used to detach the lateral border of the prostate and the neurovascular bundle from the perirectal fat. An interfascial nerve-sparing approach is accomplished with a combination of sharp dissection

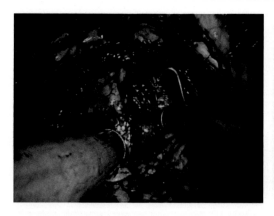

Fig. 24.17 Back-bleeding suture is placed at the anterior aspect of the base of the prostate

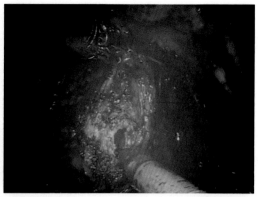

Fig. 24.19 The anterior bladder neck is incised and the Foley catheter is seen in the lumen

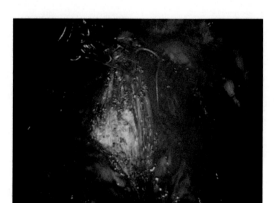

Fig. 24.18 The base of the prostate is elevated prior to anterior bladder neck dissection

and robotically applied Hem-o-lok clips (Figs. 24.25, 24.26, and 24.27). Assistant retraction with the suction device and/or marionette sutures allows for placement of Hem-o-lok clips to the vascular pedicles and smaller vessels attached to the neurovascular bundles.

Urethral Dissection and Division

The 8-mm monopolar shears are used to incise the ligated dorsal vein complex, exposing the underlying urethra (Figs. 24.28 and 24.29). The urethra is transected without cautery (Fig. 24.30). The tip of the urethral catheter is withdrawn, and the posterior urethral wall is transected sharply. Complete dissection of the

prostate apex is accomplished in a retrograde fashion; the prostate is released and placed in a 10-mm entrapment bag (Fig. 24.31).

Pelvic Lymph Node Dissection

A standard lymph node dissection is performed in the identical manner to the standard robot-assisted laparoscopic prostatectomy (RALP) technique. External iliac nodal tissues, as well as nodes from the obturator fossa, are included in the dissection. The specimen is removed with a laparoscopic grasper that is introduced through the SILS port (5-mm trocar removed) or a 12-mm assistant port.

Ureterovesical Anastomosis

The 8-mm robotic needle drivers in the left and right hand are used to complete the vesicoureteral anastomosis. Two sutures of 2-0 poliglecaprone 25 (Monocryl) on an RB-1 needle are placed in a semicircular "running" fashion starting from the 6 o'clock position toward the 12 o'clock and then tied together (Figs. 24.32 and 24.33). A 20F Foley catheter is inserted under vision into the bladder before completion of the anastomosis. The anastomosis is tested by instilling 100 ml of saline into the bladder to ensure water tightness. The prostate is extracted

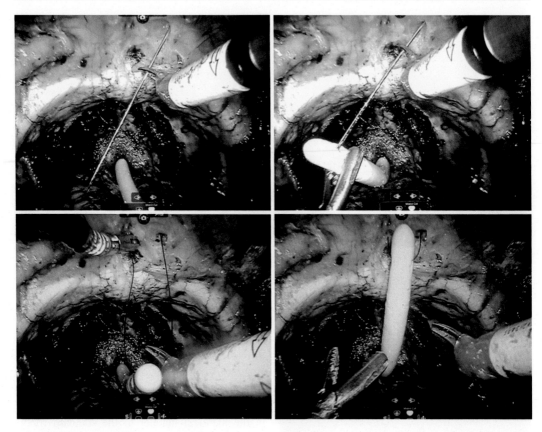

Fig. 24.20 The Foley catheter is elevated in a marionette fashion

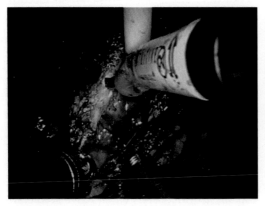

Fig. 24.21 Posterior bladder neck dissection

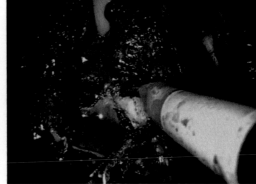

Fig. 24.22 Posterior bladder neck dissection

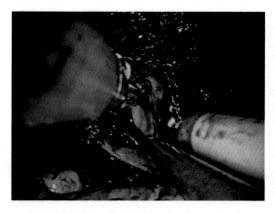

Fig. 24.23   Seminal vesicle dissection

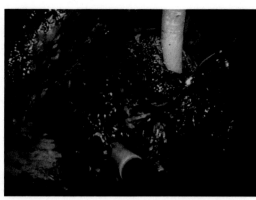

Fig. 24.26   Left neurovascular dissection

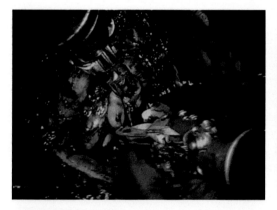

Fig. 24.24   Placement of Hem-o-lok clip via robotic clip applier at the seminal vesicle artery

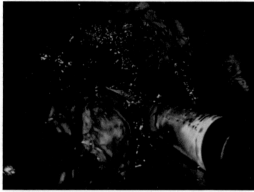

Fig. 24.27   Right neurovascular dissection

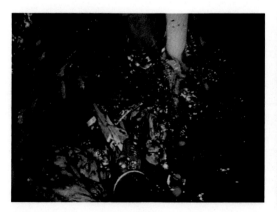

Fig. 24.25   Control of the left vascular pedicle

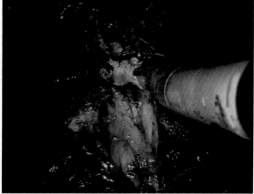

Fig. 24.28   Incision of dorsal vein

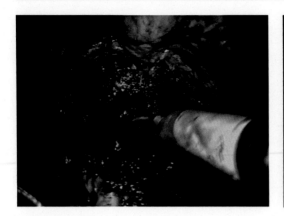

Fig. 24.29 Athermal apical dissection

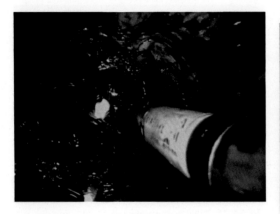

Fig. 24.30 Incision of urethra with underlying Foley catheter visible

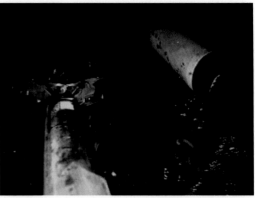

Fig. 24.31 Prostate placed in laparoscopic entrapment bag

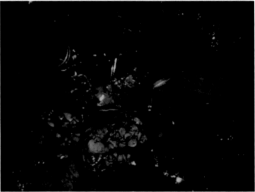

Fig. 24.32 Initial placement of suture in the posterior bladder neck

after the robot is de-docked and the SILS port or 12-mm camera trocar is removed (Fig. 24.34). A Jackson-Pratt drain is placed in the pelvis and exited through either a separate fascial stab or one of the 8-mm trocar fascial defects. The drain is brought out via the same skin incision (Fig. 24.35).

Tips and Tricks

All steps of traditional RALP can be duplicated, but certain modifications will be necessary on a case-by-case basis. Flexibility between a 0 and 30° lens looking upward must be maintained to

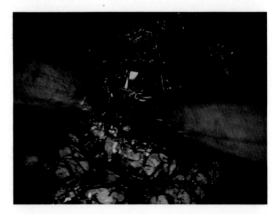

Fig. 24.33 Suture placed at the 6 o'clock position in the urethral mucosa

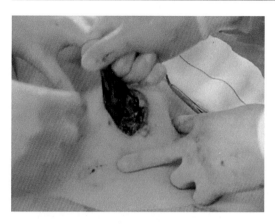

Fig. 24.34 Prostate extraction

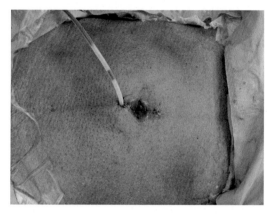

Fig. 24.35 Final closure appearance

avoid instrument clashing. Additionally, repositioning the scope out of the path of the instruments is needed under certain circumstances and must be communicated to the assistant. Instrument crossing does not occur when the robotic cannulae are slightly staggered, ensuring that they are not in parallel.

Early in the experience, it was preferred to use an 8-mm instrument in the right hand and a pediatric grasper in the left hand to maximize the benefits of each instrument, but by staggering the 8-mm trocars, an improved range of motion can be achieved with the standard robotic

instrumentation and the pediatric instruments may not be needed. An additional benefit of using an 8-mm robotic instrument is the ability to use the robotic Hem-o-lok clip applier. This allows the operating surgeon to place clips and overcomes the clashing encountered by the assistant. More important, use of the robotic clip applier has allowed for the replication of our nerve-sparing technique that we perform during traditional RALP. In non-nerve-sparing cases, a 5-mm harmonic scalpel can be used, but it must be recognized that this instrument does not articulate or deflect and can be challenging at times. Fortunately, the use of this device is purely optional, and the pedicles can be controlled with either Hem-o-lok clips or suture ligation.

References

1. Desai MM, Aron M, Berger A, et al. Transvesical robotic radical prostatectomy. BJU Int. 2008;102:1666–9.
2. Kaouk JH, Goel RK, Haber GP, et al. Robotic single-port transumbilical surgery in humans: initial report. BJU Int. 2009;103:366–9.
3. Barret E, Sanchez-Salas R, Kasraeian A, et al. A transition to laparoendoscopic single-site surgery (LESS) radical prostatectomy: human cadaver experimental and initial clinical experience. J Endourol. 2009;23:135–40.
4. Kaouk JH, Goel RK. Single-port laparoscopic and robotic partial nephrectomy. Eur Urol. 2009;55:1163–70.
5. Stein RJ, White WM, Goel RK, Irwin BH, Haber GP, Kaouk JH. Robotic laparoendoscopic single-site surgery using GelPort as the access platform. Eur Urol. 2010;57:132–7.
6. Barret E, Sanchez-Salas R, Cathelineau X, Rozet F, Galiano M, Vallancien G. Re: initial complete laparoendoscopic single-site surgery robotic assisted radical prostatectomy (LESS-RARP). Int Braz J Urol. 2009;35:92–3.
7. Kaouk JH, Goel RK, Haber GP, Crouzet S, Desai MM, Gill IS. Single-port laparoscopic radical prostatectomy. Urology. 2008;72:1190–3.
8. Clayman RV, Kavoussi LR, Soper NJ, et al. Laparoscopic nephrectomy: initial case report. J Urol. 1991;146:278–82.

Part V

Outcomes and Future Directions

Complications of Laparoendoscopic Single-Site Surgery in Urology

25

Idir Ouzaid, Vishnuvardhan Ganesan, and Georges-Pascal Haber

Introduction

Laparoendoscopic single-site surgery (LESS) as an evolution of the conventional laparoscopic approach, in the pathway of minimally invasive surgery, should be evaluated comparatively to widely accepted procedures. According to a multi-institutional compilation of cases [1], most LESS procedures (86 %) were performed in the upper urinary tract, with most of these being extirpative or ablative (84 %).

According to IDEAL recommendations [2], the steps to evaluate a new surgical technology are (1) an "innovation step" in which the surgical innovation is described for the first time; (2) a "development step" in which the surgical innovation is evaluated in a small group of patients to refine or modify the precise technique; and (3) an "exploration step" in which the safety and effectiveness of the surgical innovation can be tested in the context of prospective, single-center, case-series study uti-

lizing a large number of cases. Only after these three steps can the effectiveness of surgical innovation be assessed (the "assessment step") against current standard of treatment in the context of randomized controlled trials or non-randomized, well-designed comparative studies.

Herein, in order to comply with the IDEAL guidelines, we summarize reported complications from procedures including radical prostatectomy, nephrectomy (radical or partial), donor nephrectomy, adrenalectomy, and pyeloplasty.

LESS Radical Prostatectomy

Minimally invasive radical prostatectomy (RP) is known to be technically challenging. The learning curve to optimize functional and oncological outcomes is steep even for the conventional approach.

After the first LESS radical prostatectomy (LESS-RP) was reported from the Cleveland Clinic [3], various LESS approaches have been reported including transperitoneal (laparoscopic, robotic assisted), preperitoneal, and transvesical (Table 25.1) [4–7]. Most studies reported initial experiences with a limited number of cases [8, 9]. While there were no reported cases of conversion from LESS to open RP, conversion to conventional laparoscopic was reported in up to 5 % of the cases with the addition of one or more trocars in up to 10 % [5].

I. Ouzaid, MD • V. Ganesan
Department of Urology, Center for Laparoscopic and Robotic Surgery, Glickman Urological and Kidney Institute, Cleveland Clinic Foundation, Cleveland, OH, USA

G.-P. Haber, MD, PhD (✉)
Associate Staff, Department of Urology, Center for Robotic and Image Guided Surgery, Glickman Urological Institute, Cleveland Clinic, Cleveland, OH, USA
e-mail: haberg2@ccf.org

© Springer Science+Business Media New York 2017
J.H. Kaouk et al. (eds.), *Atlas of Laparoscopic and Robotic Single Site Surgery*, Current Clinical Urology, DOI 10.1007/978-1-4939-3575-8_25

Table 25.1 Complications of LESS radical prostatectomy

Study	Number of patients	Conversion to open (%)	Conversion to lap (%)	Additional port (%)	Intraoperative complication (%)	Postoperative complication (%)	Grade 1–2 (%)	Grade 3–5 (%)
Caceres [4]	31	0	0	0	0	19.4	6.45	12.9
White [5][a]	20	0	5	10	0	20	15	5
Jiang [6]	20	0	0	5	0	20	20	0
Gao [7][b]	16	0	0	0	0	31.25	31.25	0

[a]Robotic LESS
[b]Transvesical LESS

Caceres and colleagues reported a series of 31 patients undergoing LESS-RP using the "Key port™" manual system (Richard Wolf GmbH, Knittlingen, Germany) [4]. In their experience, the large median lobe did not pose a specific problem. However, they used an additional lateral port for retraction. The average operative time and the estimated blood loss (EBL) were 207 min (range 120–390) and 258 ml (range 200–500), respectively. Postoperative complications were reported in 20 % of the cases. One patient required reintervention with a single-port umbilical left colostomy due to a rectal lesion that presented on day 2 as peritonitis. The patient developed hypercapnia with respiratory acidosis and needed to be admitted into the intensive care unit. Authors assumed this last complication was related to long operating time (390 min) and occurred in the first case of the series. After a mean follow-up of 20 weeks (range 12–27), continence recovery was observed in 33.3 %.

Using a robotic-assisted LESS approach, White et al. reported a slightly shorter time (187.6 min, range 120–300) and a reduced EBL (128.8 ml, range 50–350) [5]. One procedure (5 %) was converted to a conventional robotic-assisted RP due to the need for more traction. An additional port was used in two procedures (10 %) because of robotic instrument clashing. The only high-grade complication (Grade 4) was urosepsis which appeared on postoperative day 45 (n = 1) and necessitated an intensive care unit admission.

Another approach of LESS-RP used a transvesical approach. This has been proved to be feasible in cadavers [10] with the rationale of improving functional outcomes in selected patients with low-risk disease. Gao et al. reported an initial experience of 16 procedures of transvesical LESS-RP [7]. Mean EBL and operative time were 130 (range 75–500) and 105 min (range 75–180), respectively. Authors did not report any major complications and low-grade complications occurred in five cases (31.5 %). Moreover, there were no positive margins in these selected low-risk patients. Continence recovery was 100 % and IIEF-6 score was greater than 18 in 75 % patients after 12 months of follow-up. However, length of stay (LOS) of this series was 12.7 days, which is much longer than LOS reported in contemporary RP series.

Ferrara and colleagues reported their comparative experience of LESS-RP (n = 10) versus conventional laparoscopic RP (n = 10). They found LESS-RP procedures took longer to be performed (on average 43 min longer) but had similar rates of positive margins and no increased rate of complications [11].

Finally, although comparative studies on LESS-RP are lacking, most studies reported a cosmesis advantage. The technique is challenging but has shown similar results in terms of disease control and complication rates in experienced laparoscopic and robotic hands. Although the advent of the robot seemed to be useful in overcoming suturing difficulties during the urethrovesical anastomosis, there is a lack of data on robotic instruments clashing and a well-assessed added value in LESS-RP.

LESS Renal Surgery

LESS renal surgery has been reported from various institutions. In a multi-institutional study that reported 1076 LESS procedures, renal surgery accounted for 65 % of the cases and included tumor or mass, cyst, nonfunctioning kidney, and living donor [1].

Some comparative studies of LESS nephrectomy and conventional laparoscopic nephrectomy available in the current literature include two randomized control studies [12, 13]. The goal was to address whether LESS nephrectomy has similar outcomes compared to conventional approach. Herein, we focus on complications.

LESS Radical Nephrectomy

The most widely adopted LESS procedures in urology are simple and radical LESS nephrectomies (LESS-RN). The feasibility and safety of this minimally invasive approach have both been well documented [14]. Table 25.2 summarizes major comparative studies of LESS-RN [12, 15–18]. The reported complication rate was reported to be less than 20 % and no conversion to conventional RN or open RN was reported in most studies.

In the matched analysis reported by Wang and colleagues, a 5-mm ancillary trocar was inserted during the first two cases of LESS-RN for tissue retraction. In one case, a conversion from LESS to standard laparoscopy occurred because of an uncontrollable hemorrhage from an inadvertent injury of an anomalous renal artery branching from the celiac trunk. The converted patient received transfusion intraoperatively. Spontaneous pneumothorax developed during the induction of anesthesia in one patient with chronic obstructive pulmonary disease. In the conventional LRN group, one patient had an intraoperative hemorrhage and received a transfusion, but surgical conversion was not needed. Postoperative bleeding developed in two patients; this was managed conservatively by transfusion [17].

A recent meta-analysis included 2 RCTs and 25 retrospective studies compiling the data of 1094 cases of LESS renal surgery [19]. In the radical nephrectomy subgroup analysis, the complication rate was similar (OR 0.80; 95 % CI 0.37–1.74 %) between LESS-RN and conventional LRN, but conversions were higher in the LESS-RN group (OR 4.88; 95 % CI 1.42–16.78). An additional trocar for liver retraction was commonly used in right nephrectomies [20–22]. Reasons for conversions included difficult retraction (33.3 % of converted cases), bleeding (26.7 %), difficult dissection (13.3 %), failure to progress (20 %), and difficult access (6.7 %). Postoperative pain measurements (OR −0.91; 95 % CI −1.63 to −0.19 %) and analgesic intake (OR −7.66; 95 % CI −13.06 to −2.27 %) favored the LESS-RN group.

LESS Partial Nephrectomy

LESS partial nephrectomy (LESS-PN) was mainly reported for small renal exophytic masses. Greco and colleagues reported the largest experience of

Table 25.2 Major comparative studies of LESS radical nephrectomy (LESS-RN) and conventional laparoscopic radical nephrectomy (LRN)

Study	LESS-RN			LRN		
	n	Complications (%)	Conversion (%)	n	Complications (%)	Conversion (%)
Park [15]	19	15.8	0	38	21.1	2.6
Seo [16]	10	10	0	12	17	0
Wang [17]	20	15	5	33	9.1	0
White [18]	10	10	0	10	10	0
Tugcu [12][a]	14	0	0	13	0	0

[a]Randomized controlled trial

LESS-PN compiling data from different institutions [23]. Median operative time and EBL were 170 and 150 ml, respectively. A clampless technique was adopted in 70 cases (36.8 %), and the median warm ischemia time (WIT) was 16.5 min. The overall postoperative complication rate was 14.7 %. The adoption of a robotic LESS technique versus conventional LESS (OR 20.92 [95 % CI, 2.66–164.64]; $p=0.003$) was found to be an independent predictor of no postoperative complications of any grade. In 117 cases (61.6 %), the surgeons required additional ports, with a standard laparoscopy and open surgery conversion rate of 5.8 % (11 of 190 cases) and 2.1 % (4 of 190 cases), respectively. The reasons for conversion to standard laparoscopy were difficulties during dissection and exposure (four cases), demanding suture (five cases), and bleeding (two cases). No case was converted to RN.

Tiu et al. compared LESS-PN in large tumors using a comparative study that included 20 patients with renal tumors >4 cm and 47 patients with renal tumors <4 cm [24].

Patients were comparable in terms of baselines demographics. Intraoperative complications were higher for patients with tumors >4 cm (10 % vs. 0 % for patients with tumors <4 cm), without reaching statistical significance ($p=0.89$). Patients with tumors >4 cm had two intraoperative complications: one patient had an intraoperative ureteric injury that was repaired with intracorporeal suturing and insertion of ureteric stent, and the other patient had a renal vein injury that was successfully controlled with intracorporeal suturing. Postoperative complications occurred in three patients with tumors >4 cm: two patients required blood transfusions (Dindo-Clavien

grade 2), and one patient had clot retention (Dindo-Clavien grade 2), which was managed with irrigation via a three-way, indwelling, urinary catheter. In seven patients with tumors <4 cm, five required blood transfusion (Dindo-Clavien grade 2); one developed urine leakage (Dindo-Clavien grade 3), which was managed with a ureteric stent; and one developed severe postoperative bleeding requiring open nephrectomy (Dindo-Clavien grade 3). Nevertheless, there was no statistical significant difference in the complication rate between the groups. Authors concluded patients with tumors >4 cm operated with LESS-PN had a statistically significant, higher mean nephrometry score, longer warm ischemia time, and longer length of stay, but there was no increased risk of adverse outcomes.

Similarly, in the meta-analysis of LESS renal surgery, authors did not find any differences in perioperative complication rate, postoperative pain, and analgesic requirements in the subgroup of LESS-PN [19].

LESS Living Donor Nephrectomy

Given the nature of the procedure, aspects of LESS donor nephrectomy (LESS-DN) that need to be considered include donor safety, graft outcome, and morbidity.

In 2008, Gill and colleagues were the first to report the feasibility and safety of LESS-DN [25]. A several case series [26–29] and one randomized trial [13] have since been published (Table 25.3). There were no documented deaths among the donors and complications ranged from 0 to 16 %.

Table 25.3 LESS donor nephrectomy

Study	n	Design	Mean WIT (min)	EBL (ml)	Complications (%)
Canes [26]	17	Comparative with C-LDN	6.1	108	12
Ganpule [27]	13	Descriptive	6.8	158	0
Gimenez [28]	40	Descriptive	3.96	107	2.5
Kurien [13]	25	RCT	7.2	84	16
Lunsford [29]	10	Comparative with C-LDN	–	50	0

RCT randomized controlled trial, *C-LDN* conventional laparoscopic living donor nephrectomy

The most recent large series compared outcomes from 135 LESS-DN with an immediately preceding cohort of 100 conventional laparoscopic DN [30]. In this study, 16 cases that were initiated via a single port required placement of multiple ports and were successfully completed with transumbilical extraction. Intraoperative causes for additional port placement included obese donors with large amounts of perirenal fat ($n=7$), gaseous intestinal distension and inability to achieve adequate abdominal domain with pneumoperitoneum ($n=4$), prior renal biopsy or other surgery with scarring ($n=2$), bleeding ($n=1$), and diaphragmatic injury repair ($n=1$). None of these cases were aborted, required conversion to an open approach, or received blood transfusion. Compared with successful single-port cases, patients requiring additional ports had similar body mass indexes (28.5; $p=0.2$) and numbers of vessels ($P=0.1$). Operative times (4.0 ± 1.0 h; $P<0.01$), blood loss (240.9 ± 150 ml; $P<0.01$), and length of stay (3.3 ± 1.3 days; $P=0.02$) were all increased. The transumbilical extraction incision was slightly increased in apparent length (4.7 ± 0.7 cm; $P<0.01$). Complications were not significantly different between any groups. No LESS-DN donor required open conversion or blood transfusion. Hernia occurred in three (2.2 %) single-port patients that required repair. In the comparative groups, a total of nine patients required hernia repair with a similar incidence in patients with multiple-port laparoscopy and transumbilical extractions (1.5 %; $p=0.7$). Authors concluded single-port approach had similar outcomes compared with all previous laparoscopic donor nephrectomies. Moreover, the 36-Item Short Form Health Surveys demonstrated no significant differences, and additional survey data revealed that single-port patients were more satisfied with cosmetic outcomes ($p<0.01$) and the overall donation process ($p=0.01$).

Finally, kidney extraction through the umbilicus [25], the single-port device [28], or the vagina [31] did not seem to be associated with substantial complications.

LESS Pyeloplasty

The first report of LESS pyeloplasty (LESS-P) came out of Desai and colleagues [32].

Soon after the first report, a comparative study matched 14 patients who underwent LESS-P with 28 patients who underwent conventional laparoscopic pyeloplasty (CL-P) [33]. Minor postoperative complications (14.3 % vs. 14.3 %; $p=1.0$) or major postoperative complications (21.4 % vs. 10 %; $p=0.18$) were similar in the two groups. In the LESS-P group, there were two minor complications (hematuria) that were managed conservatively and three major complications including urine leak ($n=2$) and acute clot obstruction ($n=1$) all of which were managed successfully with percutaneous nephrostomy tube placement. Tugcu and colleagues reported a randomized trial of LESS-P ($n=19$) and CL-P ($n=20$) without any significant differences in terms of intraoperative or postoperative complication rate between the two groups [34]. Of note, one patient who underwent a LESS-P had prolonged urine leakage that resolved spontaneously within 5 days after indwelling a Foley catheter. Postoperative pain, the use of analgesics, time to return to normal activities, and cosmesis satisfaction were significantly lower in patients who underwent LESS-P compared with those who underwent CTL-P. However, LESS-P showed a longer operative time.

Due to the lack of proper intra-abdominal instruments triangulation, LESS suturing appears to be extremely demanding, even for a skilled laparoscopic surgeon [1]. LESS suturing is considered the most challenging step of LESS pyeloplasty [35] with an increased risk of urinary fistula formation and a subsequent increased risk of ureteropelvic junction recurrence. Best et al. reported a urinary anastomotic leak in 11 % of patients and the frequent need to use an auxiliary 3- or 5-mm port to achieve proper instrument triangulation for correct suturing [36]. Consequently, Kaouk et al. [1] reported the feasibility of robotic single-port pyeloplasty (R-LESS-P) on two patients using 5-mm surgical instruments and a gel-port platform for the access. In an attempt to assess the added value of R-LESS-P as compared to LESS-P, Olweny and colleagues compared robotic and conventional LESS ($n = 10$ in each group) [37]. The mean operative time was significantly longer for R-LESS-P (226 vs. 188 min; $p = 0.007$). Conventional LESS-P alone required an accessory port for the anastomosis in ten of ten cases. Two conversions to standard laparoscopy and two postoperative complications occurred in three of ten patients in the LESS-P group, compared with no conversions and one postoperative complication in the R-LESS-P group ($p = 0.26$). The added value of the R-LESS-P is not well established partly because of small cohort of patients and the lack of quantification of subjective outcomes such as instrument clashing and maneuverability.

The largest series for LESS-P was reported in a multi-institutional cohort of 140 patients [38]. Overall, R-LESS-P was applied in 31 patients (22.1 %). A single 2–3 mm accessory port was used in 44 patients (31.4 %), and a single 5–12 mm accessory port was added in 9 patients (6.4 %), whereas 10 patients (7.1 %) were converted to conventional multiport laparoscopy. No patients required conversion to open surgery, nor were any intraoperative complications reported. The overall 90-day postoperative complication rate was 18.6 %, of which 7.8 % were Clavien grade 3 or greater.

LESS Adrenalectomy

A variety of approaches to LESS adrenalectomy (LESS-AD) with different advantages and disadvantages have been described since this approach was first used in 2005 [39–46].

Hirano and colleagues reported one of the initial series of retroperitoneal LESS-AD route in 54 patients [39]. The procedure was completed in all patients but one. Intraoperative or postoperative complications were observed in 12 patients (22.2 %). Intraoperative complications consisted of pneumothorax in three cases (5.6 %) during dissection of the retroperitoneal space using a balloon dilator and hemorrhage necessitating blood transfusion in four cases (7.4 %), one of which was converted to open surgery because of uncontrolled bleeding. Postoperative complications consisted of fulminant hepatitis (1.9 %), pulmonary thrombosis (1.9 %), and superficial wound infection (5.6 %). The patient with fulminant hepatitis died from hepatic failure on postoperative day 14 (mortality rate 1.9 %).

Comparison between transperitoneal and retroperitoneoscopic approaches using a single-site access did not show any difference in a small comparative study [41]. Interestingly, retroperitoneoscopic LESS-RA versus conventional retroperitoneoscopic adrenalectomy in the largest case-control matched study that included 47 patients in each group reported an overall complication rate of 8.5 % and 6.4 %, respectively. Operative time was longer for LESS-RA (56 ± 28 min versus 40 ± 12 min; $p < 0.05$). However, pain medication and hospital stay favored the LESS-RA approach [43]. This study confirmed the outcomes of studies with smaller sample size [47].

A recent review of the literature about LESS-AD concluded that the feasibility and safety of LESS adrenalectomy have been demonstrated. Only long-term follow-up outcomes will prove its benefits over conventional laparoscopy and define the role and the oncological safety of LESS adrenal surgery [46].

Conclusion

Available data in the literature showed promising outcomes of LESS surgery especially in terms of postoperative pain, analgesics requirement, and a substantial cosmesis advantage without compromising safety. Specifically, conversion rates are very low and adding a 5-mm or smaller port overcame retraction challenges in most cases. Using the robotic LESS, although it is cumbersome, seemed to add more ergonomics during suturing, but comparative studies are lacking in the current literature to better define the role of the robot in LESS procedures.

Although the reported studies showed promising outcomes, reports are mostly initial experiences from high-volume centers, and prospective controlled trials are awaited for the majority of the procedures.

References

1. Kaouk JH, et al. Laparoendoscopic single-site surgery in urology: worldwide multi-institutional analysis of 1076 cases. Eur Urol. 2011;60(5):998–1005.
2. McCulloch P, et al. No surgical innovation without evaluation: the IDEAL recommendations. Lancet. 2009;374(9695):1105–12.
3. Kaouk JH, et al. Single-port laparoscopic radical prostatectomy. Urology. 2008;72(6):1190–3.
4. Caceres F, et al. Safety study of umbilical single-port laparoscopic radical prostatectomy with a new DuoRotate system. Eur Urol. 2012;62(6):1143–9.
5. White MA, et al. Robotic laparoendoscopic single-site radical prostatectomy: technique and early outcomes. Eur Urol. 2010;58(4):544–50.
6. Jiang C, et al. Extraperitoneal transumbilical laparoendoscopic single-site radical prostatectomy using a homemade single-port device: 20 cases with midterm outcomes. World J Urol. 2014;32(3):829–36.
7. Gao X, et al. Single-port transvesical laparoscopic radical prostatectomy for organ-confined prostate cancer: technique and outcomes. BJU Int. 2013;112(7):944–52.
8. Kumar P, et al. Laparoendoscopic single-site surgery (LESS) prostatectomy – robotic and conventional approach. Minerva Urol Nefrol. 2010;62(4):425–30.
9. Silberstein JL, Power NE, Touijer KA. Laparoendoscopic single site (LESS) radical prostatectomy: a review of the initial experience. Minerva Urol Nefrol. 2011;63(2):123–9.
10. Desai MM, et al. Transvesical robotic radical prostatectomy. BJU Int. 2008;102(11):1666–9.
11. Ferrara V, et al. SILS extraperitoneal radical prostatectomy. Minerva Urol Nefrol. 2010;62(4):363–9.
12. Tugcu V, et al. Laparoendoscopic single-site surgery versus standard laparoscopic simple nephrectomy: a prospective randomized study. J Endourol. 2010; 24(8):1315–20.
13. Kurien A, et al. First prize: standard laparoscopic donor nephrectomy versus laparoendoscopic single-site donor nephrectomy: a randomized comparative study. J Endourol. 2011;25(3):365–70.
14. Merseburger AS, et al. EAU guidelines on robotic and single-site surgery in urology. Eur Urol. 2013; 64(2):277–91.
15. Park YH, et al. Comparison of laparoendoscopic single-site radical nephrectomy with conventional laparoscopic radical nephrectomy for localized renal-cell carcinoma. J Endourol. 2010;24(6):997–1003.
16. Seo IY, Lee JW, Rim JS. Laparoendoscopic single-site radical nephrectomy: a comparison with conventional laparoscopy. J Endourol. 2011;25(3):465–9.
17. Wang L, et al. A matched-pair comparison of laparoendoscopic single-site surgery and standard laparoscopic radical nephrectomy by a single urologist. J Endourol. 2012;26(6):676–81.
18. White MA, et al. Robotic laparoendoscopic single-site radical nephrectomy: surgical technique and comparative outcomes. Eur Urol. 2011;59(5):815–22.
19. Fan X, et al. Laparoendoscopic single-site nephrectomy compared with conventional laparoscopic nephrectomy: a systematic review and meta-analysis of comparative studies. Eur Urol. 2012;62(4): 601–12.
20. Greco F, et al. Laparoendoscopic single-site and conventional laparoscopic radical nephrectomy result in equivalent surgical trauma: preliminary results of a single-centre retrospective controlled study. Eur Urol. 2012;61(5):1048–53.
21. Mir SA, et al. Minimally invasive nephrectomy: the influence of laparoendoscopic single-site surgery on patient selection, outcomes, and morbidity. Urology. 2011;77(3):631–4.
22. Raman JD, Bagrodia A, Cadeddu JA. Single-incision, umbilical laparoscopic versus conventional laparoscopic nephrectomy: a comparison of perioperative outcomes and short-term measures of convalescence. Eur Urol. 2009;55(5):1198–204.
23. Greco F, et al. Laparoendoscopic single-site partial nephrectomy: a multi-institutional outcome analysis. Eur Urol. 2013;64(2):314–22.
24. Tiu A, et al. Feasibility of robotic laparoendoscopic single-site partial nephrectomy for renal tumors >4 cm. Eur Urol. 2013;63(5):941–6.
25. Gill IS, et al. Single port transumbilical (E-NOTES) donor nephrectomy. J Urol. 2008;180(2):637–41; discussion 641.
26. Canes D, et al. Laparo-endoscopic single site (LESS) versus standard laparoscopic left donor nephrectomy: matched-pair comparison. Eur Urol. 2010;57(1):95–101.
27. Ganpule AP, et al. Laparoendoscopic single-site donor nephrectomy: a single-center experience. Urology. 2009;74(6):1238–40.
28. Gimenez E, et al. Laparoendoscopic single site live donor nephrectomy: initial experience. J Urol. 2010;184(5):2049–53.
29. Lunsford KE, et al. Single-site laparoscopic living donor nephrectomy offers comparable perioperative outcomes to conventional laparoscopic living donor nephrectomy at a higher cost. Transplantation. 2011;91(2):e16–7.
30. Barth RN, et al. Single-port donor nephrectomy provides improved patient satisfaction and equivalent outcomes. Ann Surg. 2013;257(3):527–33.
31. Kaouk JH, et al. Transvaginal hybrid natural orifice transluminal surgery robotic donor nephrectomy: first clinical application. Urology. 2012;80(6):1171–5.
32. Desai MM, et al. Scarless single port transumbilical nephrectomy and pyeloplasty: first clinical report. BJU Int. 2008;101(1):83–8.
33. Tracy CR, et al. Perioperative outcomes in patients undergoing conventional laparoscopic versus laparoendoscopic single-site pyeloplasty. Urology. 2009;74(5):1029–34.
34. Tugcu V, et al. Laparoendoscopic single-site versus conventional transperitoneal laparoscopic pyeloplasty: a prospective randomized study. Int J Urol. 2013;20(11):1112–7.

35. Gill IS, et al. Consensus statement of the consortium for laparoendoscopic single-site surgery. Surg Endosc. 2010;24(4):762–8.

36. Best SL, et al. Complications during the initial experience with laparoendoscopic single-site pyeloplasty. BJU Int. 2011;108(8):1326–9.

37. Olweny EO, et al. Perioperative comparison of robotic assisted laparoendoscopic single-site (LESS) pyeloplasty versus conventional LESS pyeloplasty. Eur Urol. 2012;61(2):410–4.

38. Rais-Bahrami S, et al. Laparoendoscopic single-site pyeloplasty: outcomes of an international multi-institutional study of 140 patients. Urology. 2013; 82(2):366–72.

39. Hirano D, et al. Retroperitoneoscopic adrenalectomy for adrenal tumors via a single large port. J Endourol. 2005;19(7):788–92.

40. Castellucci SA, et al. Single port access adrenalectomy. J Endourol. 2008;22(8):1573–6.

41. Agha A, et al. Single-incision retroperitoneoscopic adrenalectomy and single-incision laparoscopic adrenalectomy. J Endourol. 2010;24(11):1765–70.

42. Jeong CW, et al. Synchronous bilateral laparoendoscopic single-site adrenalectomy. J Endourol. 2010;24(8):1301–5.

43. Walz MK, Groeben H, Alesina PF. Single-access retroperitoneoscopic adrenalectomy (SARA) versus conventional retroperitoneoscopic adrenalectomy (CORA): a case-control study. World J Surg. 2010;34(6):1386–90.

44. Yuge K, et al. Initial experience of transumbilical laparoendoscopic single-site surgery of partial adrenalectomy in patient with aldosterone-producing adenoma. BMC Urol. 2010;10:19.

45. Shi TP, et al. Laparoendoscopic single-site retroperitoneoscopic adrenalectomy: a matched-pair comparison with the gold standard. Surg Endosc. 2011;25(7):2117–24.

46. Rane A, et al. Laparoendoscopic single site (LESS) adrenalectomy: technique and outcomes. World J Urol. 2012;30(5):597–604.

47. Ishida M, et al. Technical difficulties of transumbilical laparoendoscopic single-site adrenalectomy: comparison with conventional laparoscopic adrenalectomy. World J Urol. 2013;31(1):199–203.

Mark W. Ball and Mohamad E. Allaf

Introduction

Laparoendoscopic single-site surgery (LESS) is an emerging platform for minimally invasive surgical therapy. Virtually every extirpative and reconstructive urologic procedure that can be performed via traditional laparoscopy has been performed with LESS [1]. While there have been many reports of LESS procedures, adoption of the technique has been somewhat limited with only 11.6 % of upper tract laparoscopic cases performed utilizing a LESS approach in a recent multi-institutional review [2]. This resistance to adoption of LESS is likely multi-factorial and includes technical, training, and evidence-based challenges. Technical challenges of LESS include adapting to a new platform and instruments. Training challenges include gaining exposure and skills by practicing urologists, as well as

M.W. Ball, MD (✉)
James Buchanan Brady Urological Institute and
Department of Urology, The Johns Hopkins
University School of Medicine, 600 N.
Wolfe Street/Marburg 134,
Baltimore, MD 21287, USA
e-mail: mark.ball@jhmi.edu

M.E. Allaf, MD
James Buchanan Brady Urological Institute and
Department of Urology, The Johns Hopkins
University School of Medicine, 600 N.
Wolfe Street/Park 223,
Baltimore, MD 21287, USA
e-mail: mallaf@jhmi.edu

integrating LESS into curricula for current trainees. Evidence challenges include demonstrating the comparative effectiveness and cost-effectiveness of LESS technology to other surgical platforms. Currently, there are active efforts to optimize LESS surgery in each of these domains. Herein, we review the current state of the field and current efforts to optimize technology, training, and evidence in LESS surgery.

Technology Perspectives

Perhaps the strongest barriers to the adoption of LESS are technical limitations. While traditional laparoscopy relies on the of principles of instrument triangulation, traction/countertraction, and in-line vision, the use of a single entry port prohibits triangulation and predisposes the operator to both internal and external instrument clashing and decreased maneuverability. As a result, innovations in instrumentation are necessary to overcome this limitation. There are three main varieties of instruments that have been developed and used to implement LESS – articulating instruments, pre-bent instruments, and needlescopic instruments.

Articulating instruments attempt to recapitulate the triangulation of traditional laparoscopy by using surgeon-controlled intracorporeal deflection. This allows the surgeon's hand to be placed apart from each other while still focusing

© Springer Science+Business Media New York 2017
J.H. Kaouk et al. (eds.), *Atlas of Laparoscopic and Robotic Single Site Surgery*,
Current Clinical Urology, DOI 10.1007/978-1-4939-3575-8_26

the instrument tips at the same point intra-abdominally [3]. Multiple models currently exist, including the Covidien Roticulator™ (Hamilton HM FX, Bermuda), Novare RealHand™ (Cupertino, CA, USA), and Cambridge Endo Autonomy Laparo-Angle™ (Framingham, MA, USA). These instruments provide up to seven degrees of freedom, as well a 360° rotation. Limitations of these instruments include their expense, as they are not reusable. Additionally, knot tying may be impaired when using these instruments due to insufficient joint forces [4]. Finally, a steeper learning curve exists in learning to use these instruments in terms of time and accuracy when compared to traditional laparoscopic instrumentation [5].

Pre-bent instruments also restore triangulation, but the deflection of the tip of the instrument is not adjustable. While these instruments, which include the HIQLS™ hand instruments (Olympus, Tokyo, Japan) and the S-portal™ series (Karl Storz, Tuttlingen, Germany), offer less degrees of freedom than the articulating instruments, they may be associated with a shorter learning curve. In a comparative study in an animal model, Stolzenburg et al. found that pre-bent instruments had increased maneuverability and ease of use compared to articulating instruments [6]. Additionally, these instruments are reusable and may be more cost-effective than articulating instruments.

Needlescopic instruments or mini-laparoscopic instruments are 3-mm or smaller instruments. The instruments are often used in ancillary capacity to the main multichannel port. They maintain the goal of a single incision as they are inserted through Veress needle ports, requiring only a skin puncture without a separate skin incision [7]. They also aid in the restoring instrument triangulation and enable increased dexterity. The Laparoendoscopic Single-Site Surgery Consortium for Assessment and Research (LESSCAR) advocates the use of ancillary 1.9-mm instruments to enhance surgeon confidence in the learning stage of LESS [8]. In a study comparing needlescopic and laparoscopic adrenalectomy, patients undergoing a needlescopic procedure had shorter surgical time,

less blood loss, shorter hospital stay, and shorter convalescence [9].

In addition to innovations in instrumentation, novel platforms are under development to optimize LESS. The Magnetic Anchoring and Guidance System (MAGS) consists of a moveable magnet that is positioned intra-abdominally and stabilized externally with a magnet placed on the abdominal wall (Fig. 26.1). The platform is placed via a single access port and allows placement and spacing of instruments uncoupled from port placement, thereby restoring triangulation and reducing instrument collision [10]. In the initial human clinical report, Cadeddu et al. successfully completed a laparoscopic nephrectomy and appendectomy using the MAGS system to anchor

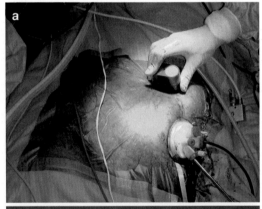

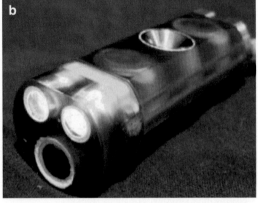

Fig. 26.1 Magnetic Anchored Guidance System (MAGS) (**a**) external magnetic on the abdominal wall controls intra-abdominal magnetic camera and (**b**) Internal component, with LED lights and camera (From Cadeddu et al. [11]. Reprinted with permission from Springer Science + Business Media)

the camera placed through a single-incision working port [11]. The authors concluded that this system resulted in fewer instrument collisions and improved working space without significantly comprising image quality.

The advent of robotic technology changed the landscape of traditional laparoscopy by enabling complex minimally invasive procedures traditionally reserved for center of excellence by the broader urologic community [12]. Similarly, there is enthusiasm that robotic technology may enable the increased utilization of LESS. The superior ergonomics, optical magnification, and surgical dexterity afforded by robotic technology may ameliorate the technical difficulties that standard laparoscopic single-site surgery presents [13]. The initial report of robot-assisted LESS in humans (RA-LESS) by Kaouk et al. in 2009 reported perioperative outcomes of three procedures utilizing the da Vinci Robotic System (Intuitive Surgical Inc., Sunnyvale, CA) – radical prostatectomy (RP),

dismembered pyeloplasty, and radical nephrectomy [14]. The authors demonstrated that RA-LESS is safe and feasible for these procedures, though further comparative series are warranted to investigate any additional benefit derived by using a single port.

The current da Vinci Robotic System is not without its limitations. The external profile of the robot is bulky, and robotic arm collisions and unfamiliar camera angles are technical obstacles that must be overcome [3, 15]. New techniques are under development to overcome these limitations. The "chopstick surgery" technique, described by Joseph et al., for example, is a technique in which the robot instruments cross intra-abdominally at the abdominal wall so that the right instrument is on the left side of the target and the left instrument is on the right [16]. Each arm is then assigned to the opposite control at the robotic console (Fig. 26.2). In a comparison to a traditional instrument configuration in inanimate trainers, the chopstick configuration resulted in

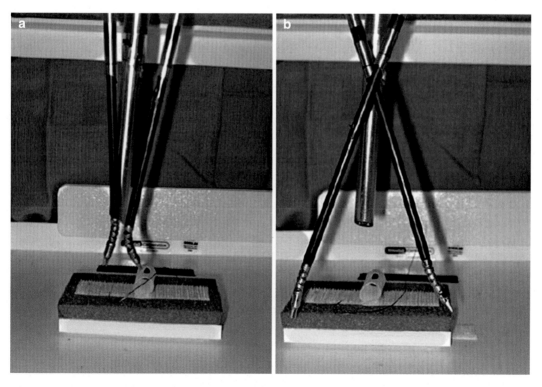

Fig. 26.2 (a) Standard LESS instrument configuration and (b) "chopstick" instrument configuration through single port (From Joseph et al. [16]. Reprinted with permission from Springer Science + Business Media)

Fig. 26.3 da Vinci
single-port system with
curved robotic cannulas,
robotic camera, and
laparoscopic assistant port
(From Kroh et al. [18].
Reprinted with permission
from Springer Science +
Business Media)

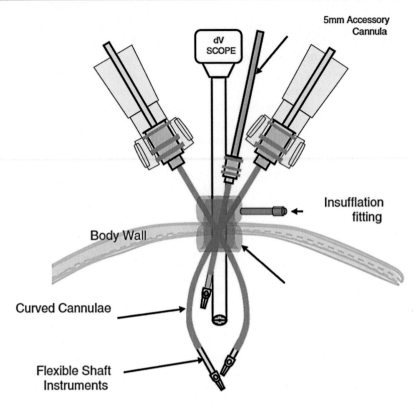

improved performance times, less instrument collisions, decreased camera manipulation, decreased clutching maneuvers, and fewer errors during all tasks.

Intuitive Surgical has released a-port system using da Vinci Single-Site instruments for use with its da Vinci Si surgical system [17] (Fig. 26.3). While limited data are currently available, Kroh et al. reported successfully performing cholecystectomy in 13 patients [18]. This platform requires further evaluation but may provide the technologic advantage to push LESS into the mainstream.

Training Perspectives

While optimizing the technical aspects of LESS is important, training surgeons to perform LESS surgery is equally paramount to increase its utilization. There is currently no formal LESS curriculum or required case numbers for residents and fellows as there are for traditional laparoscopy or robotics. Similarly, there is no formalized

accreditation system for practicing surgeons to become certified in LESS. However, the need for such a system is felt by urologists in practice. Rais-Bahrami et al. studied the current state of LESS by surveying practicing urologists. While 44.7 % of the 422 respondents reported performing LESS surgery, 75 % had only performed less than ten LESS cases. The majority thought that LESS should be integrated into residency and fellowship and supported a credentialing process for urologists performing LESS procedures [19].

Attempts to incorporate LESS into resident training thus far have been successful. Joseph et al. evaluated the incorporation of LESS into a surgical curriculum by evaluating the performance of seven chief residents in performing 49 LESS cholecystectomies [20]. While the early cases included conversion to standard laparoscopy and had slightly longer operative times, operative time returned to historic laparoscopic times by the fifth case. The authors concluded that LESS training could safely be incorporated into residency training with little impact on operating room efficiency.

Other investigators have proposed their own LESS curricula. Müller et al. described porcine surgeries that could be used as training for LESS including single-port and single-incision cholecystotomy and nephrectomy [21]. From their experience with these models, they conclude that the traditional "Halstedian" training models of training surgeons should be abandoned for one that educates the entire surgical team. They too advocate for the need to incorporate LESS training into residency programs.

For the surgeon who has already completed residency, no formal guidelines or accreditation process exists for LESS training. Several societies, however, have weighed in with recommendations for adopting LESS for the urologist in practice. The Endourological Society NOTES and LESS Working Group and the European Society of Urotechnology NOTES and LESS Working Group suggest that a surgeon should regularly perform standard laparoscopic procedures before transitioning to LESS. Additionally, first transitioning from standard laparoscopy to a reduced port laparoscopic approach may allow the surgeon to become more comfortable with less working ports before transitioning solely to LESS [22].

Similarly, the Laparoendoscopic Single-Site Surgery Consortium for Assessment and Research (LESSCAR) offers a suggested stepwise training schedule of LESS surgery. The consortium recommends beginning with inanimate training with LESS instruments, followed by hands-on training in animal models, observation of live LESS procedures, and finally performance of LESS surgery in a proctored and mentored setting [8].

Outcomes Perspectives

The final barrier to the widespread adoption of LESS, and an important avenue for its future development, is to support its use with evidence from well-conducted trials and studies. Specifically, the questions that should be answered are defining the ideal patients for LESS, demonstrating what the benefits of LESS

are over traditional laparoscopy and robotic-assisted laparoscopy, and analyzing the cost of LESS in comparison to other approaches.

Several studies have sought to compare LESS to traditional laparoscopy, though most have been case-control studies. The first such study by Raman et al. compared 11 LESS nephrectomies and 22 traditional laparoscopic nephrectomies [23]. No differences between the two groups were observed for length of stay, analgesic use, complications rate, operative time, or transfusion requirements, though blood loss was lower in the LESS group. The authors concluded that the advantage of LESS was limited to cosmesis. Similar case-control studies comparing LESS and conventional laparoscopy for pyeloplasty [24] and adrenalectomy [25] also demonstrated similar results.

In contrast, Canes et al. compared 18 patients undergoing laparoscopic and LESS donor nephrectomy and found improvements in postoperative convalescence, including days off work, days to 100 % recovery, and day of oral pain medication [26]. The conflicting results of these retrospective studies are likely due to selection bias and highlight the need for higher-quality prospective studies.

A few randomized studies have been performed evaluating LESS. Kurien et al. performed a randomized study of LESS and standard laparoscopic donor nephrectomy [27]. Overall, the LESS cohort was associated with increased perceived difficulty by the surgeon, longer warm ischemia time, decreased hospital stay, and improved pain scores after 48 h. Operative time, complications, patients reported quality of life, cosmetic scores, and estimated GFR at 1 year were similar between groups.

Tugcu et al. also performed a prospective, randomized study of LESS and laparoscopic pyeloplasty in 39 patients, with mean follow-up of 19.7 months [28]. A LESS approach was associated with lower visual analog pain scale and postoperative analgesic use, as well as improved patient satisfaction and faster return to normal activities.

The disparate outcomes of these LESS studies highlight the need to define patients who benefit the most from LESS. It has been suggested that patients undergoing reconstructive procedures (e.g., pyeloplasty) may benefit more than patients undergoing extirpative procedures where larger extraction incisions are necessary [29]. However, objective criteria to evaluate this idea are lacking.

Further clinical studies are needed to help LESS gain acceptance – namely, answering the questions of ideal patient selection, objective benefits of LESS over laparoscopy and robotics, and cost-effectiveness are a priority. Additionally, further comparative studies of RA-LESS are needed as interest in this field is rapidly growing.

Conclusion

The field of LESS surgery continues to mature. While its short past has seen the development of novel instrumentation, preliminary training modules, and encouraging clinical studies, its future is sure to contain advancements in all three of these areas. The future of LESS is bright, and further advancement may lead to more widespread adoption.

References

1. Kaouk JH, Autorino R, Kim FJ, Han DH, Lee SW, Yinghao S, et al. Laparoendoscopic single-site surgery in urology: worldwide multi-institutional analysis of 1076 cases. Eur Urol. 2011;60(5):998–1005.
2. Irwin BH, Rao PP, Stein RJ, Desai MM. Laparoendoscopic single site surgery in urology. Urol Clin North Am. 2009;36(2):223–35. ix.
3. Autorino R, Cadeddu JA, Desai MM, Gettman M, Gill IS, Kavoussi LR, et al. Laparoendoscopic single-site and natural orifice transluminal endoscopic surgery in urology: a critical analysis of the literature. Eur Urol. 2011;59(1):26–45.
4. Jeong CW, Kim SH, Kim HT, Jeong SJ, Hong SK, Byun SS, et al. Insufficient joint forces of first-generation articulating instruments for laparoendoscopic single-site surgery. Surg Innov. 2013;20(5):466–70.
5. Tuncel A, Lucas S, Bensalah K, Zeltser IS, Jenkins A, Saeedi O, et al. A randomized comparison of conventional vs articulating laparoscopic needle-drivers for performing standardized suturing tasks by laparoscopy-naive subjects. BJU Int. 2008;101(6):727–30.
6. Stolzenburg JU, Kallidonis P, Oh MA, Ghulam N, Do M, Haefner T, et al. Comparative assessment of laparoscopic single-site surgery instruments to conventional laparoscopic in laboratory setting. J Endourol. 2010;24(2):239–45.
7. Soble JJ, Gill IS. Needlescopic urology: incorporating 2-mm instruments in laparoscopic surgery. Urology. 1998;52(2):187–94.
8. Gill IS, Advincula AP, Aron M, Caddedu J, Canes D, Curcillo 2nd PG, et al. Consensus statement of the consortium for laparoendoscopic single-site surgery. Surg Endosc. 2010;24(4):762–8.
9. Gill IS, Soble JJ, Sung GT, Winfield HN, Bravo EL, Novick AC. Needlescopic adrenalectomy – the initial series: comparison with conventional laparoscopic adrenalectomy. Urology. 1998;52(2):180–6.
10. Zeltser IS, Bergs R, Fernandez R, Baker L, Eberhart R, Cadeddu JA. Single trocar laparoscopic nephrectomy using magnetic anchoring and guidance system in the porcine model. J Urol. 2007;178(1):288–91.
11. Cadeddu J, Fernandez R, Desai M, Bergs R, Tracy C, Tang SJ, et al. Novel magnetically guided intra-abdominal camera to facilitate laparoendoscopic single-site surgery: initial human experience. Surg Endosc. 2009;23(8):1894–9.
12. Patel HD, Mullins JK, Pierorazio PM, Jayram G, Cohen JE, Matlaga BR, et al. Trends in renal surgery: robotic technology is associated with increased use of partial nephrectomy. J Urol. 2013;189(4):1229–35.
13. Rane A, Tan GY, Tewari AK. Laparo-endoscopic single-site surgery in urology: is robotics the missing link? BJU Int. 2009;104(8):1041–3.
14. Kaouk JH, Goel RK, Haber GP, Crouzet S, Stein RJ. Robotic single-port transumbilical surgery in humans: initial report. BJU Int. 2009;103(3):366–9.
15. Wedmid A, Llukani E, Lee DI. Future perspectives in robotic surgery. BJU Int. 2011;108(6 Pt 2):1028–36.
16. Joseph RA, Goh AC, Cuevas SP, Donovan MA, Kauffman MG, Salas NA, et al. "Chopstick" surgery: a novel technique improves surgeon performance and eliminates arm collision in robotic single-incision laparoscopic surgery. Surg Endosc. 2010;24(6):1331–5.
17. Haber GP, White MA, Autorino R, Escobar PF, Kroh MD, Chalikonda S, et al. Novel robotic da Vinci instruments for laparoendoscopic single-site surgery. Urology. 2010;76(6):1279–82.
18. Kroh M, El-Hayek K, Rosenblatt S, Chand B, Escobar P, Kaouk J, et al. First human surgery with a novel single-port robotic system: cholecystectomy using the da Vinci Single-Site platform. Surg Endosc. 2011;25(11):3566–73.
19. Rais-Bahrami S, Moreira DM, Hillelsohn JH, George AK, Rane A, Gross AJ, et al. Contemporary perspectives on laparoendoscopic single-site surgery in urologic training and practice. J Endourol. 2013;27(6):727–31.
20. Joseph M, Phillips M, Farrell TM, Rupp CC. Can residents safely and efficiently be taught single incision laparoscopic cholecystectomy? J Surg Educ. 2012;69(4):468–72.
21. Muller EM, Cavazzola LT, Machado Grossi JV, Mariano MB, Morales C, Brun M. Training for laparoendoscopic single-site surgery (LESS). Int J Surg. 2010;8(1):64–8.
22. Gettman MT, White WM, Aron M, Autorino R, Averch T, Box G, et al. Where do we really stand

with LESS and NOTES? Eur Urol. 2011;59(2): 231–4.

23. Raman JD, Bagrodia A, Cadeddu JA. Single-incision, umbilical laparoscopic versus conventional laparoscopic nephrectomy: a comparison of perioperative outcomes and short-term measures of convalescence. Eur Urol. 2009;55(5):1198–204.

24. Tracy CR, Raman JD, Bagrodia A, Cadeddu JA. Perioperative outcomes in patients undergoing conventional laparoscopic versus laparoendoscopic single-site pyeloplasty. Urology. 2009;74(5): 1029–34.

25. Jeong BC, Park YH, Han DH, Kim HH. Laparoendoscopic single-site and conventional laparoscopic adrenalectomy: a matched case-control study. J Endourol. 2009;23(12):1957–60.

26. Canes D, Berger A, Aron M, Brandina R, Goldfarb DA, Shoskes D, et al. Laparo-endoscopic single site (LESS) versus standard laparoscopic left donor nephrectomy: matched-pair comparison. Eur Urol. 2010;57(1):95–101.

27. Kurien A, Rajapurkar S, Sinha L, Mishra S, Ganpule A, Muthu V, et al. First prize: standard laparoscopic donor nephrectomy versus laparoendoscopic single-site donor nephrectomy: a randomized comparative study. J Endourol. 2011;25(3):365–70.

28. Tugcu V, Ilbey YO, Sonmezay E, Aras B, Tasci AI. Laparoendoscopic single-site versus conventional transperitoneal laparoscopic pyeloplasty: a prospective randomized study. Int J Urol. 2013;20(11):1112–7.

29. Best SL, Tracy CR, Cadeddu JA. Laparoendoscopic single-site surgery and natural orifice transluminal endoscopic surgery: future perspectives. BJU Int. 2010;106(6 Pt B):941–4.

Index

© Springer Science+Business Media New York 2017
J.H. Kaouk et al. (eds.), *Atlas of Laparoscopic and Robotic Single Site Surgery*,
Current Clinical Urology, DOI 10.1007/978-1-4939-3575-8